Psychoanalysis and Narrative Medicine

SUNY series in Psychoanalysis and Culture

Henry Sussman, editor

Psychoanalysis

and

Narrative Medicine

Edited by

Peter L. Rudnytsky and Rita Charon

STATE UNIVERSITY OF NEW YORK PRESS

Published by
STATE UNIVERSITY OF NEW YORK PRESS, ALBANY

© 2008 State University of New York

For information, contact State University of New York Press,
www.sunypress.edu

Production and book design, Laurie Searl
Marketing, Anne M. Valentine

Library of Congress Cataloging-in-Publication Data

Psychoanalysis and narrative medicine / edited by Peter L. Rudnytsky, Rita Charon.
    p. ; cm. — (SUNY series in psychoanalysis and culture)
    Includes bibliographical references and index.
    ISBN 978-0-7914-7351-1 (hardcover : alk. paper)
    ISBN 978-0-7914-7352-8 (pbk. : alk. paper)
1. Narrative medicine. 2. Psychoanalysis. I. Rudnytsky, Peter L. II. Charon, Rita. III. Series.
    [DNLM: 1. Narration. 2. Psychoanalysis. 3. Medicine in Literature. WM 460.5.C5 P974 2008]

RC48.P79 2008
616.89'17—dc22

                                                                    2007016955

10   9   8   7   6   5   4   3   2   1

To my sister Betsy, who looks at life from both sides
—PLR

To my mother, in love and out of time
—RC

Contents

Acknowledgments

My most tangible debt is to the Thomas H. Maren Foundation, and especially to Emily Sabah Maren, for welcoming the idea of this conference and for providing the financial support that made it possible. Sarah Mallonee, my editorial assistant on *American Imago* from 2001–2004, was the Ariel of our tempest. Her successor, Kristen Smith, expedited the journey from revel to page, not least by her compilation of the index. Cheryl believed in my rough magic. I am grateful to all those who came to the University of Florida to participate in the conference. Lynn Gamwell and Silvia Ivanova of the Binghamton University Art Museum graciously provided the image of Freud's drawing of the spinal ganglia and spinal cord of petromyzon that adorns the cover. My thanks also to James Peltz for giving this volume—a successor to *Psychoanalyses/Feminisms*—a home at SUNY Press, and to Henry Sussman for again lending his imprimatur to my work.

—PLR

All of my work in narrative medicine stems from ongoing generative collaborations at Columbia, especially with Sayantani DasGupta, Craig Irvine, Eric Marcus, David Plante, Maura Spiegel, and Patricia Stanley, the members of the National Endowment for the Humanities project on narrative medicine. I also thank all the editors and contributors to *Literature and Medicine* who are together inventing and deepening a field of urgent inquiry.

—RC

Earlier versions of the introduction and of chapters 4, 8, 9, 14, and 16 appeared in the Fall 2004 issue of *Literature and Medicine* and are reprinted here with the permission of The Johns Hopkins University Press: Peter L. Rudnytsky, introduction, as "A Multiple Birth: Pyschoanalysis and Narrative Medicine," *Literature and Medicine* 23, no. 2 (2004): 252–64; Terrence E. Holt, "Narrative Medicine and Negative Capability," *Literature and Medicine*

23, no. 2 (2004): 318–33; Fred L. Griffin, "The Fortunate Physician: Learning from Our Patients," *Literature and Medicine* 23, no. 2 (2004): 280–303; Lisa J. Schnell, "Learning How to Tell," *Literature and Medicine* 23, no. 2 (2004): 265–79; Neil Scheurich, "Reading, Listening, and Other Beleaguered Practices in General Psychiatry," *Literature and Medicine* 23, no. 2 (2004): 304–17; Geoffrey Hartman, "Narrative and Beyond," *Literature and Medicine* 23, no. 2 (2004): 334–45. Chapter 10, "Imagining Immunity," by Ed Cohen, appeared as "Metaphorical Immunity: A Case of Biomedical Fiction," in *Literature and Medicine* 22, no. 2 (2003): 140–63, © The Johns Hopkins University Press. Portions of chapter 1 and Rita Charon's afterword appear in her *Narrative Medicine: Honoring the Stories of Illness* (New York: Oxford University Press, 2006), and are reprinted here by permission.

Introduction

PETER L. RUDNYTSKY

"Chance and the prepared mind." This aphorism favored by the psychologist Henry Murray best captures the serendipitous set of circumstances that led to the conference on "Psychoanalysis and Narrative Medicine" I organized at the University of Florida on February 19–22, 2004. A long-standing interest in psychoanalysis prompted me to propose a conference on this topic to the Thomas H. Maren Foundation, which responded with a munificence that allowed me to build my field of dreams without cutting any corners.

If my yoking of psychoanalysis and narrative medicine had in it an element of pragmatism, since a conference on psychoanalysis alone would not have been compatible with the mission of the Maren Foundation, this improvised theme now seems to me in retrospect to have been a stroke of genuine inspiration. It was after I had announced the title of the Gainesville conference that narrative medicine made its splash in the popular media in October 2003 with an article in *The New York Times* and a feature on National Public Radio. The conference, moreover, proved to be a "first" in two important respects. Not only was it the first conference ever on narrative medicine with an open call for papers, but it was also the first time that narrative medicine had been conjoined with psychoanalysis, thereby creating the opportunity for a new interdisciplinary dialogue. By bringing together individuals with backgrounds in psychoanalysis, the humanities, and the health care professions, the conference in Gainesville can be said to have forged a new intellectual community.

In designing the program, one of my primary objectives was to get away from the status consciousness that is too often the bane of the academic world. Although my budget permitted me to invite an extraordinary list of featured speakers—Rita Charon, Sander L. Gilman, Bennett Simon, Jody

Messler Davies, Mark Solms, Abraham Verghese, Jeffrey Berman, Norman Holland, David B. Morris, Lynn Gamwell, Geoffrey Hartman, and Frans de Waal—I also set up seminars, each of which was co-directed by two of the invited speakers. In these seminars, all the conference participants who wished to offer papers could have them discussed in a small-group format. The papers were posted on our Web site as they came in, assigned to a seminar several weeks before the conference, and members were asked to read the other papers in their group before arriving in Gainesville. Unfortunately, a family emergency prevented Jody Davies from attending at the last minute, and her place on the program was ably filled by Vera Camden, whose paper had initially been slated for inclusion in one of the seminars. Excursions to the Harn Museum of Art, led by Lynn Gamwell, to see a special exhibition of photographs of Freud's apartment at Berggasse 19 taken in 1938 by Edmund Engleman, shortly before the emigration of the Freud family from Vienna to London, rounded out the bill of cultural fare.

Besides receiving financial support from the Maren Foundation, one further way in which chance merged with design is that the conference was sponsored jointly by *Literature and Medicine*, co-edited by Rita Charon and Maura Spiegel, and *American Imago*, of which I am the editor and Vera Camden is a co-editor. In this cooperation between our respective journals, both of which are published by The Johns Hopkins University Press, I again discerned an emblem of the interdisciplinary synergy I hoped to achieve; and five of the papers included in the present volume—those by Lisa Schnell, Fred Griffin, Neil Scheurich, Terrence Holt, and Geoffrey Hartman—as well as an earlier version of this introduction, first appeared as a cluster in the Fall 2004 issue of *Literature and Medicine*.

ᴥ

Although I am not a scholar of narrative medicine, I believe that in proposing a conjunction with psychoanalysis I was inviting this exciting new discipline to claim an insufficiently acknowledged portion of its own history. For whereas narrative medicine arose from a desire to bring "literary competence" (and the benefits of literary study generally) within the purview of the medical school curriculum, it is, of course, psychoanalysis that is known as the "talking cure," and thus distills the essence of what narrative medicine is all about. From the standpoint of psychoanalysis, conversely, an alliance with narrative medicine offers the prospect of basking in the reflected glory of this revival of humanism within the bastions of science, and thereby strengthening its own position both intramurally within the mental health profession and in American culture at large.

In tracing the psychoanalytic genealogy of narrative medicine, three prominent names come to my mind. The first, inevitably, is Freud. Freud's fundamental theoretical contribution is to have elucidated the influence of unconscious mental processes, and the defenses against them, on the whole of human life, while his greatest invention is of a new kind of human relationship—that between analyst and patient—in which people can seek a "soul-cure" through exploring the meaning of their often painful experiences with a trained professional in a secular context. Although Freud was himself a neurologist before he became a psychotherapist, he insisted that "psychoanalysis is not a specialized branch of medicine" (1927, 252), but rather belonged to psychology; and that the education of future analysts should "include branches of knowledge which are remote from medicine and which the doctor does not come across in his practice: the history of civilization, mythology, the psychology of religion, and the science of literature" (1926, 246).

Without Freud, there would have been no psychoanalysis, but in at least one important respect he impeded rather than abetted the contemporary rapprochement with narrative medicine. I refer to his notorious recommendation that the analyst should cultivate an "emotional coldness" and model his technique on that of "the surgeon, who puts aside all his feelings" (1912, 115) while performing an operation. Whereas it has been a principal thrust of narrative medicine to encourage physicians genuinely to listen to their patients, and in doing so to learn to look upon them not simply as a bundle of symptoms but as fellow human beings, Freud's own espousal of a surgical model of psychoanalytic therapy paradoxically steered his movement in the opposite direction, a wrong turn from which it is only now finally being rescued.

The other two psychoanalysts who can be regarded as progenitors of narrative medicine, Georg Groddeck and Michael Balint, are central figures in the relational tradition that has, in my understanding, succeeded in rectifying many of Freud's mistakes, including his minimizing of the need for genuine compassion and empathy on the part of the analyst in order for emotional healing to take place in the patient. Both Groddeck and Balint were closely associated with Sándor Ferenczi, Freud's great Hungarian disciple, who—as Paul Stepansky (1999) has shown in his study of the vicissitudes of the surgical metaphor in Freud's work—effected the "only bona fide transformation" (89) in Freud's conception when Ferenczi redefined the analyst not as a surgeon but as an obstetrician:

> The doctor's position in psychoanalytic treatment recalls in many ways that of the obstetrician, who also has to conduct himself as passively as possible, to content himself with the post of onlooker at a natural proceeding, but who must be at hand in the critical moment with the forceps in order to complete the act of parturition that is not progressing spontaneously. (1919, 182–83)

While reserving the right to use the "forceps" of active intervention as a last resort, Ferenczi exhorts the analyst to adopt a stance of wise passiveness, though this should not be misunderstood to mean being aloof or devoid of human sympathy.[1]

Ferenczi's admonition was heeded by Groddeck, the maverick director of a sanatorium in Baden-Baden who cheerfully called himself a "wild analyst" and who in his masterpiece, *The Book of the It* (1923), recounted how, in 1909, he "took over the treatment of a severely ill woman who compelled me to become an analyst" (264). Because the patient "saw in me the mother," Groddeck gradually came to renounce the practice of "authoritative, infallible, fatherly suggestion" that he had learned from his mentor Ernst Schweninger, and instead of being an "active, meddling doctor" he sought to become "a passive tool" who placed himself at the patient's disposal (266–67).

As a result of this conversion experience, Groddeck discovered that he himself was being healed by his encounter with his patient: "Then suddenly I stood before the odd fact that I am not treating the patient, but that the patient is instead treating me; or to translate it into my language, that the It of my neighbor seeks so to transform my It, indeed so transforms it, that it becomes serviceable to its purposes" (267). Groddeck summarizes his emphasis on the mutuality of the relationship between analyst and patient, which makes him a founder of contemporary relational thinking, with the affirmation that "it is not the doctor who is the essentially active partner, but the patient. The doctor's chief enemy is hubris" (1926a, 126). And because in every healing relationship there should come "a strange turning point where the patient becomes the doctor and decides himself what he is to do with the doctor's services and even whether he wants to accept them at all" (1928, 215), it follows that if the therapeutic process breaks down for any reason, "the doctor will have to tell himself: I have made a mistake; what matters then is to find out what kind of mistake it was and to discuss it honestly with the patient without any embarrassment or attempt at apology" (1926b, 225–26).

In the history of psychoanalysis, Groddeck is best known for the concept of the "It," that primal source of the psyche-soma, underlying even the unconscious, of which the "I" is no more than an inescapable mirage or symptom. In German, Freud's "id" is also called *das Es*, while his "ego" is *das Ich*, but James Strachey's decision to translate these ordinary German words into English with their Latin equivalents, rather than as "it" and "I," accurately captures the difference between Freud's pseudoscientific structural theory and Groddeck's unabashedly subjective vision of the power of the It to shape human life.

Whereas I revere Groddeck both for his attempt to deflate the hubris of physicians—whether they be psychoanalysts or medical doctors—and for his appreciation of the unconscious dimensions of physical illness, he is attacked by the late Susan Sontag in *Illness as Metaphor* (1978) precisely because he ascribes diseases to internal causes and thereby seems to hold the patient responsible for his or her own suffering. "Such preposterous and dangerous views," she rails, "manage to put the onus of the disease on the patient and not only weaken the patient's ability to withstand the range of plausible medical treatment but also, implicitly, direct the patient away from such treatment" (47). Ironically, despite her own eminence as a writer, Sontag's critique of Groddeck reflects her inability to appreciate the positive contributions of either psychoanalysis or narrative medicine. For the main thesis of her book is that "illness is *not* a metaphor, and that the most truthful way of regarding illness—and the healthiest way of being ill—is one most purified of, most resistant to, metaphorical thinking" (3). Contrary to Sontag, however, it is not necessary to lay down the potent weapons of Western biomedicine, or, in Lou Andreas-Salomé's words, to look upon "the sick man as a criminal to be punished" (Freud and Andreas-Salomé 1966, 138), to recognize that even a physical illness will be given unconscious meanings by the person who suffers from it, and that the metaphors one fashions are likely to affect the outcome of the psyche-soma's efforts at self-healing. In her resistance to seeing illness as a metaphor, Sontag in effect counsels patients supinely to entrust themselves into the hands of their supposedly godlike physicians, and thereby spurns what there is to be learned not only from Groddeck but also from both Freud and Rita Charon.

Unlike Groddeck, who was Ferenczi's friend and contemporary, Balint was his most outstanding pupil; and when he left Budapest for London in January 1939, six years after Ferenczi's death, Balint provided a living link between the Hungarian and British schools of psychoanalysis. Together with W. R. D. Fairbairn, D. W. Winnicott, Marion Milner, John Bowlby, and others, Balint became a mainstay of the Independent tradition in British psychoanalysis, which is the most fertile seedbed of contemporary relational thought. Balint's theoretical contributions include a refutation (1937) of Freud's misguided notion of primary narcissism, and the elaboration of his own model of the "basic fault" (1968); but his most important achievement in the present connection is to have pioneered in introducing psychoanalytic principles into the practice of general medicine. He developed his ideas out of group seminars conducted in the 1950s at the Tavistock Clinic, and his book, *The Doctor, His Patient, and the Illness* (1964), inspired a far-flung movement of "Balint groups" that continues to the present day.

Written in nontechnical language for practicing internists, who are seen as mediating between the patient and the specialist, *The Doctor, His Patient, and the Illness* is founded on the premise that "by far the most frequently used drug in general practice [is] the doctor himself," yet "no guidance whatever is contained in any textbook as to the dosage in which the doctor should prescribe himself" (1964, 1). Among the many valuable insights in the book is that "in general practice the real problem is often the illness of the whole person" (39), and diagnosis constitutes a movement from an "unorganized" to an "organized" state through a process in which patients "*offer or propose various illnesses* . . . until between doctor and patient an agreement can be reached, resulting in the acceptance by both of them of one of the illnesses as justified" (18). As Balint stresses, "*if you ask questions, you get answers— and hardly anything else*" (133); and the doctor must therefore above all simply "learn *to listen*" (121). This ability, he adds, "*is a new skill, necessitating a considerable, though limited, change in the doctor's personality.*" By learning to listen to what may be unconscious in the patient, moreover, "the doctor will start listening to the same kind of language in himself." In the psychoanalytic terminology that Balint introduces only in his appendices, the doctor is being encouraged to monitor his or her *countertransference* to the patient. As a practical matter, a cultivation of the ability to listen entails shifting the doctor-patient relationship away from the "pattern of a physical examination" because such an objectification of the patient "inactivates the processes [the doctor] wants to observe as they can happen only in a two-person collaboration" (121).

Despite the burgeoning interest in narrative medicine, I suspect that many physicians who may already be convinced of the need to listen empathically to their patients, as well as of the desirability of enhancing "literary competence" as a part of medical education, have not yet recognized the extent to which this symbiotic relationship between literature and medicine is triangulated by psychoanalysis. As a modest first step, I would encourage teachers of courses in narrative medicine to consider including psychoanalytic texts on their syllabi. Not only does the psychoanalytic literature contain classics well worth reading for their own sakes, but the theoretical framework of psychoanalysis provides a language for describing the experiences that occur in everyday life, but can be observed in heightened form in highly charged relationships such as those between doctors and their patients. And it surely would not be amiss to bring psychoanalysts into the ongoing conversations between humanists and health-care providers.

Although there is perforce some overlap in their concerns, I have divided the chapters in this book into four sections. The first, "Contextualizing Narrative Medicine," serves as a portal for the entire collection. Pride of place belongs to Rita Charon who, in "Where Does Narrative Medicine Come From? Drives, Diseases, Attention, and the Body," recapitulates both the origins and bedrock principles of this new way of honoring "the complexities of the self's relation to the body in which it lives." Describing how she was first "visited" by the phrase "narrative medicine," Charon notes that its "grammatical kinship to such names as nuclear medicine and internal medicine" allows her inspired coinage to "say with more directness than can a phrase such as 'literature and medicine' that this is a bona fide field of medicine in which you can specialize and still be a doctor."

Of particular interest to readers of this volume will be Charon's reflections on the similarities and differences between narrative medicine and psychoanalysis, particularly with reference to their relations to the body. It is certainly true, as Charon notes, that the work of the internist or surgeon requires "corporeal contact"—indeed, the inflicting of pain—in a way that is prohibited to the analyst, though Charon likewise stresses the degree to which communication between analyst and patient takes place through "the bodily experiences of passion and drives." From my relational perspective, I would question Charon's contention that "the goals of treatment start with freeing the patient's libidinal energy," while "emotional or existential" aims have only a secondary importance. Uninhibited sexual gratification, however great its intrinsic reward, is no guarantee of happiness in life, and it is not uncommon for promiscuity to be the symptom of an underlying "emotional or existential" conflict. Still, Charon's insistence on the body as an "integument" that at once connects us to and separates us from other human beings remains powerfully evocative, and her example of how "a shadow story of severe congestive heart failure" elicited by a physician's questioning contradicts a patient's protestations of being in good health shows the body to be an agent of unconscious communication in the most radical sense.[2]

As Rita Charon can be credited with having created the discipline of narrative medicine, so Sander L. Gilman has in his immensely productive and wide-ranging career carved out his own distinctive field as a literary and cultural historian of the representations of disease and pathology. In a *tour de force*, his "Desire and Obesity: Dickens, Endocrinology, Pulmonary Medicine, and Psychoanalysis" takes the character of Joe, the "Fat Boy" in Dickens's *Pickwick Papers*, as the nodal point for an investigation into the stereotype of obesity in the nineteenth and twentieth centuries. As Gilman shows, Dickens at once exploited and subverted the conventional "image of the stupid fat man," and his character remained a standard point of reference in the subsequent medical literature on obesity, especially in children. Gilman's paper is a feast of many courses, but perhaps the most delectable portion is the concluding section on Hilde Bruch, a German-Jewish physician who, after fleeing the Nazis, came to the United States, where she underwent a training analysis with Frieda Fromm-Reichmann and "popularized the diagnosis of anorexia nervosa." Citing Bruch's 1973 book, *Eating Disorders*, which offers a psychodynamic rather than an organic explanation for Joe's so-called "Pickwickian Syndrome," Gilman reminds us that issues of gender and race are never far from the surface in the readings and misreadings generated by this singularly persistent—and pernicious—stereotype.

The depth and breadth of Sander Gilman's work find a worthy sequel in that of our two Holts. Richard Lewis Holt's "Pinel and the Pendulum" itself juxtaposes two Foucaults, J.-B. and Michel, and the pendulum suspended in 1751 by the former in the Pantheon with the metaphor of the pendulum as it pertains to the conflicting forces that bisect Holt's chosen field of psychiatry. Holt's chapter leads into an extended meditation on Philippe Pinel, best known for having in 1795 unchained the patients in his asylum Le Bicêtre, and a reading of Pinel's landmark text of 1801, A *Treatise on Insanity*. Although Pinel advocated the "moral" treatment of insanity, Holt makes it clear that this Enlightenment ideal was by no means "immune to empirical scrutiny and validation." And though Pinel not only unchained but also listened to his patients, and thereby introduced "the patient utterance as a legitimate object of study," his position at the apex of "both the physical and discursive spaces of insanity" exemplifies Holt's point that "it was an institution, the asylum, that gave rise to Pinel's novel psychiatric perception," as much as "a new way of looking at the mentally ill" can be said to have created "new powers and institutions." In thus using Pinel to demonstrate that "the modern medical gaze is as much about power as it is about knowledge," Holt circles back to Michel Foucault, whose *Histoire de la folie* he had in his pocket as he walked from La Salpêtrière to the Pantheon during his student days in Paris.

Terrence E. Holt first gained a PhD in English literature before qualifying as a medical doctor. Drawing on his scholarly training, Holt in "Narrative Medicine and Negative Capability" offers an incisive cultural history of narrative medicine. As Holt argues, its cultivation of confessional writing has antecedents in the New Journalism of the 1960s. Through its rejection of "Olympian objectivity," this "reinserting [of] the first-person singular point of view into journalism" risked indulging in "the voyeuristic pleasures of participation without any of the guilt." Yet, Holt contends, as a paradigm of "the mixed motives and shameful pleasures that accompany the most virtuous acts," such a "contradictory fragmentation of impulse" is "an inevitable part of ethical discourse" that paradoxically "offers a ground that actually enables a practical ethics of care."

Any examination of medical autobiographies, Holt continues, turns not simply on the doctor-patient relationship, but above all on the relationship with the audience that consumes these often harrowing tales of fallibility and even incompetence. For Holt, as one schooled in poststructuralism, narrative medicine is less a "response to contemporary pressures in medicine" than it is a "particularly revealing example of the fissures and paradoxes that necessarily result whenever we tell ourselves any story of the 'I.'" Fittingly, Holt concludes with an autobiographical vignette of his own about an occasion when, as an exhausted resident, he had ordered the discontinuance of a pump that had kept one of his cardiac patients alive. Reminded of his father's death a decade earlier under "nearly identical" circumstances, Holt sobbed to himself while simultaneously thinking about how soon he could get away for lunch and of the many other patients for whom he was also responsible. Far from being troubled by this "splitting," however, Holt experienced it as a truthful liberation that enabled him to respond in the moment of crisis both as a detached medical professional and as a human being united in grief with the dying woman and her family. Such a capacity for "entertaining two seemingly opposed responses" Holt attributes to his training "not as a doctor, but as a reader," and he equates it with what the poet-physician (and tuberculosis victim) John Keats two centuries ago called "negative capability."

Our four chapters in "Psychoanalytic Interventions" include three by practicing psychoanalysts with a profound literary sensibility, and one by a scholar with a deep knowledge of psychoanalysis. In "'The Past Is a Foreign Country': Some Uses of Literature in the Psychoanalytic Dialogue," Vera Camden takes off from Freud's references to Oedipus and Hamlet to contend that "narrative functions like the repressed core that will inevitably return, however disguised, to haunt the science of psychoanalysis." The heart of her paper is an extended case history of a deeply traumatized woman, haunted by the childhood memory of having had to drown kittens in a bucket of water and crying hysterically as she saw their excrement in the water. Mrs. F.'s analysis was flooded by anal material, including bouts of diarrhea that interrupted her sessions, and chaotic dreams that it was Camden's task to "clean up." Listening to Mrs. F. reminded Camden of L. P. Hartley's novel, *The Go-Between*, in which the narrator is similarly traumatized by the "foreign country" of his past. Although Camden did not divulge her countertransferential associations directly to her patient, they did inform how she worked with Mrs. F., and the changes they were able to effect together in her psychic landscape. It may not require being an English professor, as Camden is, to be a gifted psychoanalyst; but Camden's chapter is a model of how the "talking cure" is indeed on every level synonymous with narrative medicine.

The theme of trauma receives more general elaboration in Bennett Simon's "It's Really More Complicated Than You Imagine: Narratives of Real and Imagined Trauma." Drawing on his previous work on both tragic drama and ancient Greek thought, as well as on his experience as a psychiatrist and psychoanalyst, Simon defines traumas as events that "at once demand to be made meaningful, yet also resist understanding." Narratives, he explains, require the dynamism of "trouble," but overwhelming trauma is precisely "not symbolizable," and may thus be known "mainly by the uncanny or despairing affects in the patient or those induced in the therapist or both." Simon marshals research by neuroscientists and developmental psychologists to bolster his point that, unlike "ordinary autobiographical memory," traumatic experiences "are initially imprinted as sensations or feeling-states that are not immediately transcribed into personal narratives." The therapist who works with traumatized patients will thus find he or she "has stepped into a mine-field without knowing it," and from a series of arresting vignettes Simon draws the conclusion that "the problem of sorting out true memories from fantasies" is "enough to drive the clinician *meshuge*."

Beginning, like Simon, with the phenomenon that "trauma evades narrative memory," Janet Sayers, in "Narrative and Feminine Empathy: James to Kristeva," focuses on the ineffable states of mystical transcendence to which the shattering experience of trauma is paradoxically akin. Whereas both narrative medicine and psychoanalysis tend to place their faith in the curative powers of speech, Sayers points to a countertradition, stemming from William James, in which it is rather the escape from language that can heal "the divided self." Sayers then explores how D. W. Winnicott, Wilfred Bion, and Julia Kristeva variously trace the roots of a "proto-narrative" capacity for empathy to the mother-infant bond. The psychoanalyst who, through reverie, assists the analysand in "digesting" otherwise inchoate data of experience—in Bion's terms, transmuting a "β-element" into an "α-element"—is recapitulating the role of the mother. To imbue experience with the resonance of a dream is likewise the task of art. In the context of her concerns with psychoanalysis and narrative medicine, Sayers's chapter brings together the questions of gender and religion, and she intimates that it may be possible to reconcile narrative with what lies before or beyond it, the wordless expanse captured in Henry James's image (invoked by Rita Charon) of the healer's "great empty cup of attention."

Our final chapter in this section, Fred L. Griffin's "The Fortunate Physician: Learning from Our Patients," expatiates on John Berger's *A Fortunate Man* (1967), a literary portrait of the life of an English country doctor, John Sassall, in order to convey in accessible language what a psychoanalyst has to offer to physicians "on the front lines of patient care." Griffin, himself a physician as well as a psychoanalyst, has recently co-founded a discussion group on narrative medicine under the auspices of the American Psychoanalytic Association, and he conceives of this chapter as a contribution to the "conversation" not only between psychoanalysts and primary care providers but also between the disciplines of psychoanalysis and narrative medicine. Without being influenced by Groddeck, Sassall concurs that "the forms in which disease are expressed are largely determined by the entire personality of the patient," and that the physician should give up a conception of himself as "a heroic figure" in order to be able to learn from his or her patients, while Griffin's own project of speaking to physicians about psychoanalysis without resorting to its esoteric terminology finds its prototype in Balint's Tavistock seminars.

Some of the most deeply affecting chapters in this book are those in the third section, "The Patient's Voice." For as both narrative medicine and contemporary psychoanalysis have cultivated a more collaborative partnership between both members of the treatment dyad, so both modalities encourage the patient to share his or her own story as an integral part of the healing process. In "Learning How to Tell," Lisa J. Schnell combines the tale of the death of her daughter Claire at eighteen months from a horrifying neurological disorder with the tale of her own psychosomatic illness arising from an unconscious identification with her daughter's plight, and Schnell weaves this exceptionally poignant dual narrative together with arrestingly original meditations on psychoanalytic theory.

Although Schnell does not cite either Groddeck or Balint, her chapter, like Griffin's, makes a compelling case for their teachings. She comes to recognize that her physical symptoms are nothing if not metaphors, caused by her "inability to pronounce *da*—to tell, to imagine, the whole of my and Claire's story." In keeping with Balint's view of diagnosis as a process of negotiation between doctor and patient, Schnell explains that she "was looking for another story, one that I could own even if I couldn't control it," and that it was her "doctor's very refusal to tell his own story about my illness that allowed me to regain my health." She reads the *fort-da* game of Freud's grandson recounted in *Beyond the Pleasure Principle* as a parable about the origins of narrative out of an experience of primordial loss, and how the ability to mourn requires that one possess "an internal space of perception," which is tantamount to acknowledging the "cognitive distance" between a thing and its linguistic representation. Thus, "learning how to tell" becomes a matter of replacing hysterical imitation that does not allow for symbolic distance with a verbal *mimesis* that at once accepts and transmutes loss.

Whereas Lisa Schnell explores how her mental anguish expressed itself through physical symptoms, Ed Cohen in "Imagining Immunity" leaps across the mind/body divide from the opposite direction. Stricken with Crohn's disease in his early teens, Cohen recounts what it has meant to him medically, intellectually, and spiritually to have grown up "in thrall to a metaphor." While not denying the efficacy of Western biomedicine, Cohen indicts the professionals who treated him because they "didn't believe that metaphor had much to do with their practices," and he attributes his own astonishing recovery from near death to the activation of his body's innate healing powers, chiefly through trances in which he visualized "wrapping a band of warm light around the surgical incisions." Cohen joins Richard Holt in paying homage to Foucault for enabling him to understand how his own experience as a patient was "enmeshed in the institutional plays of power/knowledge," and his chapter likewise dovetails with Janet Sayers's reflections on the symbiotic relations between narrative understanding and intimations of transcendence.

What I find perhaps most impressive about Cohen's chapter, as about Schnell's, is its seamless transition from spellbinding autobiography to scintillating theoretical analysis. He traces the concept of "immunity" to its origins in Roman jurisprudence, showing how by the end of the nineteenth century its metaphorical power had displaced the earlier view of healing as "a natural manifestation of the organism's inherent elasticity" (and its connection to the universe as a whole) with a definition of medicine as "a powerful weapon in the body's necessary struggle to defend itself from the world." As Cohen argues, both the triumphs and the limitations of Western biomedicine can be understood in terms of the way the metaphor of immunity has supplanted that of healing, with the consequence that the patient is reduced to being a passive tool in the hands of doctors and researchers. Echoing my own critique of Susan Sontag's attempt to eradicate metaphor from medicine, Cohen asks us to imagine what it might mean "to affirm healing *as* metaphor." One dividend would be the rehabilitation of the "placebo effect," which, as Cohen notes, is ironically excluded from biomedicine "not because it is *not* effective but precisely because *it is*." For Cohen, in short, metaphor is a "transformational technology" that should open all of us to "a potentially productive kind of not-knowing, a kind of not-knowing that asks us to engage imaginatively with the organisms-that-we-are in the service of our vitality and aliveness."

For Kimberly R. Myers, the journey chronicled in "A Perspective on the Role of Stories as a Mechanism of Meta-Healing" began somewhat later in life when, as a graduate student, she was diagnosed with inflammatory bowel disease. After what she calls "the fall (from health)," Myers found that the literature she had always appreciated "intellectually and philosophically" now took on a "new significance" in its visceral demonstration that she "was not alone in facing life-altering bodily change." Impelled by the need to "restore a sense of agency in the face of my loss of control," Myers borrowed from alternative medicine the notion of "meta-healing," which she defines as "a means of healing that occurs in observing the healing of others." In what was "probably the most vulnerable moment of my life," Myers admitted to the students in her course on literature and medicine that a pathography she had asked them to read was actually her own illness narrative, a revelation that transformed their communal bond and inspired the students to break-throughs in their final projects.

Following her participation in a 2002 National Endowment for the Humanities Institute on "Medicine, Literature, and Culture," Myers issued a call for pathographies from academics in any discipline. The response was overwhelming. In her interactions with the more than ninety people who submitted illness narratives, Myers was faced not simply with the normal tasks of an editor but also with the ethical responsibility "to witness the stories." Despite her belief in "meta-healing," Myers—struggling with her own chronic illness—found "the sheer magnitude of fear and grief recounted within these pages" almost more than she could bear, leading her to compare herself to Holden Caulfield vainly "trying to catch everybody who was about to go over the cliff." Still, she did not allow her physical and emotional distress to deter her from her commitment, which has borne fruit in a volume entitled *Illness in the Academy: A Collection of Pathographies by Academics*. As Myers writes no less wisely than courageously, "[T]he gift in simply being there is valuable not because it is *easy*, but precisely because it is so difficult. Venturing into the shadowlands full force is the gift one gives not only to another, but also to oneself."

Unlike the other contributions to this section, Jean S. Mason's "The Discourse of Disease: Patient Writing at the 'University of Tuberculosis'" is not a first-person illness narrative. Rather, in an impressive piece of scholarship, Mason sifts the largely overlooked archive left behind by patients at Saranac Lake, New York, the sanatorium founded in 1884 by Dr. Edward Livingston Trudeau, who had himself been diagnosed with tuberculosis before discovering the salubrious effects of this Adirondack Mountain locale. In its mingling of patients and practitioners, as well as its integration of "patient care, scientific research, medical training, and patient rehabilitation," what Mason denominates the "university of tuberculosis" became "an exemplary model of community-based health care." Given that the treatment of TB imposed "long hours of enforced idleness," many patients turned to writing as a means of passing the time. Their productions ranged from bare-bones diaries to published collections of poetry by such gifted authors as Herbert Scholfield, Adelaide Crapsey, and John Theodore Dalton, to the entrepreneurial gold mine of *Trotty Veck Messages*, collections of witty inspirational passages in prose and verse (named after a character in Dickens's "The Chimes") the sales of which increased from an already impressive four thousand copies in 1916 to an astounding four million copies fifty years later.

In addition to presenting these and other intrinsically interesting texts (including the aptly named *Trouble Book of Isabel Smith*), all of which attest to "the therapeutic power of writing" confirmed by up-to-date psychological research, Mason reflects on the ways that patient narratives combine with clinical records and scientific reports to describe the medical encounter from different perspectives. Each of these sources contributes integrally to "a multidimensional discourse of disease," though narrative medicine would encourage us to give priority to the "inherently metaphoric" writings of patients. Mason quotes Anne Hunsaker Hawkins, co-director of the NEH Institute that came along so opportunely for Kimberly Myers: "Not only, then, does pathography restore the phenomenological and the experiential to the medical encounter, but it also restores the mythic dimension that our scientific, technological culture ignores or disallows."

The chapter by Jeffrey Berman provides a ready transition into our final section, "Acts of Reading." Like Kimberly Myers, Berman in "The Teaching Cure" addresses what takes place in the classroom, and he picks up where Jean Mason leaves off by doing so initially through a close reading of May Sarton's 1961 novel, *The Small Room*. As emerges from his masterful exposition, *The*

Small Room is "one of the most moving academic novels about how a teacher's empathy makes a difference in her students' lives," and it explores profoundly the dynamics of transference and countertransference in teacher-student relationships, though Berman shares Fred Griffin's inclination to eschew potentially arcane terminology in bringing his psychoanalytic sensibility to bear on Sarton's text.

From a detailed examination of *The Small Room*, the plot of which hinges on whether a student who has been caught plagiarizing at an all-female college should be expelled or given psychological counseling (at a time when the latter option was not routinely available on campuses), Berman proceeds to reflect more generally on the personal element in teaching, concurring with Sarton that teachers show their true greatness by being "humble and respectful" toward students. In a series of landmark books, Berman (1994; 1999; 2001; 2005) has advocated a pedagogy of "risky writing," the success of which depends on the teacher's capacity to create "a safe and empathic classroom." Through connecting their academic work with what is going on in their lives, students reach "not simply intellectual understanding but emotional understanding as well"; and in licensing his fellow teachers to pose the unanswerable question of "how to live," Berman eloquently vindicates his conviction that "literature and psychoanalysis are two of the best ways to learn more about ourselves and others and to preserve these provisional truths for those who come after us."

The next two chapters, both by thoughtful and literate psychiatrists, raise theoretical questions about reading prompted by the convergence of psychoanalysis and narrative medicine. Neil Scheurich's "Reading, Listening, and Other Beleaguered Practices in General Psychiatry" is written from the standpoint of someone concerned that the "core values" shared by both literature and psychotherapy have become endangered both in his own professional domain and in contemporary culture generally. Ironically, as Scheurich points out, even as medicine as a whole has seen a modest broadening of its vision beyond the technical, psychiatry, now largely divorced from psychoanalysis, "seems increasingly reduced to a biological understanding of human experience." As Scheurich argues, reading and psychotherapy, as well as the use of literature in psychiatric training, "all share common justifications stemming from the virtues of narrative form," and thus what is ultimately at stake in narrative medicine is the classic problem of how to defend literature against the charges of irrelevance or even dangerousness that go back to Plato.

Scheurich enlists many prominent thinkers who have responded to the attacks on both literature and psychotherapy, but his chapter is at bottom a personal plea in favor of the values of *autonomy, complexity, curiosity,* and *patience* shared by proponents of "serious reading and listening," notwithstanding the differences between these endeavors. While renouncing the "fantasy" that there is some "ultimate justification" that "will magically open the eyes of the indifferent," Scheurich retains the hope that literature can be used in the education of future psychiatrists "not merely to gain a clinical 'pearl' or two," but rather to induce them "to *care* about literature and the values it embodies, and to see that these same values also underlie the mixed status of psychiatry as both liberal art and science."

In "Uncertain Truths: Resistance and Defiance in Narrative," Schuyler W. Henderson offers a commentary on Michel Houellebecq's *Atomized* and John Kennedy Toole's *A Confederacy of Dunces*. He does so in the context of a searching interrogation of how behavior that most mental health professionals would classify as "resistance" can from the standpoint of the counternarratives told by those deemed to be "sick" or "mad" be affirmatively described as "defiance." To label something as "resistance," as Henderson notes, is to "put the power of knowledge squarely in the hands of another," rather than in the hands of the patient himself or herself. Whereas resistance explains the phenomena in question almost completely in terms of personal psychology, moreover, "defiance is a consciously articulated ideological position" that insists, with Houellebecq in his novel, that the very "privileging of the individual, along with his or her experience and narrative," is itself "historically derived and socially sanctioned," and hence must be subjected to a transpersonal critique. According to Houellebecq, the same period of modernity that gave birth to the ideals of "personal freedom" and "human dignity" has been "characterized by decline and destruction"; and thus, in Henderson's extrapolation, "psychology and therapy, rather than offering a solution, are themselves seen as part of the problem."

Despite his sympathy for "the deepened understanding of illness and the ill person" afforded by "the resistant/defiant text," Henderson is not an advocate of "anti-psychiatry." Although he recognizes that people with schizophrenia in the United States "not only do not do better . . . compared to other countries, but are worse off than they were thirty years ago," this indictment of the inflated claims of the pharmaceutical industry is counterpoised by Henderson's reminder that the celebration of defiance in *A Confederacy of Dunces* must be weighed against "the resounding caveat of Toole's suicide." The unwritten books by this author dead by his own hand at the age of thirty-two are no cause for celebration. In the end, Henderson leaves us with a measured plea for a "complex negotiation" or "dialogue where the narrative can be read with and against the counternarrative," as "any notion of 'progress' requires such dialogue," while he remains vigilant to the ever-present "risk that during this dialogue an appropriation of the counternarrative can occur." The most that can be said is that "resistance is an obstacle to insight, while defiance is an obstacle to abuse," and the desirability of being able to tolerate the uncertainty generated by these antithetical perspectives is one of the enduring lessons still to be learned from reading Freud.

Since the theme of trauma has run like a red thread through this book, it seems fitting that our final chapter should be Geoffrey Hartman's "Narrative and Beyond." Modestly acknowledging his "own limited roles of teacher, reader, and occasional interviewer of Holocaust witnesses," one of the leading literary critics of our time seeks in his "*membra disjecta*" to offer the outlines of a "poetics of narrative medicine." Like Lisa Schnell, who takes her epigraph from one of his essays, Hartman appeals to Aristotle's analysis of the cathartic effects of art—a concept linked to psychoanalysis through the "cathartic method" employed by Freud as a way station between his practice of hypnotic suggestion and of free association, and mediated by the medical interpretation of Aristotle's controversial notion put forward by Jacob Bernays (the uncle of Freud's future wife) in 1857.³ And as for Neil Scheurich both reading and psychotherapy are not religious but "spiritual practices inasmuch as they entail attention to the moment, a slowing of onrushing time, and observation of discipline and ritual that impose some order upon chaos," so too for Hartman the great gift of literary seminars (and, I would add, of psychoanalytic sessions) is that they furnish "the time to think freely, to explore the very process of interpretation, without having to do it in a state of emergency," while the indispensable notions of "bearing witness" and "testimony" must be invoked without "carrying, necessarily, a religious overtone."

The range of reference in Hartman's essay extends from Tolstoy to television, from the poetry of Celan, Donne, and Milton to the experiments of Stanley Milgram. In no less productive dialogue with Terrence Holt and Fred Griffin, Hartman concurs with Holt's postmodern emphasis on the inevitable fracturing of subjectivity by citing Arthur Frank's *The Wounded Storyteller* on the "variety of illness narratives that exist," and in particular on the irreconcilability of the perspectives of physician and patient, which enforces the conclusion that "the claim of a 'sovereign consciousness' may have to be given up." And yet, Hartman also lends credence to Griffin's humanistic definition of the "fortunate physician" when he observes that the physician who displays "narrative competence" will be one who, "despite the constraint of time, cultivates an empathy that ideally seeks to being forth the patient's own understanding, even self-discovery." Indeed, "what seems of paramount importance" to Hartman in the mysterious process of healing is "the element of trust."

Hartman closes his sinuous meditation by drawing attention to an Israeli study of Holocaust survivors, who were found to be "chronic patients in mental hospitals" in disproportionate numbers compared to the general population. Strikingly, their experiences of persecution were often not noted on their medical charts, and the possible traumatic etiology of their psychopathology was thus disregarded. In response, a group of psychiatrists undertook what Hartman describes as "a story cure, or more precisely, a testimony cure," by soliciting from these elderly individuals a videotaped autobiography that could then be studied by other people as well as viewed by the patients themselves.

Hartman insists that this experiment has an intrinsic value above and beyond any demonstrable practical effects, yet the results have been promising even when measured by "recognized scientific parameters." According to the authors of the study, "it has been suggested that the testimonial method alleviates many chronic symptoms by transforming the painful trauma story into a cathartic experience and document which could be useful to other people." Hartman observes that this remark "points clearly to the potential of narrative medicine," but, somewhat surprisingly in my opinion, he nowhere mentions the psychoanalytic underpinnings of the entire project undertaken by Rita Charon and her colleagues.

In particular, when Hartman goes on to urge that "more could be done in the medical humanities with different aspects of literature, not only its narrative component," and that the physician who practices narrative medicine should strive to be "sensitive also to non-narrative, apparently inconsequential or lyrical moments, surprises in the narrator's mood and mode," one might have expected him to note that this type of "listening with the third ear" is precisely the province of the psychoanalyst. To continue with Hartman's own lyrical words: "One learns to respect fragments of speech, abrupt figurations, shifts, jump-cuts, mixed genres. It also means . . . to respect what does not fit. For there may be more than one story struggle to emerge, as in a multiple birth."

As the truths of the unconscious are no less powerful for going unrecognized, or being uttered only obliquely, so in coupling "narrative" (medicine) with "beyond" Geoffrey Hartman uncannily invokes psychoanalysis without mentioning its name. In "Material and Metaphor: Narrative Treatment for the Embodied Self," Rita Charon brings this volume full circle by performing the analytic function of making the unconscious conscious. Looking back at her opening presentation in light of the experience of the conference itself and the other papers gathered here, Charon in her afterword again takes up the interplay between body and language in medical practice, where the physician not only may but must touch his or her patients, and in analytic therapy, where physical contact is prohibited. She aligns this contrast with that between the pivotal role of transference in psychoanalysis, in which "the analyst operates on the metaphorical and not the material level," and the way that the medical doctor "enters the lives of patients guilelessly, open-faced, as himself or herself." Despite this "disidentity," Charon has come to see with increasing clarity how the ordinary doctor, like the analyst, "is confronted by materiality saturated with metaphor" on a daily basis, and must draw on all the resources of both heart and mind "to divine, imagine, follow allusions to what the matter is." Although practitioners of both mental and physical healing have much to gain from this new interdisciplinary conjunction between psychoanalysis and narrative medicine, the ultimate beneficiaries promise to be the patients themselves—that is, each one of us—who have the right to expect not only "diagnostic accuracy and appropriate medical management," but also, and above all, "recognition and company on their journeys of illness."

NOTES

1. My comments here concerning Ferenczi and Groddeck draw on the more extended discussions in my *Reading Psychoanalysis* (2002).

2. Charon cites Freud's statement in *The Ego and the Id* that "the ego is first and foremost a bodily ego," and her remarks on this topic could be profitably supplemented by Didier Anzieu's (1985) psychoanalytic work on the "skin ego."

3. I have translated salient portions of Bernays's *Fundamentals of Aristotle's Lost Essay on the "Effect of Tragedy"* in the Fall 2004 issue of *American Imago*, guest-edited by Nicholas Rand, *The Growth of the Unconscious, 1750–1900.*

REFERENCES

Anzieu, Didier. 1985. *The skin ego: A psychoanalytic approach to the self.* Trans. Chris Turner. New Haven: Yale University Press, 1989.

Balint, Michael. 1937. Early developmental stages of the ego. Primary object-Love. In *Primary love and psychoanalytic technique*, 90–108. London: Maresfield Library, 1985.

———. 1964. *The doctor, his patient, and the illness.* Rev. ed. Madison, CT: International Universities Press, 1972.

———. 1968. *The basic fault: Therapeutic aspects of regression.* New York: Brunner/Mazel, 1979.

Berman, Jeffrey. 1994. *Diaries to an English professor: Pain and growth in the classroom.* Amherst: University of Massachusetts Press.

———. 1999. *Surviving literary suicide.* Amherst: University of Massachusetts Press.

———. 2001. *Risky writing: Self-disclosure and self-transformation in the classroom.* Amherst: University of Massachusetts Press.

———. 2005. *Empathic teaching: Education for life.* Amherst: University of Massachusetts Press.

Ferenczi, Sándor. 1919. On the technique of psychoanalysis. In *Further contributions to the technique and practice of psychoanalysis*, ed. John Rickman, trans. Jane Isabel Suttie, 177–89. New York: Brunner/Mazel, 1980.

Freud, Sigmund. 1912. Recommendations to physicians practicing psychoanalysis. In *The standard edition of the complete psychological works*, ed. and trans. James Strachey et al., 12, 111–20. London: Hogarth Press, 1953–1974.

———. 1926. *The question of lay analysis.* S.E., 20, 183–250.

————. 1927. Postscript to *The question of lay analysis*. *S.E.*, 20, 251–58.

Freud, Sigmund, and Lou Andreas-Salomé. 1966. *Letters*. Ed. Ernst Pfeiffer. Trans. William and Elaine Robson-Scott. New York: Harcourt Brace Jovanovich, 1972.

Groddeck, Georg. 1923. *Das buch vom es: Psychoanalytische briefe an eine freundin*. Frankfurt: Ullstein Sachbuch, 1978.

————. 1926a. Headaches. In *Exploring the unconscious*, trans. V. M. E. Collins, 119–30. London: Vision Press, 1989.

————. 1926b. Treatment. In Groddeck 1977, 222–34.

————. 1928. Some fundamental thoughts on psychotherapy. In Groddeck 1977, 211–21.

————. 1977. *The meaning of illness: Selected psychoanalytic writings*. Ed. Lore Schacht. Trans. Gertrud Mander. London: Maresfield Library, 1988.

Rudnytsky, Peter L. 2002. *Reading psychoanalysis: Freud, Rank, Ferenczi, Groddeck*. Ithaca: Cornell University Press.

Sontag, Susan. 1978. *Illness as metaphor*. New York: Farrar, Straus and Giroux.

Stepansky, Paul E. 1999. *Freud, surgery, and the surgeons*. Hillsdale, NJ: Analytic Press.

PART I

Contextualizing Narrative Medicine

ONE

Where Does Narrative Medicine Come From?

Drives, Diseases, Attention, and the Body

RITA CHARON

A FORTY-EIGHT-YEAR-OLD Dominican man visits me for the first time, having chosen my name at random from his Medicaid Managed Care plan book. He has been suffering from dizziness and chest pain and, he tells me, he fears for his heart. As his new internist, I tell him, I have to learn as much as I can about his health. "Could you tell me whatever you think I should know about your situation?" I ask him. And then I do my best to not say a word, to not write in his medical chart, but to absorb all that the patient emits about himself—about his life, his body, his fears, and his hopes. I listen not only for the content of his narrative but for its form—its temporal course, its images, its associated subplots, its silences, where he chooses to begin in telling of himself, how he sequences symptoms with other life events. After a few minutes, the patient stops talking and begins to weep. I ask him why he cries. He says, "No one has ever let me do this before."[1]

In this emerging form of medical interviewing, I am developing new skills to achieve what I think of as the diastolic position—relaxed, absorbing, accepting, oceanic, filling. Like the heart, this position alternates with and mutually requires the systolic position—vectored, muscular, propulsive. One may but need not gender these positions. The heart beats. Either function can be deranged—diastolic dysfunction, we have learned, is as severe a handicap as systolic dysfunction. Good cardiac function absolutely requires both.

THE ROOTS OF NARRATIVE MEDICINE

As an internist, I have been given specified and quite circumscribed duties toward those in my care. I attend to the patency of the blood vessels, the inflation of the lungs, the integrity of the skin. I listen for, in the inspired words of Felix Guyot (1937), the silence of health.[2] As Lewis Thomas said somewhere: If you were put in charge of your own liver, you'd be dead in a day. And so, the internal-medicine ideal of the body is that of the BMW: the barest whirr of parts well-oiled, the confident ignorance to which one can consign the workings of the insides. If something goes wrong, signals flash on the dashboard, the silence is broken by the sounds—the complaints, as we call them—of disease.

It is only when the body complains that we have something to do. Medicine is based on symptoms, and symptoms reflect derangement of function, that is to say, disease. However much some of us like to pay attention to preventing disease or, even a greater reach, being well, the tremendous armature of medicine—NIH, training, everyday practice—is vectored, systolically, toward fixing what is broken. The body is not Virginia Woolf's (1926) smudged and rosy pane of the soul; it is the messenger of molecules gone awry. With near delight do doctors rub their hands together in the presence of disease, or at least rare or unusual diseases—zebras, we call them—because we can behold the perfect in the negative image of the diseased. It is only when something breaks that it becomes visible. Genetic mistakes or acquired damage become the portal through which, in the obverse, medical scientists behold the order of the universe. Disease is the cost—paid, of course, by someone else—of medical knowledge.

But that is not the kind of hearing that my Dominican patient with dizziness and chest pain needs from me. The internist's choice ought not be between the silence of health and the utterance of disease. There are other kinds of communications to be heard. They, too, come from the body. But the body is heteroglossic, is it not? The poor internist has only been trained in one tongue—the tongue of complaint. I think narrative medicine came about in order to teach doctors the language of pleasure, the language of loss, the language of life, and to help them come to understand that these discourses, too, speak of health. What they speak of is *salient* to the work of the general internist, the pediatrician, the busy surgeon examining a belly, the obstetrician sounding a uterus.

Looking with a critical and catholic eye at the emerging field of narrative medicine reveals its disparate roots—literature and medicine, the so-called medical humanities, primary care, relation-centered care, patient-centered care, and biopsychosocial medicine. These several movements are different ways to honor the complexities of the self's relation to the body in which it lives, and they all in one way or another circle around language, telling, relation, and the imagination. They are all roads toward correcting the undue simplemindedness of biomedicine. Biomedicine has become paltry, limited, conceptually cramped, even as it takes pride in its dazzling complexity and daring. The poverty of medicine is in the dimensions of the figural, the connotative, the meaningful. As doctors and scientists rub their hands in glee in front of their various zebras, sick people are being abandoned left and right, not because their doctors do not recognize their molecules but because they cannot apprehend their narratives.

The name "narrative medicine" visited me as I was working on an essay for a medical journal and could not decide between calling it the narrative hemisphere of medicine or the narrative dimensions of medicine. I realized all of a sudden that if you took the narrative out of medicine, there would be very little left. What would be left in the non-narrative hemisphere? Not research, which always starts with a story; not teaching, which relays tradition; and not clinical care, which, ideally anyway, unfolds in time, attends to the singular, seeks causality and tries to tolerate contingency, requires intersubjective connection, and raises ethical issues between teller and listener. All these features of what we call medical practice—temporality, singularity, intersubjectivity, causality and contingency, and ethicality—are bedrock narrative features. You find them in the tables of contents of the narratology textbooks of Seymour Chatman (1978), Gérard Genette (1972), Shlomith Rimmon-Kenan (2002), Percy Lubbock (1957), and E. M. Forster (1949).

These are the enduring features of how stories are built, and these are the subterranean but nonetheless enduring features of medical knowledge and practice. So the phrase *narrative medicine* came to me as a way to designate medicine practiced with the narrative competence to acknowledge the urgency of time, to value the singularity of patients and self, to seek the causality and to tolerate the savage contingency of disease, to dare to forge an intersubjective connection to sick people, and to fulfill the ethical duties incurred by hearing the stories of illness. I appreciated the grammatical kinship to such names as nuclear medicine and internal medicine. As a nominal phrase, it can say with more directness than can a phrase such as "literature and medicine" that this is a bona fide field of medicine in which you can specialize and still be a doctor.

The roads that narrative medicine have so far traveled began with its roots in humanities and medicine and in general practice. We have joined with literary scholars, novelists, poets, chaplains, oral historians, health professionals of all kinds, artists, and patients to examine the discourse of health care, to teach professionals and trainees about what patients go through, to attend to the interior of those who practice medicine, nursing, or social work, and to develop the competence to recognize, absorb, interpret, and be moved by the stories of self and other. Narrative medicine has evolved as a means to honor the stories of illness, whether told by the patient, family member, doctor, or nurse. More sharply, it has become a way to probe the *narrativity* of disease, of health, of healing, and of the relation between the sick person and the one who tries to help. The Program in Narrative Medicine at Columbia directs research in the mechanisms and outcomes of narrative training for health professionals, oversees the teaching of medical interviewing skills in the medical school, supports Writers-in-Residence at the medical school (including, of late, Michael Ondaatje and Susan Sontag), provides required courses at the medical school in humanities disciplines, and coaches training seminars in writing and reading for faculty and staff of the medical center.

Unlike such movements as humanism in medicine and professionalism in medicine, narrative medicine provides *methods*. It is not enough to exhort doctors to be humanistic or professional. One has to show them how to achieve such complex goals. Methods developed and sharpened in English departments, creative writing workshops, and oral history projects *work* to teach close reading, reflective writing, and bearing witness to others' suffering. We are slowly coming to see that these are the skills that medicine now lacks, these abilities—I call them collectively *narrative competence*—to get the news from stories, to cohere the booming buzzing world so that it makes sense, to value the tellings themselves and the position of the witness. We are accruing evidence that narrative training is helpful for health professionals and students, but we are at the very beginnings of understanding what really happens when one offers them these methods.[3] We have convened an intensive study seminar of Columbia faculty from a variety of humanities and clinical departments, funded by the National Endowment for the Humanities, to investigate the mechanisms, the intermediates, and the consequences of narrative training for health professionals. What happens that accounts for the benefit of reading and writing in medicine? Our NEH deliberations are generating the hypotheses that narrative training increases learners' capacities to attend to the narratives of patients, to represent that which occurs in clinical practice, and—by virtue of conferring form in the act of representation—to examine these situations once they have been rescued from formlessness. Guy Allen, a psychoanalytic scholar at the University of Toronto, proposes that personal narrative writing functions as a playground, a Winnicottian transitional object, allowing True Self to emerge from False Self and enabling the teller to navigate the shoals between self and non-self. Whether as a transitional object or through another mechanism, we find that narrative writing enables health professionals and patients to join together collaboratively, to build community, to enter affiliation with one another toward the work of healing.

Narrative medicine from the start has been a very practical field, never theorizing outside a praxis, be it in patient care or medical education or doctorly reflection. We offer narrative skills to health professionals and students not as civilizing veneer—how cute, a doctor who writes poetry—but as means to increase their clinical effectiveness. Although one runs the instrumental risk of seeming to flatten the intrinsic value of reading and writing by virtue of focusing on the improvements in clinical performance that occur as a result of narrative training, we believe that this field has first to declare its *usefulness* within the clinical setting if it wants health professionals to make time for it and to choose it against all the other skills competing for time and effort.

PSYCHOANALYSIS AND NARRATIVE MEDICINE?

What, though, is the relation between narrative medicine and psychoanalysis? They are both forms of talking cure; they rest on shared beliefs about the nature of health or well-being; they include interior aspects of patient and professional in the work of healing; and they respect the intersubjective dimensions of healing relationships. But what are the dividends of putting them side by side?

A young psychoanalyst paid me a visit in my writing studio. He had read something about narrative medicine on our Web site or in *The New York Times*, and he wanted to learn more about it. We started off on a rocky course because when he looked at my bookshelves—the Henry James criticism section—he said, "I read James in high school." A little on my guard, I then listened as he explained that all I said about narrative medicine was already known in psychoanalysis and in fact was entirely derivative. "Well, but," I countered, still smarting from his diminishment of my author, "narrative medicine has the body."

He disagreed, saying that analysis, too, has the body. The body of the analysand can often give clues to the analyst that words cannot—in gestures, position, expressions, and the like. He said that the analyst will as a matter of course attend to the patient's physical presence while trying to understand his or her experience and conscious or unconscious material. Although his answer was all too meager and foreclosed the disagreement, I admired and chose to sustain the argument. A few weeks later, at a conference at Bellagio on "Narrative, Pain, and Suffering" hosted by David Morris, I related this conversation and wondered aloud to the gathered pain medicine specialists and narratologists whether my visitor was right that narrative medicine was just a synonym for psychoanalysis. Internist Eric Cassell bellowed, "RITA, WE HAVE THE BODY." And he proceeded rather scathingly to dismiss the similarities between the two fields because of the overriding engagement by narrative medicine with corporeal experiences of pain and suffering. The bodily illness, Cassell seemed to be saying, alters the talk and the relation between the two parties, and, I think more to the point, alters the *point* of the encounter. Now, happy in an odd and irrational way that the slight to James had been paid back, I could contemplate with my medical colleagues what it might mean to put these two fields together.

I think both Cassell and I were wrong, not that narrative medicine does not have the body because indeed it does, but that psychoanalysis does not. And my young visitor was far too limited in his conception of what the body does in treatment. Maybe he did not read enough James. Here is Milly Theale in *The Wings of the Dove* after her first visit to Sir Luke Strett, the physician in the novel:

> So crystal clean the great empty cup of attention that he set between them on the table. . . . His large, settled face, though firm, was not, as she had thought at first, hard; he looked, in the oddest manner, to her fancy, half like a general and half like a bishop. . . . She had established, in other words, in this time-saving way, a relation with it; and the relation was the special trophy that, for the hour, she bore off. It was like an absolute possession, a new resource altogether, something done up in the softest silk and tucked away under the arm of memory. (1902, 231)

James figures Milly's transferential relationship with the doctor's body, his face, as a physical object with sensual dimensions, and he realizes that *memory has arms*. The body is right in there, from the start, as transference develops. Known to many as a cerebral and virginal writer, James undergoes the most hazardous passion, the wildest ecstasy, the most daring offering of body and surrender of self. If he couches or hedges his scenes of desire, it is only as a testament to their absolute peril.

He called it "the great empty cup of attention." How did he know about that emptiness? How did he know that, to perform healing by one of the other, one has to empty oneself of thought, distraction, and goals? One has to donate oneself as the amphora, the clay vessel that resonates with the sound of the breath, the sound of the self. In a remarkable early essay, Roy Schafer writes, "Generative empathy may be defined as the inner experience of sharing in and comprehending the momentary psychological state of another person, . . . experiencing in some fashion the feelings of another person" (1959, 345). He cites Christine Olden's statement that "the subject temporarily gives up his own ego for that of the object" (344). Do we not feel exhilarated when we can achieve this empty attention, when we can place ourselves at the disposal of the other, letting the other talk *through* us, ventriloquizing, finding the words in which to say that which cannot be said? This attention has profound implications for narrative medicine, for it is the method through which we enact our professional duty.[4] Developing the capacity for attention may be the main reason that serious close reading is good for health professionals—we allow ourselves as readers to be taken up by the author or the text, in the fashion of Georges Poulet (1969) and congener reader-response theorists. We donate ourselves to the demands of form and of plot. And as Norman Holland (1968; 1975) has discovered, this process simultaneously clarifies and reveals the self—its characteristic modes of coping with tension, its dispositions toward meaning making. Attention may be the pivotal value in all our work—to attend gravely, silently, absorbing oceanically that which the other says, connotes, displays, performs, and means.

But it is Sir Luke's face that forms the link with Milly. Is it the body that functions as the amphora? The body is at the same time the vehicle through which we experience sameness with the other human being and the separateness of the integument. As we sit together, we sit apart. The merging of empathy is tempered by the discreteness conferred by the delimiting skin. The body, that is to say, is *required*. We all know that the experience of analysis is a *highly* corporeal one. Like the reader who silently mouths the words on the page or the little girl who learns to dance by standing on her father's dancing feet, the analysand takes in *nothing* if not through his or her body. We perform our drives. We enact our instincts. It is not enough to think them or imagine them. They require the presence of matter—our bodily matter, James's softest silk—to become visible, graspable, treatable.

The work of treatment takes place within the playground of transference, the bodily experiences of passion and drives toward the analyst, experienced directly in the body of the patient. The analyst too would be *absent* were it not for his or her body. Freud kept reminding us that his work began with drives. "The ego is first and foremost a bodily ego," he writes in *The Ego and the Id* (1923, 26). The goals of treatment are anterior to any emotional or existential ones. The goals of treatment start with freeing the patient's libidinal energy. The emotions and life choices will follow from the release of instinctual energy for personal use.

And yet the metaphorical dimensions of the thought that followed in Freud's wake obscured the fundamentally *bodily* realm in which he found—or placed—symptom, diagnosis, and treatment. The theoretical writings of contemporary psychoanalytic scholars in literary studies and cultural studies seem sometimes to suggest that psychoanalysis is an abstract venture, grounded, if in anything, in discursive notions of the imagination. Whether Freudian or Lacanian, the formulations that have accrued currency in present-day postmodern scholarship—and I am thinking here decidedly of the nonclinical theorizing—treat power and discourse, identity and difference, and whether or not the unconscious is structured like a language and not the elemental drives and physical instincts revealed in successful clinical treatment. Even the work of such scholars as Judith Butler and Eve Kosofsky Sedgewick treats the body as a conceptual category. Only when transference becomes alive in the analysand's body can it dwell in the self and lead to change. Transference happens between the body of the patient and the body of the analyst. Anything symbolic that might precede the physical stage of transference is foreplay.

THE BODY AND THE SELF

If psychoanalysis reminds us of the corporeal dimensions of insight, narrative medicine reminds us of the metaphorical dimensions of illness. The body is *not* transparent, however good the MRI may get. The body—and by metonymic shift, the patient—is not seeable as an object. It is as opaque and explosive a body that sits in the internist's office as is the one that sits or reclines in the treatment session. That the internist *thinks* it is transparent is the problem. That he or she has not been trained to appreciate its opacity is the *real* problem.

I had a patient, a fifty-one-year-old man, who developed terrible headaches and was convinced that he had a fatal brain tumor. He discovered—to his great astonishment and sadness—that he felt ready and even eager to die. He found the prospect of an early death to be a release, a wished-for escape from life. It was through this physical symptom and his response to it that he uncovered a serious depression. He is now in treatment and no longer suicidal.

He comes to mind here because his body *told* him something his self did not know. Illness occasions the telling of two tales at once, one told by the "person" and the other told by the body of the self. How the body communicates its tale is very mysterious. Sometimes its signals are very clear—my left knee hurts since I ran thirteen miles or a sore throat tells me I'm getting the flu. Sometimes its signals are obscure, like the paralysis suffered by Freud's hysterical patients. Even though the body is material, its communications are always representations, mediating the sensations and the meanings ascribed to them. It is sometimes as if the body speaks a foreign language, relying on bilingual others to translate or interpret or in some way make transparent what it means to say.

The self depends on the body for its presence, its location. Without the body, the self cannot be uttered. Without the body, the self cannot enter relation with others. Without the body, the self is an abstraction. Religious scholar John Hull, who became blind in midlife, says that without vision, "I often feel I am a mere spirit, a ghost, a memory" (1990, 25). "This is such a profound lostness" (145). Anthropologist Robert Murphy experienced fleeting neurological symptoms of muscle spasms and numbness of his feet. Eventually, he learned that a tumor had grown around his spinal cord from the level of his neck to mid-chest, compressing the cord and eventually causing quadriplegia. Murphy bends all his skills and conceptual powers as an anthropologist to write a "participant-observer" report on himself, called *The Body Silent* (1990). He understands this dual nature of the body:

> People in good health take their lot, and their bodies, for granted; they can
> see, hear, eat, make love, and breathe because they have working organs
> that can do all those things. These organs, and the body itself, are among

the foundations upon which we build our sense of who and what we are, and they are the instruments through which we grapple with and create reality. (12)

Poised between world and self, the body simultaneously undergoes the world while emanating to that world its self. Or again, the body is simultaneously a receiver with which the self collects all sensate and cognate information about what lies exterior to it and a projector with which the body declares the self who lives in it. The body is the copulative term that bridges self to world.

We are beginning to realize the metaphorical generativity of the body. Ed Cohen (2003) has written about the complex healing metaphors of the body, including the pluripotence of the word *immunity*. The body is probably equaled only by Shakespeare or the Bible in its allusive powers. One need not exceed the body to utter almost anything of value about life. For example, I am currently working on an essay entitled "The Clitoral Brain." What I mean to point to by that phrase is the fact that the body, in all its fecundity, can represent almost anything one cares to represent. It is the master mediator of our passions, the sacred fount of trope. Both merging and keeping separate, this body combines its diastole and systole, ever not explaining but *living* our human situation.

But it is also the harbinger of dread. In a routine medical interview tape-recorded and transcribed in linguistic research, an internist meets a patient for the first time.[5] The patient is a sixty-five-year-old former truck driver who has had to take early retirement for a variety of symptoms. (In what follows, D = doctor, P = patient, tabulated utterances represent interruptions, and square brackets represent inaudible utterances.)

D: You wake up at night short of breath?

P: Right.

D: You do. How long has that been going on?

P: I think about a year. I be sleeping . . .

    D: Uh-hunh . . .

P: Where for [. . .] pretty much out of nowhere, and all of a sudden I wake up and I can't get my breath back and I sit up.

D: And how often has that happened in the last year? Is it, you know, once a month, every week, every night?

P: Not every night, not every night. I figure maybe once a week, some-time every two weeks, it all depends, you know it varies.

D: Un-hunh, so and then you, and then what happens?

P: I set up. I'm in pretty good shape.

D: Un-hunh.

P: I be alright, you know.

D: How long does it take before you, your, your breathing calms down?

P: Maybe about five minutes.

D: Five minutes. Anything else when that happens, do you sweat a lot, or . . . ?

P: Once in a while I might break into a sweat, if it be real warm, but that don't happen too often.

D: Most of the time, what about chest pain when that happens, do you have chest pain or not?

P: No, no, no.

D: You're not . . .

P: Not . . .

D: Okay. And, um, uh, uh, do you sleep with one pillow, more than one pillow?

P: Three pillows I sleep on.

D: Three pillows. How long you been doing that?

P: Past two or three years.

D: Past two or three years.

    P: Since I quit work.

D: Is that because your breathing is easier on two or three pillows?

P: In a way, yes. It helps.

D: It does.

P: Un-hunh.

The patient seems to be trying to tell a story of himself as a strong working man who drove a produce truck until retirement age, leaving his job only when his leg gave way but who continues to be "in pretty good shape." The doctor interferes with this story, eliciting instead a shadow story of severe congestive heart failure told unwittingly by the patient. Although the patient does not know the significance of his nighttime breathlessness and his reliance on three pillows for comfortable sleep, the doctor does. In effect, the patient's body tells the doctor—over the patient's shoulder, as it were, whispering out of his hearing—about his heart disease. The patient's statement of health—"I be alright, you know"—is overpowered by the voice of his own body. In effect, the body colludes with the doctor to negate what the patient says.

In the analyst's office, the body of the patient takes center stage. It is not the body of symptoms that signify disease, but the body of drives and instincts signifying libidinal health, or a potential return to health. In the internist's office, the patient's body that presents itself is one of hidden frailty, bad news to be delivered. "I'm sorry to have to tell you this, but you have end-stage congestive heart failure. You have a 20 percent chance of being alive in five years." The double vision that internists develop is one of impending death. All we see when we look into the distance is defeat—not pleasure, not freedom, but death. This is true.

Another important feature of medical practice is illuminated by placing it beside psychiatric or psychoanalytic treatment. It is the case that I can touch the bodies of my patients. I must. I must inevitably inflict pain on them. I do things to them that no one else is allowed to do. I handle my patients' bodies, I fondle them, I stroke them. I percuss them, I palpate them, I inject them. Surgeons do worse. We have *not at all* thought about the implications of this corporeal contact in our work, and I simply bracket that thought for future work.

What the analytic situation makes clear to the narrative medicine situation is the centrality of relation. "Non-narrative medicine," whatever that might be, dispenses with the transference. It overlooks it. It pretends to universality, that is, the belief that any doctor would do the same thing as any other doctor. It dismisses the personal investment in and love of the patient. When we introduce narrative methods to medicine, we are encouraging health professionals to examine their deep attachments to patients. Here is a short poem written by a social worker in Narrative Oncology, where doctors, nurses, and social workers on the inpatient oncology unit gather to read to one another what they have written about their clinical work:

> I look at you in the bed, a child
>> you think you are a man.
> You are fading away,
>> now only your eyes seem to enlarge.
> You ask when you can go home,
>> go back to your life.
> This is your life now.
> Your family members stand mute
>> awaiting answers that are not there.
>
> I will stay the course with you.

We find it is helpful for health professionals and students to reconcile themselves to their tremendously powerful feelings of love and attachment to their patients. The casual use of the word "countertransference" that has sprung up in medicine is usually reserved for feelings of hatred or distaste that we all occasionally experience toward patients, especially those with revolting diseases. And yet the positive countertransference of medicine is tremendously magnetic. Here is a third-year medical student's entry in the Parallel Chart, a place where students are encouraged to write those aspects of their care of patients that do *not* belong in the hospital chart, in which she has merged, in imaginative identity, with a woman dying of AIDS:

> The day you started to bleed out I ran to the lab with a tube of your blood to find out how many platelets you had left. I told the lab lady that it had to be STAT, STAT, STAT because you were bleeding. She STAT, STAT, STAT-ed her way to the automated blood count machine and promptly put your tube in line behind eight others. I said No!—My blood—I meant your blood—goes in first—and I managed to get us six tubes ahead on the conveyor belt. As the row of purple tops advanced, I watched the tubes ahead of ours be picked up and stirred by the science-fictiony robotic arm. Then it disappeared into the machine and the computer screen told us that someone named Melissa Brand had 110,000 platelets. I never thought there was such a thing as "platelet envy"—but when your count came back as 2,000, I found that I was very resentful of Melissa Brand.[6]

I think that one of the most urgent goals of narrative medicine is to reveal to health care professionals the extent of their positive regard for patients under their care. The corollary goal is to let them understand the power of this transferential relation to improve health. This is vital. The time I spend with a patient, over decades, equals what an analyst might spend with an analysand over years. If I see a patient every two or three months for a half hour at a time and a couple of times a day when she is hospitalized, and this goes on for twenty-five years, and all those phone calls in between and letters to housing, to the disability board, to Medicaid, to get her off jury duty, I have amassed the equivalent of the analytic hours of a couple of years, at least.

We ordinary doctors, I am trying to suggest, can reformulate the goals of everyday medicine in view of psychoanalytic lessons about attention, drives, and relationships. Complicating our notions of the body helps us to do so. Acknowledging the medical transference that develops between us and our patients likewise aids us in this effort. We can all try to achieve the oceanic absorptive position, intercalating and giving *lift* and singularity to our vectored actions on the patient's behalf. We can recognize the human meaning and consequences of disease along with its mechanisms and molecular implications, and we can accept that recognizing them is a necessary ingredient to our care. We can bear witness to patients' suffering as we try to diagnose and treat their diseases.

What will my Dominican man and I do together? My pact is that I will husband his health while I offer an absorptive space and reflective surface to try to *represent* him for his view. His stress test revealed ischemic heart disease, and so we will embark together on treatment, on improving his health, on living within the limitations imposed by his circulatory anatomy. I prepare for a long life with him—I will get to know his unit number by heart, the names of all his kids and grandkids, his chest x-ray, his LDL, his ejection fraction, his fears, his hopes. Knowing more or less what is in store for him (for I have seen it before), I can illuminate the future of his body while we *find* together a future of attachment and investment. What we generate together in our relation is something of substance, a "special trophy," an "absolute possession" for both of us that matters, that counts, that contributes to his health and well-being and, as a dividend, to mine. Through the attention I donate and the authenticity he displays, we grow together in knowledge, in action, and in grace, hoping for the best, making it out together.

NOTES

1. This description has been published in my "Narrative and Medicine" (2004, 862–64).

2. When I gave this lecture at the Psychoanalysis and Narrative Medicine conference, I wrongly attributed the phrase "the silence of health" to René Dubos. In a marvelous and telling collaborative act, Norman Holland came up with the actual source.

3. See DasGupta and Charon (2004) for a report of some outcomes of narrative writing for medical students.

4. The literature on attention is a vast and most varied one, including philosophers Iris Murdoch, Simone Weil, Gabriel Marcel, and Martin Buber; psychologists of mindfulness; religious scholars who write on contemplative states in Zen practice, mystical Christianity, and the Jewish Kaballah; literary scholars Roland Barthes and Sharon Cameron; aesthetic theorists John Berger and Susan Sontag; and such novelists as Marcel Proust and James.

5. This transcript is derived from a linguistic research project in Ageism and the Clinical Encounter completed at Columbia University, funded by the Andrus Foundation and AARP, with Columbia University Institutional Review Board approval as well as signed informed consent from patients and providers giving permission to the researchers to cite anonymously from the transcripts for educational purposes.

6. Permission has been granted by the author to publish this excerpt of the Parallel Chart. The name Melissa Brand is an alias.

REFERENCES

Allen, Guy. 2002. The "good-enough" teacher and the authentic student. In *A pedagogy of becoming*, ed. Jon Mills, 141–76. Amsterdam: Rodopi.

Charon, Rita. 2004. Narrative and medicine. *New England Journal of Medicine* 350:862–64.

Chatman, Seymour. 1978. *Story and discourse: Narrative structure in fiction and film.* Ithaca: Cornell University Press.

Cohen, Ed. 2003. Metaphorical immunity: A case of biomedical fiction. *Literature and Medicine* 22:140–63.

DasGupta, Sayantani, and Rita Charon. 2004. Personal illness narratives: Using reflective writing to teach empathy. *Academic Medicine* 79:351–56.

Forster, E. M. 1949. *Aspects of the novel.* London: E. Arnold.

Freud, Sigmund. 1923. *The ego and the id.* In *Standard edition of the complete psychological works,* ed. and trans. James Strachey et al., 19, 3–66. London: Hogarth Press, 1953–1974.

Genette, Gérard. 1972. *Narrative discourse: An essay in method.* Trans. Jane Lewin. Ithaca: Cornell University Press, 1980.

Guyot, Felix. 1937. *Yoga: The silence of health.* New York: Schocken Books.

Holland, Norman. 1968. *The dynamics of literary response.* New York: Columbia University Press, 1989.

———. 1975. *5 readers reading.* New Haven: Yale University Press.

Hull, John. 1990. *Touching the rock: An experience of blindness.* New York: Vintage Books.

James, Henry. 1902. *The wings of the dove.* In *The New York edition: The novels and tales of Henry James.* Vol. 19. New York: Charles Scribner's Sons, 1909.

Lubbock, Percy. 1957. *The craft of fiction.* New York: Viking Books.

Murphy, Robert. 1990. *The body silent: The different world of the disabled.* New York: Norton.

Poulet, Georges. 1969. Phenomenology of reading. *New Literary History* 1:53–67.

Rimmon-Kenan, Shlomith. 2002. *Narrative fiction: Contemporary poetics.* Second ed. London: Routledge.

Schafer, Roy. 1959. Generative empathy in the treatment situation. *Psychoanalytic Quarterly* 28:343–73.

Woolf, Virginia. 1926. On being ill. In *The moment, and other essays,* 9–23. New York: Random House, 1974.

TWO

Desire and Obesity

Dickens, Endocrinology,
Pulmonary Medicine, and Psychoanalysis

SANDER L. GILMAN

DICKENS AND THE PHYSIOGNOMY OF OBESITY

THE IMAGE of the obese man is one that seems quite fixed in the worldview of nineteenth-century Anglophone high culture. His stereotype permeates the metaphors (and thus the minds) of even the most radical of thinkers of the time. Thus, on October 16, 1851, Frederick Douglass, abolitionist and fighter for women's rights, announced that *"The [New York] Herald*, in noticing the [Liberty Party National Convention] nominations, thus exhibits its innate vulgarity: 'Mr. D. is white, which shows some progress during the past year even with the old Liberty party.' We do not see what complexion has to do with a man's fitness for an office requiring an active and a well informed mind; but we do see, that gross obesity, as tending to induce mental stupidity, as coarseness of feeling, might seriously disqualify a man for such an office" (8). In this world of stereotypical physiognomic equivalents, obesity is a sign of mental vacuity and of an insensitivity of emotional response. The stupidity and crudity of emotions that Douglass gestured at were those of the senior James Gordon Bennett, the corpulent and conservative editor of *The New York Herald.*

Being fat is identical to being unreceptive to the realities of the world about one. It is a sign of the impairment of one's intelligence and emotions. Thus, at the beginning of the nineteenth century William Wadd, the Surgeon-Extraordinary to the Prince-Regent, stated that "if the Goddess of Wisdom were to grow fat, even she would become stupid. . . . Fat and stupidity, says the accomplished Lord Chesterfield, are looked upon as such inseparable companions that they are used as synonymous terms" (1829, 53). While this is an ancient parallel, it is also clear that the assumption that body size reflects mental acuity and emotional life was not simply a commonplace in the culture of the nineteenth century, but was also contested in unusual ways.

The most evident literary encapsulation of the image of the stupid fat man seems to be found in Charles Dickens's *The Pickwick Papers* (1836). This is the last great eighteenth-century novel of travel, making Dickens the heir of Fielding and Smollett (see Klienberger 1981). But it is also the first Victorian novel inasmuch as, as V. S. Pritchett noted, the desire for food replaces the "eighteenth-century attitude to sex in the comic unity of Dickens" (1966, 313). In *Tom Jones*, food is a path to sex; in Dickens it seems to be a substitute for it. The representation of desire is made socially acceptable by being placed at the table rather than in the bed. Yet desire remains the hallmark of what is truly human.

Dickens uses his readers' expectations as to which characters should or should not be able to experience desire as well as what the appropriate object of desire should be in order to critique the very notion of the lack of an emotional (and intellectual) life for the obese. The shift in imagining desire plays upon the physiognomy of the characters as a means of undermining these expectations. In Dickens's early *Sketches by Boz* (1833–1836), he presents the notion that if "the agitation of a man's brain by different passions" (qtd. in Tytler 1982, 253–54) can shape his skull, so too can it shape the form and function of his street-door knocker. Many years ago, I (1978; see also Vega-Ritter 2003) tracked this social/physiognomic phenomenon in Dickens's work on insanity, showing how his representation of the insane provided a critique of the assumptions concerning madness in the world of the reformed asylum. Relying on the physiognomic presuppositions of his time (and the rise of psychiatric photography pioneered by his friends), Dickens was able to provide readers with insight into their own visual expectations of insanity.

What is striking is that when one turns to *The Pickwick Papers* to examine the question of obesity, not only is the question of physiognomy central to the author's concern but there is an explicit critique of the prevailing assumptions concerning our ability to read the physiognomy of the obese as opposed to the merely corpulent. From the standpoint of a contemporary reader (and viewer of the "Phiz" illustrations by Hablot K. Browne), everyone in *The Pickwick Papers* is fat. (One can note that the initial images of Pickwick by Robert Seymour, who committed suicide in 1836, had more in common with the body of Don Quixote than that of Sancho Panza [see Johannsen 1956]). Juliet McMaster (1987) argues convincingly that Dickens presents two kinds of "fat": The first is Mr. Samuel Pickwick (and his middle-class friends) who is, to use her words, "fat-cheery" instead of "fat-bloated" (25; see also Huff 2000). Pickwick (and his friends) is plump and "charged with energy, solar or otherwise. He bursts, he beams, he bulges. . . . His fatness . . . is scarcely even heavy" (McMaster 1987, 88). But the "fat-bloated" form of obesity seems to be incorporated in Mr. Wardel's "boy," his servant, Joe. He is "better known to the readers of this unvarnished history by the distinguishing appellation of the fat boy" (Dickens 1836, 338) whose body mirrors his soul, or so it seems.

Joe, the comic parallel to Mr. Pickwick's clever (and thin) servant Sam Weller, is defined in the novel by his blank expression, huge appetite, and ability to avoid work by falling asleep instantaneously. He is a version of Sancho Panza except that all of the Quixotes in this novel are "fat-cheery" except him. He is regularly described as snoring "in a low and monotonous sound." Joe is comic because of his girth and what it implies:

> "Come along, Sir. Pray, come up," said the stout gentleman. "Joe!—damn that boy, he's gone to sleep again.—Joe, let down the steps." The fat boy rolled slowly off the box, let down the steps, and held the carriage door invitingly open. Mr. Snodgrass and Mr. Winkle came up at the moment. "Room for you all, gentlemen," said the stout man. "Two inside, and one out. Joe, make room for one of these gentlemen on the box. Now, Sir, come along," and the stout gentleman extended his arm, and pulled first Mr. Pickwick, and then Mr. Snodgrass, into the barouche by main force. Mr. Winkle mounted to the box, the fat boy waddled to the same perch, and fell fast asleep instantly. (Dickens 1836, 61)

In this description, we are presented with the stereotype that "Fat Boys" such as Joe move their buttocks comically (like an animal) and that they are lazy, falling asleep whenever they cease moving as a sign of their almost medieval sinful sloth and stupidity. Joe is *seen* as fat, and fat means that he is mentally "slow" and without the appropriate emotional responses. But what that actually means in Dickens's world of false appearances is not at first quite clear.[1] And that is reflected in the very nature of how he is seen. Sam Weller calls him "young dropsy" (340), ironically seeing his sleepiness as a reflection of illness. Pickwick calls him a "young opium eater" (344). He is a freak, a body that "had never [been] seen in or out of a traveling convoy" (675). His is a truly obese body, unlike that of the bourgeois characters. And it is seen as neither healthy nor "normal."

The Fat Boy in Dickens's novel seems to be ill, as one commentator in a Philadelphia African-American newspaper of the 1860s noted about obesity:

> A voracious appetite, so far from being a sign of health, is a certain indication of disease. Some dyspeptics are always hungry; they feel best when they are eating, but as soon as they have eaten they enter torments, so distressing

in their nature, as to make the unhappy victim wish for death. . . . Multitudes measure their health by the amount they can eat; and of any ten persons, nine are gratified at an increase of weight, as if mere bulk were an index of health; when in reality, any excess of fatness is, in proportion, decisive proof of existing disease; showing that the absorbents of the system are too weak to discharge their duty; and the tendency to fatness, to obesity, increases, until existence is a burden, and sudden death closes the history. (*Christian Recorder* 1864, 12)

Obesity for the Victorian was an illness unto death.

But is Joe truly ill in this sense? Gail Turley Houston notes: "Dickens expects the reader to differentiate between Pickwickian gentlemanly gusto and the ludicrous gorging of the poverty-stricken hangers-on such as . . . the fat boy" (1994, 21). Thus, Mr. Pickwick when awakened by the first rays of the sun "was no sluggard . . . he sprang like an ardent warrior from his tent-bedstead" (Dickens 1836, 75). He is plump but quick of body and mind—and therefore healthy and wise. But Joe's "illness" is clearly not physiological but "social," not an illness of his own making but a reflection of the society's perception of obesity. What differentiates Joe from Mr. Pickwick is the work's definition of true masculinity.

Indeed, the boundary that defines the masculine seems to run along the fault line of obesity in the Anglophone nineteenth century. In the Victorian epic of Canada, *Idomen; or, the Vale of Yumuri* (1843), by Maria del Occidente (i.e., Maria Gowen Brooks, 1794/5–1845), the protagonist is described as follows:

> His age at this time was twenty-three years;
> his stature much exceeded six feet, and his figure,
> though still supple and slender, had attained
> enough of obesity to give that roundness
> of surface so much admired by painters.
>
> The ancient Romans, sometimes fed their
> gladiators with a chosen food, to make them
> look more beautiful;—but here, what tints and
> contour had been refined by a process of nature,
> from the snowy earth of Canada! (25)

"The Stranger's" body is full and yet masculine, formed by his experience on the frontier. Here is the male body in all its glory, just "obese" enough to be attractive. This clearly is not the body of the Fat Boy, who never seems to be the object of anyone's desire.

There is one odd but effective moment very early in *The Pickwick Papers* where Mr. Wardel's "boy" Joe's inferior mental and emotional status is drawn into question. Joe accidentally observes an attempted seduction take place in the garden. Mr. Tracy Tupman is wooing the "spinster aunt" (Dickens 1836, 94) Rachael Wardle, an odd match even in the world of Pickwick, for "young men, to spinster aunts, are as lighted gas to gunpowder." Joe observes them, and the seducer looks at Joe being "perfectly motionless, with his large circular eyes staring into the arbour, but without the slightest expression on his face that the most expert physiognomist could have referred to astonishment, curiosity, or any other known passion that agitates the human breast. Mr. Tupman gazed on the fat boy, and the fat boy stared at him; and the longer Mr. Tupman observed the utter vacancy of the fat boy's countenance, the more convinced he became that he either did not know, or did not understand, anything that had been going forward" (89). This is a clear misapprehension.

For, of course, Joe has understood all too well. As Tupman walks off, "there was a sound behind them, as of an imperfectly suppressed chuckle. Mr. Tupman turned sharply round. No; it could not have been the fat boy; there was not a gleam of mirth, or anything but feeding in his whole visage." His fat physiognomy is unreadable, but he knows what he has observed and turns it to his own advantage! Later he turns to his employer's aged mother, to whom he wishes to reveal all. She is initially frightened at his desire to speak because he had been marked by a silence that reflected his girth. She protests that she had always treated him well and given him enough to eat. He responds with the emotionally ambiguous statement: "I wants to make your flesh creep" (93). In revealing what he has seen in all of its detail, with all of its "kissin' and huggin'," he shows that not only does he recognize ill-placed desire but he can also tell the story for his own betterment. (The reader first meets a similar character in a similar mode in the *Sketches by Boz* when a "corpulent round-headed boy" peeps through a keyhole [1833–1836, 371].)

In Wilhelm Ebstein's (1884) late Victorian study of obesity, the first standard medical presentation of obesity as a physiological problem, the author quotes the eighteenth-century German essayist Georg Lichtenberg who says that "there be people with such plump faces that they may laugh under their fat, so that the greatest physiognomist shall fail to notice it, while we poor slender creatures with our souls seated immediately beneath the epidermis, ever speak a language which can tell no lies" (11). Joe seems to be inscrutable in his obesity, but the tale he tells will make all notice him. He tells stories that will indeed "make your flesh creep," but at his own pace and in his own time. James Joyce knows the power of this moment when in the Scylla and Charybdis chapter of *Ulysses* he has John Eglinton say that Stephen Dedalus "will have it that Hamlet is a ghost story. . . . Like the fat boy in Pickwick he wants to make our flesh creep" (1922, 154; see Bowen 1997). And our flesh does creep at these ghost stories because of the anomalous nature of the narrator, our seemingly stupid and insensitive Fat Boy.[2]

This is the reader's introduction to Joe at the very beginning of the novel. His stories may make the characters' flesh creep only because they seem not to be able to read his face. For Fat Boys' physiognomy seems not to mirror their character. And yet at the very conclusion of the novel, Dickens returns to the same scene in a different setting. Joe stumbles into another seduction, now of age-appropriate individuals, seeing Mr. Augustus Snodgrass with his arm about his beloved Emily Wardle's waist.

> "Wretched creature, what do you want here?" said the gentleman, who it is needless to say was Mr. Snodgrass.
>
> To this the fat boy, considerably terrified, briefly responded, "Missis."
>
> "What do you want me for," inquired Emily, turning her head aside, "you stupid creature?"
>
> "Master and Mr. Pickwick is a-going to dine here at five," replied the fat boy.
>
> "Leave the room!" said Mr. Snodgrass, glaring upon the bewildered youth.
>
> "No, no, no," added Emily hastily. "Bella, dear, advise me."
>
> Upon this, Emily and Mr. Snodgrass, and Arabella and Mary, crowded into a corner, and conversed earnestly in whispers for some minutes, during which the fat boy dozed.
>
> "Joe," said Arabella, at length, looking round with a most bewitching smile, "how do you do, Joe?"
>
> "Joe," said Emily, "you're a very good boy; I won't forget you, Joe."
>
> "Joe," said Mr. Snodgrass, advancing to the astonished youth, and seizing his hand, "I didn't know you before. There's five shillings for you, Joe!"
>
> "I'll owe you five, Joe," said Arabella, "for old acquaintance sake, you know"; and another most captivating smile was bestowed upon the corpulent intruder.
>
> The fat boy's perception being slow, he looked rather puzzled at first to account for this sudden prepossession in his favour, and stared about him in a very alarming manner. At length his broad face began to show symptoms of a grin of proportionately broad dimensions; and then, thrusting half-a-crown into each of his pockets, and a hand and wrist after it, he burst into a horse laugh: being for the first and only time in his existence.
>
> "He understands us, I see," said Arabella.
>
> "He had better have something to eat, immediately," remarked Emily.
> (Dickens 1836, 685–86)

Joe certainly understands. He understands the moment of seduction he has observed. He certainly understands the double sense of Arabella's statement that she will not forget him, a two-edged statement that has to do with monetary reward but also an acknowledgment of him as a human being. He may be "slow" but he clearly understands the sexual tension in the room and the power that that grants him. His physiognomy is completely readable by all. He smiles and he laughs, as for once he is in control of the situation; or is he?

And the company sends the servant Mary off with Joe to make sure that he does not again expose lovers to the forces of social control. It is the laughter (that had also signaled Joe's first sense of awareness in his observation of the earlier seduction) that makes them anxious. They immediately sit down to feed Joe's appetite. Mary's feeding of Joe is to draw his attention away from the desire shown by the lovers, and Joe unexpectedly offers Mary some of the food with which she was bribing him:

> The fat boy assisted Mary to a little, and himself to a great deal, and was just going to begin eating when he suddenly laid down his knife and fork, leaned forward in his chair, and letting his hands, with the knife and fork in them, fall on his knees, said, very slowly—
> "I say! How nice you look!"
> This was said in an admiring manner, and was, so far, gratifying; but still there was enough of the cannibal in the young gentleman's eyes to render the compliment a double one.
> "Dear me, Joseph," said Mary, affecting to blush, "what do you mean?"
> The fat boy, gradually recovering his former position, replied with a heavy sigh, and, remaining thoughtful for a few moments, drank a long draught of the porter. Having achieved this feat, he sighed again, and applied himself assiduously to the pie. (686)

The question of Joe's unexpected attraction to Mary startles the reader in Dickens's use of the image of the cannibal. He ironically has us see the Fat Boy reducing Mary from an object of erotic desire to one of gustatory pleasure. Yet the "heavy sigh" points to a very different desire. He knows what object of desire is available to him. Following this exchange, Joe returns to Pickwick with a note from Emily Wardle. He comments to Sam Weller about the servant girl Mary (in whom Weller is more than interested), "'I say,' said Joe, who was unusually loquacious, 'what a pretty girl Mary is, isn't she? I am SO fond of her, I am!' Mr. Weller made no verbal remark in reply; but eyeing the fat boy for a moment, quite transfixed at his presumption, led him by the collar to the corner, and dismissed him with a harmless but ceremonious kick" (712–13). Even Fat Boys can show desire! And here V. S. Pritchett's claim of the transformation of the erotic into the pleasures of the table is undermined by our recognition that Joe's motivations are much more complex than merely gustatory. His desire for status (in reporting the first seduction) and our awareness of his potential for love in the latter case change how Joe is seen both within the text and by the reader. Masculinity is not canceled by what has been apostrophized in the novel as pathological obesity. Joe can desire and can express this desire.

Yet there is the unstated question of whether the Fat Boy can have desire, whether he can be a sexual being. In 1859, the British colonial surgeon W. G. Don, reporting from India, presented the case of a twelve-year-old "Hindoo

boy, known in the streets of Bombay under the soubriquet of the 'Fat Boy'"
(363). The echo of Dickens in this colonial report is clear. Don's "Fat Boy" had
become very fat at the age of two until "his whole body is now encased in an
immense mass of solid adipose tissue, which hangs in pendulous folds over his
chest and hips, and the flexures of his limbs." At twelve he is forty-eight and
a half inches tall, weighing 206 lbs. He seems in good health except for "a difficulty breathing," but his "appearance is extremely odd" as he "walks with difficulty, and when tired rests himself by leaning his pendulous abdomen against
a wall." While he seems normally developed for a twelve-year-old, "the genital organs, however, are not larger than those of an infant, while the testes are
very small, and seem either to be undeveloped or to have become atrophied."
He is, however, "highly intelligent." Here the unstated "secret" of the Fat Boy
seems to be revealed. Can Victorian Fat Boys have sexual desire? Or is their
physiognomy the hidden secret of their seeming lack of desire?

The idea that the fat man's physiognomy was misread and that the
"rules" of physiognomic interpretation led to flagrant abuses was a topic
before Dickens. Thomas Love Peacock (1785–1866) in his *Crotchet Castle*
(1831) presents the reader with Dr. Folliet, who, while quoting Greek poetry
to a nightingale, is attacked by two armed robbers and drives them off with
his walking stick. He is able to do so in a rage, because he imagines them
looking at him and thinking that he is an easy target because he appears to
be a fat, old man:

> One of them drew a pistol, which went off in the very act of being struck
> aside by the bamboo, and lodged a bullet in the brain of the other. There
> was then only one enemy, who vainly struggled to rise, every effort being
> attended with a new and more signal prostration. The fellow roared for
> mercy. "Mercy, rascal!" cried the divine; "what mercy were you going to
> show me, villain? What! I warrant me, you thought it would be an easy mat-
> ter, and no sin, to rob and murder a parson on his way home from dinner.
> You said to yourselves, doubtless, 'We'll waylay the fat parson (you irrever-
> ent knave) as he waddles home (you disparaging ruffian), half-seas-over
> (you calumnious vagabond).'" And with every dyslogistic term, which he
> supposed had been applied to himself, he inflicted a new bruise on his
> rolling and roaring antagonist. "Ah, rogue!" he proceeded; "you can roar
> now, marauder; you were silent enough when you devoted my brains to dis-
> persion under your cudgel. But seeing that I cannot bind you, and that I
> intend you not to escape, and that it would be dangerous to let you rise, I
> will disable you in all your members . . ." (1831, 364; see Hewitt 1971; Mul-
> vihill 1983)

His fat only appears not to be masculine; in reality he is "plump," not fat—
and dangerous, too. His anger, like Joe's desire, may be masked by a misreading of the body but reveals itself in his actions. Fat Boys can indeed mislead!

JOE AND THE OBESITY OF CHILDREN

The image of the active, angry plump middle-class man is quite the opposite of that of the servant Joe, whose fat seems to have "its customary association with inertia" (McMaster 1987, 88). Joe, however, became a case study of pathology that overrode Dickens's much more complex image of limitation and awareness. It was read as an example of the obesity of youth. As Edward Jukes noted in 1833: "Fat, when moderately diffused over the body, indicates a sound state of health, and an easy disposition, gives a symmetry to the figure, and (which by many is valued more than all these) it contributes much to the beauty of the countenance; but on the contrary, where it accumulates to excess, it becomes an absolute disease, and is frequently the cause of death, particularly in habits where some chronic disorder has preceded it, or where acute attacks of disease have been aggravated by its presence" (287). The causes, according to Dickens's contemporary, are either "occasioned by indulging in the use of highly nutritious foods" or, as in the case of the Fat Boy, "a peculiarity of constitution predisposing to this state" (289–90). Fat Boys can be a separate class (in both senses of the word), born to be fat. Dickens's Fat Boy has no childhood; he is the product of his class and the immediate world in which he lives. Dickens wrestles with the question of the meaning of inheritance as his world comes to be that of Herbert Spencer's struggle of the fittest and Darwin's evolutionary model. In the *Pickwick Papers* Dickens rejects the very notion of a child being able to inherit acquired characteristics, so that Joe could not be the son nor the father of obese men (Morgentaler 2000, 35). Joe inhabits his own world and is neither degenerate nor the son of degenerates.

In the Enlightenment, Christoph Wilhelm Hufeland had captured in his extraordinarily popular *The Art of Prolonging Life* (1797, 1:169) a social explanation for adult obesity.[3] Fat is simply bad for Hufeland and the Enlighteners because most people eat much more than they need. "Immoderation" is one of the prime causes of early death (2:43). Invoking the Aristotelian golden mean, they believed that eating too much and eating too richly will kill you. "Idleness" is also a cause (2:64). Human beings have lost their natural ability to determine how much we need by childhood overindulgence. Natural man, notes Hufeland, in plowing the fields has purpose, exercise, and food appropriate to long life. "His son becomes a studious rake; and the proportion between countrymen and citizens seems daily to be diminished" (2:217). The fat child is now the father (and mother) of the fat adult. Indeed, Hufeland places at the very beginning of his list of things that will certainly cause early death a "very warm, tender, and delicate education" in childhood in which children are stuffed "immoderately with food; and by coffee, chocolate, wine, spices, and such things" (2:9). Not sin but middle-class overindulgence begins to be seen as the force that creates Fat Boys. In the nineteenth century the "science" of diet seemed to replace the morals of diet. The hidden model remained the same: the normal, reasonable man was always contrasted with the Fat Boy and always to the Fat Boy's detriment. And the reward for the thin man was life, life extended, while the fat man died young and badly.

Unlike the pampered children of Hufeland's middle class, fat children came to be seen as primal beings through the lens of the various models of evolutionary theory that dominated the world of Dickens. They were considered throwbacks to the world of the primitive. They lacked a specific sense of "masculinity" that was inherent to Victorian ideas of manliness (Tosh 1999, 4). Louis Robinson, in the middle-class journal *The Nineteenth Century*, asked: "Why should babies be so fat, when the children of their pithecoid ancestors must have been lean? . . . The suicidal swallowing capacity of the modern baby is an inheritance from the habits of the crawling cave-dweller" (1891, 831). An anonymous wag in *Punch* replied:

> Baby boy, whose visage chubby
> Doting mother marvels at,
> Full of health, albeit grubby—
> Why are you so fat?
>
> How unlike your rude forefather—
> Prehistoric, pithecoid!
> Who with nuts he chanced to gather
> Filled his aching void . . .
>
> No! but later generations
> Come, in which the infant staves
> Hunger off by dint of rations
> Picked up in the caves.
>
> Holding future meals in question,
> Grasping all with eager fist,—
> To the mill of his digestion
> Everything is grist.
>
> Consequently, you, who follow
> Him in lack of self-control,
> With atavic impulse swallow
> Dirt, and pins and coal. (1903, 203)

By the end of the century post-Darwinian fat was the product of an evolutionary development, which gave purpose to actions in the past but which had by now become atavistic.

Fat had a true function, at least in our distant past, but today such Fat Boys are primeval throwbacks, unable to function in contemporary society. In such a Darwinian reading, Joe's body is different from that of Pickwick and all of the other plump, middle-class adventurers in Dickens's novel. His body comes to be read not merely as a symptom of his class (Sam Weller's body is the body of the healthy and wily servant), but as an example of the physiognomy of the primitive that haunts this world of work. Joe is the "Fat Boy," the young man, who, unlike Sam Weller, will never be able to accomplish anything because of his girth. He is a curiosity, kept by Mr. Wardle precisely because of this fat. It is the worker who has a lack of will because of his ancestry and background. At the extreme, it is the worker as alcoholic and criminal. Here, it is the worker as Fat Boy, condemned to live out his desires because of his physical inheritance.[4]

Indeed, William Thomas Moncrieff dramatized *The Pickwick Papers* under the title *Sam Weller or The Pickwickians* (1837) so quickly that Dickens was able just as quickly to satirize him as "the literary gentleman" in *Nicholas Nickleby* in 1839. Moncrieff (1850) presented Joe as the exemplary *British* somnambulist in a ditty sung in the British music halls during the 1840s, well before the Darwin craze:

> Don't disturb yourself, pray—'tis but Joe, the Fat Boy,
> Who was never known any one's rest to destroy.
> I've come here quite by chance, so, for company's sake,
> I'll just sing you a song—it will keep me awake.
> For we are all noddin', nid, nid noddin',
> We are all noddin', abroad and at home.
> People scold because sometimes I sleep in the day,
> Although I might answer, so do they—
> For I think I can prove, if you'll list to my rhymes,
> Every one of them may be caught nodding at times.
> Yes, they all noddin', nid, nid noddin',
> They are all noddin', abroad and at home.
> The Parson, who tells us to watch and to pray,
> And will not on Sundays at home let us stay,
> Nods at church o'er his sermon, and makes us, the elf,
> Nod long ere it's finished as much as himself.
> For they are all noddin', nid, nid noddin',
> They are all noddin' to church when they come.
> Both Houses of Parliament nod, too, you'll find—
> When one party speaks, to sleep t'other's inclin'd—
> One nods till the other side's said all their say,
> And as for the Speaker, he nods right away.
> For they are all noddin', nid, nid noddin',
> They are all noddin' to the House when they come.
> Young folks, when the old folks to nod are inclin'd,

And her lover's entreating that she will be kind,
That she neither may grant nor deny him the bliss,
Will appear to nod, too, while he steals a sweet kiss.
Fur they are all noddin', nid, nid noddin',
They are all noddin' at our house at home.
But I'm getting quite tir'd—no doubt you're so too—
Ya-aw! I really beg pardon—I'll bid you adieu,
'Tis high time, for I scarce my eyes open can keep,
And I'm sure that I must have walk'd here in my sleep!
For we are all noddin'—yaw-aw!—nid, nid noddin'—
We are all noddin'—yaw-aw!—to the end when we come!
[*Yawns—sinks into chair—falls asleep—snores, and is carried off,*
first having a nightcap put on him.]

For Moncrieff everyone has a bit of "Joe" in him, the primitive hidden within.
And this is tied to social norms, including rituals of seduction and desire. But
it is the lover who mimes sleep in order to permit the seduction. What is
sham here is inherent to the makeup of the Fat Boy. It is a sign of his being a
throwback to the world of the primitive. Joe is Moncrieff's exemplar of fat;
his obesity is present in him to a greater extent than anyone else and from his
very inception.

In the early nineteenth century there was a concern about the association between childhood obesity and moral character. The medical literature
(Wadd 1829, 131–36) expressed some anxiety regarding the overfeeding of
infants in the nursery. However, fat babies were seen as healthy babies both
in earlier periods and until the late twentieth century. Indeed, one of the
decisive works on pediatric illness, Johannes Joachim Becher's posthumous
Medicinische Schatz-Kammer of 1700, lists the entire range of diseases that
were seen to befall children (including syphilis), but obesity is never mentioned. Yet after the Enlightenment, when the child became the father to the
man, obesity in children was a topic of medical interest, prompted by the
desire to distinguish between healthy fat and the risk of morbidity. In a standard handbook (Immermann 1879, 445), cases of morbid obesity in children
between 1815 and 1845 are used to document these rare occurrences. In
American popular fiction after Dickens the "Fat Boy" appears as a set character. In 1863 Stephen C. Massett produces one to characterize the homespun nature of his frontier characters:

> [O]n one side of the house, upon a piece of canvas, was displayed a painting
> of a "Fat Boy." Immediately upon entering, the showman, pointing with his
> short stick to a perfect mountain of fat, proceeded as follows: "Master Vil-
> liam Fiddes—or the Hinfant Goliath. He is the seventh son of Joel (that's
> me) and Helizabeth Fiddes, who is industrious and respectable persons, as

resides in Manchester, which was in the month of November he was born. He is only six years of age, and is considered one of the greatest venders wich this world as ever produced by the Supreme Being. Ladies and gentlemen, when this Fenominer of nature were born, he had four regular teeth, and very shortly after that possessed twenty-two teeth. He is a remarkable helthy child when he is well, and is very amusing, and possessed of very pretty features. (Show the gents your leg, Billy.) His food consists of a common and wholesome description, and is generally boiled in hot water, as the doctor says his hinside requires soft things, and is considered the greatest wonder of the world. It would be morally unpossible to describe everything belonging to this great wonder of nature, as he is endowed with every necessary qualification vich adorns the human frame, as such should be produced, and is mild, sensible, and pleasant. (172–73)

This Fat Boy is displayed as a freak but is actually no more "freakish" than the other characters inhabiting Massett's world, including his own father.

Even at the beginning of the twentieth century, the public health concern about children's bodies was with malnutrition and the diseases associated with it in children—not with obesity (Dutton 1908, 64–65). To be sure, the beautiful (fat) baby contests became part of the eugenics movement to assure a healthy breeding stock of human beings delighted in the fat baby (Stern 2002). However, through the 1930s and 1940s, fat babies became more and more pathologized as they were seen as the origin of fat (and sick) adults. In this, there was a decisive shift away from moral degeneracy as the cause of obesity.

By the beginning of the twentieth century, the universal argument that fat babies suffered from illness—either endocrine imbalance or neurosis—provided the means of defining them as ill. A debate followed between those who argued that obesity was a product of external (exogenous) forces, represented by the work of Carl von Noorden (1900), who saw most obesity as exogenous, and those who saw it as a symptom of a physiological pathology.[5] The latter picked up the work of Alfred Froehlich (1901), who had described a case of pituitary tumor in a fourteen-year old man with massive obesity and sexual infantilism.[6] "Froehlich's syndrome" became the catchword for all physiological theories of obesity. Thus, Israel Bram (1943) advocated thyroid extract as a treatment for all cases of obesity. More importantly, it drew an absolute line between sick and healthy children and was seen to have predictive force.

JOE'S FURTHER LIFE IN MEDICINE

Joe does have a life beyond nineteenth-century popular culture. Various pirated versions of the tale of Joe as well as Toby jugs with his visage circulated in the wake of his initial popularity.[7] This was equally true of the medical literature, which adopted Joe as the litmus test for obesity. In 1893, *The Lancet* (citing an American case study) reported on a "case of narcolepsy." A soldier who had regularly fallen asleep was accused of dereliction of duty because he had fallen asleep at his post. It was revealed that he seemed "well nourished and all his organs were apparently healthy. Mentally he did not seem to be lacking, although 'not very bright' best described his condition" (100). He had fallen asleep on horseback while on parade as well as frequently falling "asleep at meals, on one occasion with a spoon in his mouth." His treatment was to be put on light duty. "Later he was placed on duty in the kitchen [where] he fell asleep and let the fire out and so delayed the meal." The author of the note concludes: "We have sometimes wondered whether Dickens had any knowledge of this as a distinct pathological condition when he described his immortal Fat Boy in 'Pickwick.'" Dickens's character seems the appropriate reference for the readers of *The Lancet* to understand the nature of the soldier's ailment, and narcolepsy seems the appropriate diagnosis for the Fat Boy's dilemma. Here the mental acuity of the soldier plays a role in his diagnosis. He is "not very bright," and that becomes part of the diagnostic category of narcolepsy. Being diagnosed with a disease, he is found innocent of a very serious breach of military discipline and transformed into a case that needs treatment.

Dickens's "Fat Boy" seems the norm for comparison in all cases. When in 1904 the parents of "The Fat Boy of Peckham," Johnnie Trundley, a five-and-a-half-year-old weighing eight stone, five pounds, are accused of violating the "Act for the Prevention of Cruelty to Children" (1894) by having exhibited him as a freak, it is Dickens's character to whom the comparison is made. The author of an editorial in *The Lancet* account notes, "every traveling showman would testify that obesity has always been as highly appreciated by the public as abnormal stature, and the youthful Trundley has had the advantage, or disadvantage, of living in an age in which notoriety is easily achieved" (106). But his celebrity, the author notes, pales in comparison to the "heroes of fiction [who] have the advantage in the matter of lasting glory, and the names of Daniel Lambert and the Fat Boy of Peckham sink into insignificance beside those of Falstaff and the Fat Boy in 'Pickwick.'" Visibility as the ultimate case study of childhood obesity is assured through the medium of literature.

In an account written by William Ord (1898) at the close of the nineteenth century the visibility still attendant to Dickens's character appears in a case of obesity associated with hypothyroidism. Ord provides an easy reference as to how one of his patients is imagined as Dickens's Fat Boy Joe. He describes a case of Grave's or Basedow's syndrome or disease, the standard labels (depending on whether you were a British or a German patient) for hypothyroidism at the close of the century. His patient, a thirty-year-old waiter, was admitted to St. Thomas's Hospital in London in 1892 suffering from the end stages of the disease. Diagnosed some six years earlier, he had developed a set of both psychological and physiological symptoms: "He began at first to feel heavy, dull and depressed, and became clumsy especially with his hands. . . . His abdomen and body generally began to swell and his face became round, puffy, and yellowish-brown with flushed cheeks, earning for him the nickname of 'the fat boy in Pickwick,' which replaced the nickname of 'Skin and Buttons' which had before the illness been bestowed upon him on account of his pale and hollow-eyed countenance." He developed a "sort of Mongolian change of physiognomy" (1246). That there are specific physiognomic manifestations associated with this disease was quite well known, having first been described in Sayyid Ismail Al-Jurjani's medieval *Thesaurus of the Shah of Khwarazm*—goiter and exophthalmoses (bulging eyes) were the most evident signs. The altered mental state, too, had become a standard part of the representation of patients suffering from this illness. Treated with thyroid extract, the patient's symptoms diminished and he was able to return to work, even though he seemed clumsier at his job as a waiter than previously. The case has a negative outcome, as the patient stopped coming to clinic for the thyroid extract and eventually became an alcoholic, dying of symptoms associated with Grave's disease in 1895. Ord's case study notes that the patient's nickname seemed to fit both his mental and physiological state. Joe was becoming a case of somatic obesity, but hypothyroidism, with its diminished mental capacity, seemed not sufficient as an etiology to explain the power of the character.

With the shift in the explanation of childhood obesity to a focus on the endocrine system, Dickens's Fat Boy became a case of Froehlich's syndrome rather than of Grave's disease. The reason for this lies in the image of the asexuality of the Fat Boy, a quality not ascribed to the traditional definition of hypothyroidism (or indeed of goiter in its historical construction). By 1953, E. Watson-Williams can dismiss "the well-known but irrelevant case of endocrine obesity recorded by Dickens" (343). But the endocrine error was not hypothyroidism but an error of the pituitary gland. As early as 1922, H. Letheby Tidy had diagnosed Joe as a case of hypopituitarism (Froehlich's syndrome) or "dystrophia adiposogenitalis" (600). In addition to its onset before puberty in the form of morbid obesity ("adiposity"), other salient features are deficiency of growth and "genital dystrophy or atrophy." The Fat Boy can have no desire because his sexual development is stunted! But, Watson-Williams observes, this does not impact on his awareness of the world or his innate intelligence. His face seems to deny this awareness. This type of hypopituitarism "may produce the appearance which was described . . . as the 'pudding-face type.'" And yet this type, exemplified by Joe, is neither intellectually nor emotionally retarded. "Many of the famous Fat Boys have belonged to this group; the Fat Boy in *Pickwick* may be considered to be an example, and Dickens was by no means inaccurate in picturing him as possessing an acute intelligence in his waking moments." Joe is suffering from a childhood somatic illness, not from a weakness of the will or mind. He has now become a somatic case study with a more specific etiology, unlike the "Hindoo Fat Boy" reported some seventy-five years earlier. Yet he too is seen as without desire (or at least without sexual capacity).

It was in the world of mid-twentieth-century pulmonary medicine that the conflict between the psychological and the metabolic etiologies of obesity, at least in regards to the Fat Boy, was momentarily resolved, in the creation of the "Pickwick Syndrome," a term coined by C. Sidney Burwell and his colleagues at Harvard in 1956.[8] This is a form of obstructive sleep apnea syndrome, the condition where people stop breathing for very short intervals during their normal sleep periods. This results in the patient having a marked loss of oxygen in the blood system and lethargy while awake. Burwell's paper presented a single case study of the "association of obesity, somnolence, polycythemia and excessive appetite," and defined a new syndrome. Despite its name, the eponymous figure was to no one's surprise not Charles Dickens's Mr. Samuel Pickwick from The Pickwick Papers, but rather Mr. Wardle's "Fat Boy," Joe.[9]

Instead of considering the societal and stigmatizing ramifications of obesity, as did Dickens, Burwell sees Joe solely in terms of his pathophysiology, and not in terms of the morality read into his body. Burwell strengthens his argument that Joe is a case study by citing William Wadd's early-nineteenth-century medical account of "corpulence." Indeed, there have been claims of a greater antiquity for this syndrome (Potvliege 1982). Burwell's single case study is of "a country tradesman aged about thirty, of a short stature and naturally of a fresh, sanguine complexion and very fat," who was suffering from the combination of symptoms that Burwell finds in Joe. The man was fifty-one years old, five feet five inches tall, and weighed 263 pounds. The salient incident in this patient's life that brought him to the hospital was the fact that he fell asleep during a poker game while holding three aces and two kings! His was neither an error of intelligence (he recognized after the fact what he had done) nor an inappropriate emotional response. He is a somatic Fat Boy. In a completely phenomenological description of the case, Burwell and his colleagues see excessive eating as both the cause and a symptom, but avoid any discussion of the etiology of his patient's (and Joe's) illness. Burwell's case is that of an adult, as are subsequent studies (Sotos 2003). Burwell cannot use a child, a real Fat Boy, for his example, as these cases were the stuff of the debate about the etiology of obesity, not its phenomenology.

Post-Freudian psychoanalysis was at the height of its American prominence in the 1950s. The debate about the nature of Joe's illness was joined by Hilde Bruch (1904–1984), who countered this rather mechanistic reading of the Fat Boy. Bruch was a German Jewish physician who escaped the Nazis to England and then America, and ended her career as Professor of Psychiatry at Baylor Medical School. Her claim to fame is that she popularized the diagnosis of anorexia nervosa and was an often-cited specialist on obesity who revolutionized the debate between those who saw exogenous or endogenous causes for obesity.[10] She provided the first complex psychological theory of obesity linking both developmental forces with the external world of the pathological family. Her interest seems to have begun with her arrival in 1934 in the United States, where she was amazed at the huge number of fat, truly corpulent children, not only in the clinics but also on the street, in the subway, and in the schools (Bruch 1957, 5). Her work on the "psychosomatic aspects of obesity" was funded by the Josiah Macy, Jr. Foundation, and the results began to appear in the 1940s and were summarized in her book of 1973, *Eating Disorders*, where she argues for a form of developmental obesity that develops through specific family interactions from birth. The core is her view of the child's struggle to develop autonomy in the family setting, a view championed by Theodore Lidz (who created the "schizophrenegenic mother") with whom she had worked in Baltimore between 1941 and 1943. Undergoing a training analysis with Frieda Fromm-Reichmann in Washington at the time, Bruch began to see more complex readings of the work on obesity that had brought her to Fromm-Reichmann's initial attention. Her work sought literary and cultural parallels for the inner life of the obese, finding the analogy between creative representation and psychological reality to be compelling.

In *Eating Disorders*, she too cites Dickens, employing the passage where Joe awakens abruptly when he is offered food:

> (Sundry taps on the head with a stick, and the fat boy, with some difficulty, roused from his lethargy.) "Come, hand in the eatables."
>
> There was something in the sound of the last word which roused the unctuous boy. He jumped up, and the leaden eyes which twinkled behind his mountainous cheeks leered horribly upon the food as he unpacked it from the basket.
>
> "Now make haste," said Mr. Wardle; for the fat boy was hanging fondly over a capon, which he seemed wholly unable to part with. The boy sighed deeply, and, bestowing an ardent gaze upon its plumpness, unwillingly consigned it to his master. (Dickens 1836, 48)

She continues, "During the 1930's and the 1940's, Joe's behavior was often cited as evidence of the sleepiness of the pituitary type of obesity. During the 1950's the eponym 'Pickwickian Syndrome' was given to the clinical picture of extreme obesity associated with alveolar hypoventilation and hypoxic somnolence. Yet I doubt Joe suffered from it. I have never seen an organically determined somnolence in which one word had such a vitalizing influence" (Bruch 1973, 137). She then provides a further case study of a four-and-a-half-year-old female child weighing ninety pounds. The child had been accidentally conceived during the war and was initially rejected by the mother

(138). For the mother, "feeding showed love and expiation of guilt" (140) for having rejected the very idea of bearing the child. The mother is a compulsive fabulator, always embellishing the tales she tells about her daughter's treatments in order to manipulate them. Bruch thus provides Joe with a surrogate childhood of rejection that explains his obesity and his desire to make our skin creep. Now, Bruch's child is female as, following World War I, the exemplary patient in questions of obesity shifted from the male (as it had been since the ancient Greeks) to the female with the construction of the image of the "New Woman." Here too it is the mother who is the cause of the obesity. Indeed, the child's obesity is a neurotic response to her mother's "unnatural" rejection of her.

Yet Bruch's initial work on obesity is little known.[11] In her dissertation of 1928, written under the renowned pediatrician Carl Noeggerath at Freiburg i. Br., she tested the stamina and lung capacity of children with the new instrumentation of the spriometer. She traced how their respiration increased with increased work (turning a weighted wheel). One of the children, Maria O., was, according to Bruch, chronically obese, weighing 58.4 kg. at the age of twelve. Her aspect was similar to that of Dickens's Joe. She "speaks tiredly and in a monotone, complains about constant tiredness and weakness of memory. There is neither determination nor a joy for work" (10). This case study provides all of the negative images about desire and work and intelligence that we have found in Dickens. In providing Joe with a childhood in her later work, Bruch offers an alternative model for exogenous obesity—one beyond the control of the individual. But it is also one that provides a further meaning for the image of the fat child beyond the moral censure of Victorian culture. In this she answers not only Burwell as well as her own early work, providing the child with a neurotic context in which her only possibility of functioning is to eat. But she also provides a rationale for the psychological state of the obese child, the absence of the love of the mother, the negation of the natural desire of the parent for the offspring. The image of the lazy, stupid fat child comes to be more differentiated in a reading of Joe—but one that needs to provide him (and all fat children, real or imagined) with a family that can neither love nor desire.

The psychoanalytic work on obesity that rested upon Bruch's model of neurosis and its family connection also saw the male patients, the Fat Boys, as more tractable. As one paper noted, while such patients "become obese partly in relation to over-nurturent influences in foetal life or early childhood," these influences "will sometimes have had neurotic determinants based in the mother, in the family, and in the specific maternal attitude to the patient as an infant" (Crisp and Stonehill 1970, 342). The fact is that the male patient does better: "[S]ome patients, despite remaining massively obese for the meantime, may have the capacity to make a more healthy social adjustment auguring better for the future. The male patient and our last case seem to demonstrate this." Joe can be saved in terms of these psychodynamic models of obesity, while his morbidly obese sisters, now the focus of the psychoanalytic literature on body size, are captured by their past. And yet at this point any reference to the literary figure vanishes, even where the scholarship quotes Bruch's work.

Joe is a case study trapped between purely physiological and psychological explanations of obesity. He is the Fat Boy who will become the fat man, or, as in the case of the patient described by Burwell, has already become him! What is striking is how the definitions of masculinity are compromised due to his obesity. Thus, the case of the "wonderfully fat boy" in Dickens forms the case material that Burwell and Bruch assembled for their argument. Yet each runs quite contrary to Dickens's own comic notion of our personal inability to read obesity and the mistakes that become inherent to this misreading.

NOTES

1. Natalie McKnight (1993) argues that social class and intelligence seem to be interchangeable categories in these texts: "The profoundly uneducated and the illiterate [are presented] in a similar fashion to the more typical idiots" (6–7; see also Davies 1977).

2. See Wainapel (1996) and Loesberg (1997), who, however, do not discuss obesity.

3. The English version, from which I quote, is a fairly accurate translation of the German original.

4. Where this comes to be clearly rejected is in the discourse of childhood and race. Thus, Rabbi W. M. Feldman (1917) rejects any model of the inheritance of acquired characteristics in looking at the Jewish child.

5. Von Noorden sees pathological metabolism as a very rare cause of obesity.

6. Froehlich's claims were very much more limited than the use to which "Froehlich's syndrome" was put in the following decades.

7. See the anonymous verse paraphrase of passages from the novel with illustrations by Thomas Nast (1870?).

8. On the "Pickwick Syndrome," see Kryger (1985); Tjoorstad (1995); and Peters (1976). This syndrome continues to be used to discuss the various implications of obesity and health. See Saibara et al. (2002).

9. On naming in medicine, see Rosenberg and Golden (1992).

10. See Heitkamp (1987); Bruch (1997); J. H. Bruch (1996); and Brumberg (1988).

11. See the trajectory marked by the following works by Hilde Bruch (1940; 1943; 1974). On contemporary views see Sobal and Maurer (1999a; 1999b).

REFERENCES

Anonymous. 1893. A case of narcolepsy. *The Lancet* 142 (July 8): 100.

Anonymous. 1903. The evolution of fatness. *Punch*, March 25, 203.

Anonymous. 1904. The fat boy of Peckham. *The Lancet* 163 (January 9): 106.

Becher, Johannes Joachim. 1700. *Medicinische Schatz-Kammer*. Leipzig: Christoff Hülsen.

Bowen, Zack. 1997. Joyce's endomorphic encomia. *James Joyce Quarterly* 34:259–65.

Bram, Israel. 1943. The fat youngster. *Archives of Pediatrics* 40:239–49.

Bruch, Hilde. 1928. Gaswechseluntersuchungen über die Erholung nach Arbeit bei einigen gesunden und kranken Kindern. Diss., Freiburg i. Br. Simultaneously published in *Jahrbuch für Kinderheilkunde* 121(1928):7–28.

——. 1940. Obesity in childhood: Physiologic and psychologic aspects of the food intake of obese children. *American Journal of the Diseases of Children* 58:738–81.

——. 1943. Psychiatric aspects of obesity in children. *American Journal of Psychiatry* (March):752–57.

——. 1957. *The importance of overweight*. New York: Norton.

——. 1973. *Eating disorders: Obesity, anorexia nervosa, and the person within*. London: Routledge and Kegan Paul.

——. 1997. Obesity in childhood and personality development. *Obesity Research* 5 (March):157–61.

Bruch, Joanne Hatch. 1996. *Unlocking the golden cage: An intimate biography of Hilde Bruch*. New York: Gurze.

Brumberg, Joan Jacobs. 1988. *Fasting girls: The emergence of anorexia nervosa as a modern disease*. Cambridge: Harvard University Press.

Burwell, C. Sidney, Eugene D. Robin, Robert D. Whaley, Albert G. Bickelman. 1956. Extreme obesity associated with alveolar hypoventilation—A Pickwickian syndrome. *American Journal of Medicine* 21:811–18.

The Christian Recorder. 1864. Philadelphia, February 27.

Crisp, A. H., and Edward Stonehill. 1970. Treatment of obesity with special reference to seven severely obese patients. *Journal of Psychosomatic Research* 14 (September):327–45.

Davies, James A. 1977. Negative similarity: The fat boy in *The Pickwick papers*." *Durham University Journal* 39:29–34.

Dickens, Charles. 1833–1836. *Sketches by Boz*. London: Oxford University Press, 1957.

——. 1836. *The Pickwick papers*. Ed. James Kinsley. Oxford: Clarendon Press, 1986.

Don, W. G. 1859. Remarkable case of obesity in a Hindoo boy aged twelve years. *The Lancet* 73 (April 9).

Douglass, Frederick. 1851. *Frederick Douglass's Paper*. Rochester, New York. October 16.

Dutton, A. Stayt. 1908. *The national physique*. London: Baillière, Tindall and Cox.

Ebstein, Wilhelm. 1884. *Die Fettleibigkeit (Corpulenz) und ihre Behandlung nach physiologischen Grundsätzen*. Sixth ed. Wiesbaden: J. F. Bergmann. *Corpulence and its treatment on physiological principles*. Trans. A. H. Keane. London: H. Grevel, 1884.

Feldman, W. M. 1917. *The Jewish child: Its history, folklore, biology, and sociology*. London: Baillière, Tindall, Cox.

Froehlich, Alfred. 1901. Ein Fall von Tumor—der Hypophysis cerebri ohne Akromegalie. *Wiener klinischer Wochenschrift* 15:883–906.

Gilman, Sander L. 1978. On the use and abuse of the history of psychiatry for literary studies: Reading a Dickens text on insanity. *Deutsche Vierteljahrsschrift für Literaturwissenschaft und Geistesgeschichte* 52:381–99.

Heitkamp, Reinhard. 1987. *Hilde Bruch (1904–1984): Leben und Werke*. Diss., Cologne.

Hewitt, Douglas. 1971. Entertaining ideas: A critique of Peacock's "Crotchet castle." *Essays in Criticism* 20: 200–12.

Houston, Gail Turley. 1994. *Consuming fictions: Gender, class, and hunger in Dickens' novels*. Carbondale: Southern Illinois University Press.

Hufeland, Christopher William. 1797. *Die Kunst das menschliche Leben zu verlängern*. Jena: Akademische Buchhandlung. [*The art of prolonging life*.] Two vols. No trans. London: J. Bell, 1797.

Huff, Joyce Louise. 2000. *Conspicuous consumptions: Representations of corpulence in the nineteenth-century British novel*. Diss., George Washington University.

Immermann, H. 1879. *Handbuch der allgemeinen Ernährungsstörungen*. Leipzig: F. C. W. Vogel.

Johannsen, Albert. 1956. *Phiz: Illustrations from the novels of Charles Dickens*. Chicago: University of Chicago Press.

Joyce, James. 1922. *Ulysses*. Ed. Hans Walter Gabler. New York: Random House, 1986.

Jukes, Edward. 1833. *On indigestion and costiveness; A series of hints to both sexes*. London: John Churchill.

Klieneberger, H. R. 1981. *The novel in England and Germany: A comparative study source*. London: Wolff.

Kryger, M. H. 1985. Fat, sleep, and Charles Dickens: Literary and medical contributions to the understanding of sleep apnea. *Clinics in Chest Medicine* 6:555–62.

Loesberg, Jonathan. 1997. Dickensian deformed children and the Hegelian sublime. *Victorian Studies* 40:625–54.

Massett, Stephen C. 1863. *"Drifting about," or, what "Jeems Pipes, of Pipesville" saw-and-did*. New York: Carleton.

McKnight, Natalie. 1993. *Idiots, madmen, and other prisoners in Dickens*. New York: St. Martin's.

McMaster, Juliet. 1987. *Dickens the designer*. Totowa, NJ: Barnes and Noble.

Moncrieff, William Thomas. 1850. The fat boy. In *An original collection of songs*. London: no pub.

Morgentaler, Goldie. 2000. *Dickens and heredity: When like begets like*. New York: St. Martin's.

Mulvihill, James. 1983. Peacock's *Crotchet castle*: Reconciling the spirits of the age. *Nineteenth-Century Fiction* 38:253–70.

Nast, Thomas. 1870? *The fat boy/from Dickens*. New York: McLoughlin Bros.

Noorden, Carl von. 1900. *Die Fettsucht*. Vienna: Holder.

Occidente, Maria del. [Maria Gowen Brooks]. 1843. *Idomen; or, the vale of Yumuri*. New York: S. Coleman.

Ord, William. 1898. The BRADSHAW lecture on myxoedema and allied disorders. *The Lancet* 152 (November 12): 1243–48.

Peacock, Thomas Love. 1831. *Nightmare abbey [and] Crotchet castle*. Ed. Raymond Wright. Harmondsworth: Penguin, 1986.

Peters, Uwe Henrik. 1976. *Das Pickwick-Syndrom: Schlafänfalle und Periodenatmung bei Adiposen*. Munich: Urban und Schwarzenberg.

Potvliege, P. 1982. Le syndrome "de Pickwick." Priorité de sa description par le duc de Saint-Simon (1675–1755). *Nouvelle Presse Médicale* 11: 2360.

Pritchett, V. S. 1966. The comic world of Dickens. In *The Dickens critics*, ed. George H. Ford and Lauriat Lane Jr., 309–24. Ithaca: Cornell University Press.

Robinson, Louis. 1891. Darwinism in the nursery. *Nineteenth Century* 30:831.

Rosenberg, Charles E., and Janet Golden, eds. 1992. *Framing disease: Studies in cultural history*. New Brunswick: Rutgers University Press.

Saibara, Toshiji, Yasuko Nozaki, Yoshihsa Nemoto, Masafumi Ono, and Saburo Onishi. 2002. Low economic status and coronary artery disease. *The Lancet* 359 (March 16): 980.

Sobal, Jeffrey, and Donna Maurer, eds. 1999a. *Interpreting weight: The social management of fatness and thinness*. New York: Aldine de Gruyter.

———. 1999b. *Weighty issues: Fatness and thinness as social problems*. New York: Aldine de Gruyter.

Sotos, John G. 2003. Taft and Pickwick: Sleep apnea in the White House. *Chest* 124: 1133–42.

Stern, Alexandra Minna. 2002. Beauty is not always better: Perfect babies and the tyranny of pediatric norms. *Patterns of prejudice* 36:68–78.

Tidy, H. Letheby. 1922. An address on dyspituitarism, obesity, and infantilism. *The Lancet* 203 (September 16): 567–602.

Tjoorstad, K. 1985. Pickwick-syndromet. Fra litteraere spekulasjoner til sovnforskning. *Tidsskr Nor Laegeforen* 115:3768–72.

Tosh, John. 1999. *A man's place: Masculinity and the middle-class home in Victorian England*. New Haven: Yale University Press.

Tytler, Graeme. 1982. *Physiognomy in the European novel: Faces and fortunes*. Princeton: Princeton University Press.

Vega-Ritter, Max. 2003. Introduction to *Charles Dickens and madness*, ed. Vega-Ritter. *Cahiers Victoriens et Edouardiens* 56:11–116.

Wadd, William. 1829. *Comments on corpulency*. London: John Ebers.

Wainapel, S. F. 1996. Dickens and disability. *Disability and Rehabilitation* 18:629–32.

Watson-Williams, E. 1953. Obesity. *The Lancet* 143 (August 15): 343.

THREE

Pinel and the Pendulum

RICHARD LEWIS HOLT

INTRODUCTION

THE HOSPITAL SALPÊTRIÈRE sprawls across the northeastern edge of Paris's sixth arrondissement as it flows into the thirteenth. A bronze statue of Philippe Pinel stands at its entrance. The statue's gaze seems endlessly distant, and its right hand is held palm downward and slightly away from the body—a gesture, one assumes, of beneficence. After all, Pinel was for the institutionalized mad[1] the great messenger of the revolutionary Enlightenment doctrines of reason, liberty, and compassion. Although he enjoyed contemporary renown as an internist, Pinel is remembered today as the asylum keeper who in 1795 unchained the patients of Le Bicêtre. This symbolic act of liberation was both more and less complete than it appears. Insofar as Pinel listened to the stories of his patients and in many of them found a healing voice, he fostered a new therapeutic gaze. But it is also true that in these reformed institutions and across society less tangible and more insidious means of control took the place of physical chains.

A short walk away from Salpêtrière, in the heart of the fifth arrondissement, Jean-Bernard Foucault's pendulum hangs in the Pantheon. Suspended in 1751 at the Paris World's Fair, it was the first terrestrial device to demonstrate the earth's rotation. Like a giant mesmerist's watch, it drew great crowds of onlookers as it traced lazily through its daily arc, rendering magically visible the world's imperceptible turning below. I took this very walk almost a decade ago. At the time, I was sharing a room in the Vietnamese student ghetto of the fifteenth arrondissement with a friend whose incipient schizophrenia was tragically materializing. It was April, colder than the Paris springtime I had expected, and I remember a twinge of disappointment at the pendulum, unmoving and less formidable than the symbol of conspiracy portrayed in Umberto Eco's then-latest novel. The pendulum of J.-B. Foucault was to my thinking a footnote, a mere curiosity. By contrast, Pinel's Salpêtrière felt powerfully alive, a center of real force in the frayed copy of Michel Foucault's *Histoire de la folie* tucked away in my jacket pocket. It was this latter Foucault whose work introduced me to Philippe Pinel's asylum. As I cut across the darkened Jardin de Luxembourg on my way home, the proximity of these eighteenth-century citizens and their instruments, both in space and in time, held no particular resonance for me. I have had little occasion to ponder any connection since. That is, until now.

I began to reconsider Pinel and the pendulum during my residency interviews. Talking with clinicians and researchers from across the country, most expressed a strong sense of optimism about the future direction of psychiatric medicine. Accordingly, it was not unusual to find myself engaged in discussions about how the burgeoning science of mind promised to revolutionize the pursuit of new clinical questions and answers. Beneath this veneer, however, I sensed a less than total embrace of biological models of mental illness, and reservations about the ostensibly atheoretical *Diagnostic and Statistical Manual of Mental Disorders, Fourth Edition* (DSM-IV). The comments I heard usually took the form of rumblings from the more experienced faculty about the pendulum having swung too far in "that" direction. The pendulum metaphor was repeated often enough that I began to suspect something more behind it than semantic currency.

At the same time, I have become aware of a historical tension in psychiatric discourse vis-à-vis the narrative offerings of its subject. This intimation of conflict has led me to question the comfort with which I had heretofore accepted as natural and navigable the spaces that receive a patient's speech act. I refer not only to the physical boundaries of the asylum, ward, clinic, and community, but also to the cognitive territories demarcated by the clinical and basic sciences. Most of all, I have begun to question the alacrity with which we place patients and their utterances into conceptual spaces: diagnoses and disease models. As I struggle with the historical and theoretical substrata of psychiatry, I cannot help but return to that memory of Paris, the coincidence of Pinel and the pendulum. And so considering the pendulum, I feel less need to trace the origins of a metaphor than to inquire more fundamentally: "What is this metaphorical pendulum, and between what extremes does it swing?"

At one extreme, psychiatry's living memory invokes the excesses of psychological expansionism, such as the political abuses of Soviet psychiatry, the dissemination and subsequent internecine struggles of postwar psychoanalysis, and the rise of the antipsychiatric movement. These events, however, are so copiously documented and commonly the subject of comment that they promise to bear little new exegetical fruit. At the other extreme, the limits of biological reductionism—the advent of the third and later editions of the *Diagnostic and Statistical Manual of Mental Disorders* and the current hegemony of psychopharmacology—are perhaps too current to be the subject of meaningful retrospective. But medicine's custodial authority over its subject, the mentally "ill," is now more than two hundred years old; and while the most recent historical iterations and institutional deployments of the pendulum theme are illustrative, they also prove somewhat limiting. In order to sustain the proposition that psychiatric modernity has been defined by deep theoretical division, we must first interrogate the discipline's conceptual foundation, then return to an earlier age to trace out the birth of this conflict. At this nexus, it is my belief that we must confront the figure of Pinel.

Widely cited as a father of psychiatry, Pinel retains an iconic status in Europe commensurate in many respects with that of Benjamin Rush in America. After an early education infused with Catholic religious teaching, Philippe Pinel (1745–1826) received his MD degree from Toulouse in 1773, and became known to Paris medical circles primarily through various scholarly publications of moderate distinction. An abiding interest in natural history led him to the Paris Botanical Gardens, where in the early 1790s he encountered scientists and physicians struggling to define their role after the dissolution of the Jacobin dictatorship. In 1793, the second year of the Republic, he was appointed as physician to the men's hospital Le Bicêtre outside Paris. Here, in collaboration with the asylum's governor, Jean Baptiste Pussin (1745–1811), Pinel devoted himself to the application of natural historical methods to the study of mental alienation. He treated and described his charges with great compassion, and through the act of removing of their shackles, Pinel quickly became a widely cited exemplar of French Enlightenment reform and reason. After a mere nineteen months at Le Bicêtre, Pinel was elevated to the directorship of La Salpêtrière, the women's asylum in Paris. From this central and highly visible position, Pinel established himself as a major intellectual force in European medicine. And while he did not relish political debate, Pinel from this point onward often found himself "forced to make choices, express allegiances, and side with or against successive ruling powers" (Weiner 1994, 233).

Pinel's *Traité médico-philosophique sur l'aliénation mentale, ou la manie*[2] (*A Treatise on Insanity*), first published in 1801, appears in many ways to be a typical humanist Enlightenment document. The subject material presented in this "textbook" was familiar to contemporary medical readers: moral therapy, diagnostic classification, asylum management and the "malconformation of the skulls of maniacs and ideots" studied in "the spirit of minute and accurate observation [for] . . . the advancement of natural knowledge" (1). Yet within this hidebound framework, the modern reader may discern the stirrings of a novel clinical gaze, along with a significant and still-resonant ambivalence regarding the ability of basic scientific reason to reveal the essential nature of unreason. And while it is not my intent to argue that Pinel is in any sense a modern psychiatrist, his work does represent a fundamental rearrangement of the conceptual field surrounding the mentally ill patient—a rearrangement that makes modern psychiatric medicine possible. Pinel molds elements of both moral therapy and basic science into his clinical method, while at the same time exposing the limitations of both in his writings. This counter-gesturing may not be revolutionary per se, but it is more than mere eclecticism, for it allows significant new forms of practice and new debates to arise. Thus, in a very real sense, Pinel is the father of a new breed of practitioner, and lays the groundwork for two centuries of struggle with the daunting provisionality of the pursuit of a science of psychopathology.

In his *Treatise on Insanity* and at the asylums of Bicêtre and Salpêtrière, Pinel reconfigures extant conceptual and methodological strains within medicine into a new type of institutional praxis. In an effort to reconcile Hippocratic tradition with positivist science, Pinel challenges the assumptions of both the English moral therapists and the Continental anatomo-pathologists. Specifically, through his focus on clinical observation, Pinel reshapes moral therapeutics from humane asylum keeping into the empirical pursuit of the laws of mental alienation. A *clinical* medical gaze thus arises that takes both the individual patient and the disease state as its subject, a gaze that introduces the patient narrative as a legitimate object of medical inquiry. Defending this gaze against the methodological and ideological preoccupation with anatomy and the brain, Pinel offers a first salvo in the still-recognizable dialectic of medical psychiatry. Pinel's ambivalence to the anatomo-pathologists and his resulting focus on clinical empiricism thus represents, in a very real sense, the first "form versus function" argument—the first swing of the pendulum—of psychiatric modernity. The endurance of this dialectic may be attributed as much to Pinel's authority as to its inherent validity, for he is by no means the first to advance the ideas of humane treatment and institutional management, or even to distinguish between somatic and psychic causation. What defines Pinel as a watershed figure is the engagement of these ideas in the context of an emerging culture of medical surveillance, a nosopolitic that asserts control over the conceptual, legal, and institutional management of the mentally ill.

In short, the present chapter will examine the dialectic of form and function that defines "modern" psychiatric nosology and then use A *Treatise on Insanity* as a primary text to explore three elements at its foundation. First, I will trace Pinel's part in the emergence of the empirical gaze from the "moral" space of the eighteenth-century asylum. Second, I will detail Pinel's position in the first form/function debate that emerges from this new empirical deployment—namely, the conflict between clinical and anatomic models of psychopathology. Specifically, Pinel's insistence upon the diagnostic and therapeutic value of narrative will be addressed. Finally, Pinel will be implicated in medicine's struggle for conceptual preeminence within the post-Enlightenment social order. In particular, I will examine the power he and others wielded over the discursive field of mental illness, a power that was initially rooted not in efficacy, but in authority. Before discussing the historical particularities of Pinel and psychiatry's pendulum, a brief definition of the pendulum itself seems in order.

FORM AND FUNCTION:
A "PENDULUM" OF PSYCHIATRIC GAZE

In *The Perspectives of Psychiatry* (1986), Paul McHugh and Phillip Slavney examine a dialectic between what they describe as formal and functional methodological approaches to the mind-brain problem:

> Forms or functions, patterns or purpose, the expression of mechanisms or meanings: a choice for one or the other seems the vital problem of explanation in psychiatry. It is the origin of most conflicts, and as a means of circumventing the brain-mind disjunction it is provocative of a fundamental dialectic in the field. That there is thesis and antithesis but no synthesis becomes clearer if the contending viewpoints are considered. (10)

Formal methodology is grounded in standardized mental operations, such as algorithms, that proceed "in prescribed ways to the goals of identification and explanation" (14). As such, it is not synonymous with biological psychiatry, but rather tends to define mental phenomena from an external perspective, through patterns, mechanisms, and discrete lesions. Functional analysis, by contrast, attempts to penetrate the subject's consciousness in order to gain insight into the meaning of pathological thought and behavioral processes. While functionalist methodology is also based upon observation and may be grounded in biological science, it possesses greater interpretive latitude than its formal counterpart. Frameworks such as George Engel's biopsychosocial model (Morgan and Engel 1969) attempt to combine these two perspectives and are certainly workable. In the end, however, the observer must privilege one gaze at the expense of the other.

The irreconcilability of the dialectic between form and function arises because they represent fundamentally different approaches to an inherent uncertainty that exists regarding the patient or subject's internal milieu, a radical otherness that renders all psychological observation inescapably provisional. For example, distinct but affiliated categories of human experience—depression and sorrow, addiction and desire, mania and bliss—are not transferable as such because they do not correspond to stable physical or metaphysical states. Instead, they are "known" only insofar as they are defined and maintained by the operational production and exchange of signs.

But even if language were more reliable, the dialectic between form and function would not be effaced, for by its very definition mental illness is a basic rearrangement of individual cognition. A stranger in a strange land, the patient experiences a rupture of perceptual *form* and the *functional* emergence of disturbing thought content simultaneously. This being the case, how does the altered mental "self" undo the alteration that most challenges the existence of its premorbid "self"? Where recovery is possible, is it defined primarily formally (by right action) or functionally (by right thinking)?

For the clinician, the form/function question additionally becomes one of causality. Depending on whether it chooses a formal or functional perspective, the psychiatric gaze will assign corresponding causality to behavioral phenomena. But the notion of causality with much of psychiatric medicine is unavoidably speculative and oblique, for its basic substrate is still more often a speech act than anything as concrete as a tissue, pathogen, or serum measurement. This means that no matter what orientation one espouses, the struggle that defines the daily endeavor of psychiatry is over the hermeneutic status to be accorded to the patient's narrative. In short, it is not the corpus of the patient, but instead his or her utterances that fill the discursive spaces of both perspectives, both extremes of the pendulum. Hence the power of that oscillating metaphor, hung upon the aspiration to an ideal still point at the center of the turning world, a mythic space in which the subterranean content of a delusion, mania, or melancholic narrative might be made manifest to the clinical gaze.

The current psychiatric observational paradigm tends to privilege the *formal* features of the narrative, sometimes at the expense of narrative content. For example, the observation that a patient's expressed ideas fail reality testing in that they are autistic and self-referential can be put forward to define a speech act as delusional. This definition can then be used, along with other data, to confirm or exclude a diagnosis of schizophrenia. One advantage of this formal diagnostic method is that it defines clear standards and limits to the interpretive templates an observer places upon phenomena. This emphasis upon diagnostic reproducibility between observers and across populations leads to high inter-rater reliability. Moreover, such standardization facilitates communication between psychiatrists, as well as to legal, lay, and other medical audiences. The rigor demanded of psychiatric nosology by formalist methodology has been critical to its rise from sectarianism. Yet despite its obvious utility, a formal emphasis often neglects validity in the pursuit of consistency, and devotes very little consideration to what a narrative may communicate about a patient's motivation, meaning, and feelings. This approach at times leads to a discouraging diminution of patient agency and an overemphasis on somatic causality, and can lead to a retreat from complex disruptions of mental integration by labeling them pejoratively as "functional."

Despite its limitations, the merit of a consistent taxonomy of the general *forms* of mental illness is self-evident. By contrast, what value to assign the *content* of melancholic, manic, or delusional speech is often problematic. Within the apparent birdsong of a particular delusion or the ravings of an individual manic there is undoubtedly communication. The notion that the patient's narrative—as well as his or her body—is psychiatry's subject does not obviate the fact that it might have a subject of its own. For the adept and insightful listener, there must certainly be some method to bring this meaning forth from obscurity. Of course, psychiatry has trod down this path before and has in the past been guilty of elaborating the rich content of the human psyche with excessive promiscuity. Mined too deeply, slips of the tongue are parlayed into an enduring literature and mythology of interpersonal conflict: Electra, Oedipus, Hamlet. The child may indeed be father to the man, but a revisionist history is often required to render the ontogeny manifest. Still, the *functional* power of the patient narrative—its ability to communicate both explicit and unconscious information about an internal world—is undeniable. As such, its interpretive limits can be difficult to judge. In order to empower, insight must be purchased with appropriate rigor, lest it become overly inclusive. The truncated and inferential communiqués of the subconscious mind too easily give rise to interpretations that aspire to wear the mantle of truth. If no psychic phenomenon is deemed beyond the functionalist gaze, its authoritative claim to define pathological thinking can all too easily grow. What begins as a therapeutic modality can turn into an exercise in philosophical density, and can even be twisted into an instrument of political will.

And so the pendulum swings. Within this new Pantheon, do the sound and fury of our internal voices signify nothing, or too much? Jean-Bernard Foucault's pendulum was a proud statement of an age's ability to unravel the universe's once-hidden meanings and motions. Installed when Pinel was five years old, it had turned through four decades before the unfortunates of Le Bicêtre were unshackled. Little did he appreciate that through its peregrinations, and his own, a discipline and its metaphor would be born. A metaphor, but also an irony, in that a later (Michel) Foucault would deconstruct the nexus of power behind Pinel's struggles over psychiatric doctrine. By this most recent swing, formalist parsimony may have initially reined in the expansionist theorizing of psychoanalysis. But like its functionalist counterpart, modern biological psychiatry's own aspirations have proven far from humble.

A NEW PANTHEON: RESHAPING MORAL THERAPEUTICS IN THE EMPIRICAL ASYLUM

The central question surrounding aberrant behavioral phenomena has changed little since ancient Greek physicians first wondered, *What does it*

mean to be mad? Arrayed with the enduring calculus of loss—the abandon-
ment of reason and balance, the loss of free will or of humanity itself—madness has forever carried with it a form of otherness. To speak authoritatively
of madness, to enter this unreasoned discursive space, has been the province
of the philosopher, the cleric, and the artist. But Western medicine has since
its inception had something to say about mental illness, even if it has not
always spoken in a manner recognizable to the modern reader as a disease
form. The empirical tradition of Hippocrates (ca. 460 BC), for example,
evolved into a largely analytic ethos by the time it passed through Galen (AD
130–201). Medieval medical interpretation relied as much upon abstract sup-
positions of truth about the essential nature of disease as upon observation of
the disease process. Mental derangement was thus seen as a supernatural phenomenon or as an imbalance of humors, and often as both.[3] To the pre-
Enlightenment mind, conceptual entities such as *dyskrasia* and demonic possession were not necessarily contradictory elements of a disease state. In
Pinel's words: "The history of insanity claims alliance with that of all the
errors and delusions of ignorant credulity; with those of witchcraft, demoni-
acal possession, miracles, oracles and divination" (1801, 47).

As a cultural and intellectual force in Western Europe, Galenic medicine
endured largely intact from its rediscovery in the eleventh century until the
Age of Reason, when a new concept of mental illness began to emerge—
madness as an "alienation" or derangement of the intellect. Pinel invokes the
Hippocratic spirit of observation and individual focus, and combines these
ancient themes with the new analytic methods of empiricism in order to render mental alienation by degrees less alien. The vantage from which Pinel
attempts this synthesis, the asylum, develops into a site for the production of
medical knowledge. This space ultimately proves schismatic, for two distinct
gazes—one psychic, the other somatic—emerge to fill its wards and color its
patients' words. Pinel's empirical asylum thus represents the structural precondition for the historical development of a dialectic between form and
function. If the dialectic's metaphoric body is a pendulum, then the recon-
figured asylum is its venue, its new Pantheon.

Positivism, based upon the assertion that only through observation and
experiment can the contingently valid proposition be raised to the level of
factual knowledge, becomes a powerful theme in Western thought at the
dawn of the nineteenth century. Across Europe, broad rejection of speculative philosophies in favor of knowledge derived from the "positive" fact
promises to direct the progress of science, history, and politics; and it leads to
a renewed emphasis on empirical methods. Liberating the community of
physicians from Galenic theory, this new empiricism represents a sea change
in the process of medical inquiry. Accordingly, a whole new breed of physi-
cian-scientist comes into being during the seventeenth and eighteenth centuries, with Pinel as a direct heir. Anatomo-pathologists such as Giovanni

Morgagni (1682–1771) sought through relentless interrogation of cadaveric anatomy to unearth a new knowledge, to catalogue the actual lesions correlating to each and every human illness, madness included. In Pinel's generation, it was Xavier Bichat who would extend this inquiry into the tissues themselves. Others in France, most notably Pierre Cabanis (1757–1808) and Étienne de Condillac (1714–1780), challenged the extent to which sense-data could escape the operational language of signs. These French thinkers echoed Locke's "sensualistic" analytic method and Hume's critique of naive empiricism. In so doing, they elaborated a concept of mind that—while able to embrace physiology—was permissive of the less concrete and more numinous operations of human passions. Similar preoccupations regarding the etiological status of the somatic and psychic dimensions of mental alienation would become central to Pinel's thought.

Driven by the quest for systems through which to order the world, the eighteenth century is also notable for its proliferation of medical taxonomies. Following in the footsteps of the eminent seventeenth-century English physician Thomas Sydenham (1624–1689), William Cullen (1712–1790) and François Boissier de Sauvages (1706–1767) produced the medical classification systems that were well known to Pinel. These works, along with his own training in natural history, guided Pinel's early studies, which are permeated with taxonomic themes. In fact, Pinel's *Nosographie Philosophique* (1798) held the distinction of being the largest work of its kind upon its publication and was a standard text of French medicine throughout his lifetime. Although their aim was a kind of standardization, these botanicals and bestiaries of disease often had little in common with one another except dizzying complexity. As we shall see, Pinel matures beyond the role of encyclopedist through his experience at Le Bicêtre. Yet in spite of Pinel's eventual departure from pure medical taxonomy, it is clear that these works represent the structural framework upon which he relies to build the first flexible clinical nosology.

In addition to classification, one of the general themes of the *Treatise on Insanity* is the "moral" treatment of insanity, a relatively new tradition in Pinel's era. To avoid possible confusion regarding nomenclature, it is important to underscore the extent to which the notion of moral treatment is imbued with not only religion, but also the scientific and political currency of the Enlightenment. Moral therapy as Pinel and others understood it was therefore not predicated upon rehabilitation through morality, but rather a belief—in the words of Pinel's most eminent student, J. E. D. Esquirol—that "the application of the faculty of intelligence and of emotions" could be enlisted "in the treatment of mental alienation" (Grob 1994, 27). Moral therapists effected cures of the mentally ill through a tightly controlled institutional setting and a rigorous work schedule rather than moral instruction per se. Restraint and humoral manipulations such as bleeding and cupping were still practiced, but such "physicking" gradually diminishes in importance as the psychic dimensions of mental illness attain causal ascendancy. The Retreat at York, founded in 1792 by Samuel Tuke and the Society of Friends, was the first and most celebrated of several well-respected Quaker institutions established on the therapeutic and humanistic model of moral and environ-mental therapy. Tuke and other noted moral therapists such as the Florentine neuroanatomist Vincenzo Chiarugi (1759–1829) and the English physician-reverend William Pargeter (1760–1810) were, in general, less interested in the taxonomic particularities of mental illness than in the salubrious effects of gentle management and appropriate surroundings.[4]

As a textbook of moral and environmental therapeutics, A *Treatise on Insanity* reflects the thinking of Pinel's contemporaries:

> The laws of human economy considered in reference to insanity as well as to other diseases, impressed me with admiration of their uniformity, and I saw, with wonder, the resources of nature when left to herself, or skillfully assisted in her efforts. My faith in pharmaceutic preparations was gradu-ally lessened, and my scepticism went at length so far, as to induce me never to have recourse to them, until moral remedies had completely failed. (Pinel 1801, 109)

Closer inspection of Pinel's writing, however, reveals deep reservations beneath this general endorsement. In particular, Pinel laments the English practitioners' lack of methodological transparency. He singles out King George's celebrated clergyman-psychiatrist Francis Willis, who "we are informed . . . cures nine lunatics out of ten. The doctor, however, gives us no insight into the nature and peculiarities of the cases in which he has failed of success." Pinel continues with the admonition, "He who cultivates the sci-ence of medicine . . . pursues a more frank and open system of conduct . . . for the benefit of his successors in the same route" (55). He then describes one of his own treatment failures, noting with remarkable detail and sensi-tivity the circumstances leading to the suicide of a young man who had come to Paris to study law.

Even more than methodological laxity, Pinel deplores the "practice of the celebrated Dr. Willis" to place "every lunatic under the control of a keeper," which leads "in many instances . . . to unbridled and dangerous bar-barity" (66). Finally, insofar as "Willis' general principles of treatment are no where developed and applied to the character, intensity and varieties of insanity" (50), they offer no robust intellectual challenge to the outmoded themes of demonic possession or theories of humoral imbalance. Because they provide no suitable foundation upon which to build a new knowledge of psychopathology, Pinel can ultimately muster but lukewarm praise for his English colleagues. Impressed more by the humane than curative value of their work, he concludes, "I have discovered no secret; but, I approve of their general principles of treatment" (49).

The significance of Pinel's critique of then-current practices of English moral therapy is twofold. First, it represents a rejection of moral therapy's status as a theoretical proposition immune to empirical scrutiny and validation. Second, it underscores Pinel's lack of interest in codifying the existing praxis of moral therapy. Rather, he is intent on moral therapeutics as a means for building a knowledge of mental illness from the ground up:

> Of the knowledge to be derived from books on the treatment of insanity, I felt the extreme insufficiency. Desirous of better information, I resolved to examine for myself the facts that were presented to my attention . . . and forgetting the empty honours of my titular distinction as a physician, I viewed the scene that was opened to me with the eye of common sense and unprejudiced observation. (108)

Pinel's goal is to achieve through "unprejudiced observation" valid, not simply internally consistent, categories. And while it is arguable that Pinel practiced a rather conventional form of moral therapy, he did so with unique nosological aspirations and observational methods:

> The successful application of moral regimen exclusively gives great weight to the supposition that, in a majority of instances, there is no organic lesion of the brain nor of the cranium. In order, however, to ascertain the species, and to establish a nosology of insanity, so far as it depends upon physical derangement, I have omitted no opportunities of examination after death. I flatter myself that my treatment of this part of the subject will not discredit my cautious and frequently repeated observation. (5)

Pinel's nosographic categories of "ideotism, dementia, melancholy and mania with or without delirium" have not endured, but his preference for clinical over anatomic data is truly novel and yields some very tangible insights. He is, for example, among the first to recognize that derangements of mood often leave cognition intact, and by suggesting that reason can be systematically engaged to help restore the broken psyche, Pinel pioneers the form of what would later become individual psychotherapy. Moreover, by imbuing the rather modest theoretical construct of moral therapeutics with empirical praxis, he engages the asylum in the positivist production of medical knowledge. From this position, Pinel sets the form/function pendulum into motion as he challenges the etiological presuppositions of the anatomopathologists with his psychological perspective.

THE PENDULUM'S FIRST ARC: ANATOMY AND NARRATIVE IN THE POSITIVIST AGENDA

Through a positivist reformation of the concept of moral therapy, Pinel established the groundwork for a new clinical gaze, an advance that marked the birth of the asylum-hospital as a site from which to produce and refine medical knowledge. Nonetheless, there was at this time little unanimity concerning the operative definition of "empiricism" and its relation to the production of medical knowledge. In postrevolutionary France the taint of ideology was inescapable.[5] As a student of Locke and Condillac, Pinel believed that presuppositionless observation represents the most absolute expression of empirico-logical economy and rigor. But he was also a trained natural historian, and as such he reserved methodological primacy for *behavioral* observation, insofar as its "truths" are only secondarily dependent upon mental operations, experimentation, and the hypothetico-deductive model. If the positivist physician aspires to build medical truth through observation, the clinic must be the privileged site of that empirical enterprise:

> [Pinel] established faithful and repeated observation as the main criteria of experimental medicine, and he saw no rupture between ancient and modern medicine, no fundamental difference between observation and experimentation, the former merging into the latter and experimentation ultimately being nothing but observation made under special conditions or restrictions. (Riese 1969, 184)

For Pinel, behind any ideology of the gaze there was first and foremost a philosophy of knowledge, and it was the asylum—not the autopsy table or laboratory—that was best suited to the advancement of a true knowledge of psychopathology.

As a moral therapist and reformer—but mostly as a *clinician*—Pinel advanced a functional psychology, a medicine whose gaze depends upon the patient narrative, against the anatomo-pathologists of his day. Theirs was a quest for the definitive lesion, whereas Pinel explored the functional derangement of the "passions." To be sure, Pinel did not deny the value of basic science; he was a skilled and respected anatomist and physiologist in his own right. He was rarely openly hostile to somatic medicine, but he did consistently reject the idea that *objects* can supersede *processes* as the cause of disease states. To this end, Pinel challenged the etiological presupposition that any particular lesion could causally outrank the clinical observation of the phenomena of mental illness: "Derangement of the understanding is generally considered as an effect of an organic lesion of the brain, consequently as incurable; a supposition that is, in a great number of instances, contrary to anatomical fact" (Pinel 1801, 3).

This point is critical, for it permanently divided the science of psychopathology after Pinel into two camps:[6] those who view mental illness as the *product* of some somatic insult, and thus amenable to the refined formalist gaze; and others who see in madness a *process* that may or may not correspond causally to physical and physiological stigmata, a diathesis whose cure may be functionally effected through the enlistment of will, reason, and personal agency. The avatars of these two camps have evolved and alternately predominated over two centuries, but like the pendulum, their fundamental tension remains unchanged in the wake of successive swings.

Examples of Pinel's challenge to the hegemony of the anatomo-pathologists show up in the least likely of places. The third section of *A Treatise on Insanity*, for example, appears to be little more than a treatment of the cranial correlates of Pinel's diagnostic categories. Physiognomy, much like phrenology in subsequent decades, was a subject of both general and scientific interest at the beginning of the nineteenth century. Supported by the scholarly studies of Greding, Haslam, and Chiarugi, "malconformations" of the human skull were thought by many to bear strong relation to disease states. Pinel, who had extensively measured mammalian skulls for classificatory purposes early in his career, disputes this claim, noting that "the heads of maniacs are not characterized by any peculiarities of conformation that are not to be met with in other heads taken indiscriminately" (1801, 123). Pinel's insistence on controlled data demonstrates the reservation with which he approached anatomic correlation and medical causation. Given his focus on clinical observation, it is perhaps not surprising that he should proceed with such abiding skepticism in his postmortem dissections. However, by associating the scientific claims of the anatomo-pathologists with the deplorable treatment of asylum inmates, Pinel extends his critique of method into an indictment of motive:

> It is a general and very natural opinion, that derangement of the functions of the understanding consists in a change or lesion of some part of the head. This opinion is, indeed, countenanced by the experimental labours of Bonnet, Morgagni, Meckel and Greding. Hence the popular prejudice that insanity is an incurable malady, and of refusing them that attention and assistance to which every infirmity is entitled. (111)

This passage does not simply expose the limits of a scientific gaze that mistakes correlations with causes; it rhetorically challenges the ability of such a gaze to reconcile itself with the progressive and humanistic agendas of positivism.

Pinel's critique of the anatomo-pathologists thus stands in stark contrast to that which he proffers against the English moral therapists. While the latter are found lacking in empirical rigor but appropriately compassionate, the former engage in the therapeutic nihilism of a weak and incomplete empiricism, a medical dogma based upon synecdoche that fails to reconstruct the entire patient. In Pinel's words, "It is a very general opinion, that mental derangement depends upon lesions of the head . . . observation is far from confirming these specious conjectures" (117). Only in the case of mental retardation is Pinel willing to trust morphology at the expense of hope. Even then, he does so "without absolutely deciding that there is an immediate and necessary connection between ideotism and the various structures which I have described" (126).[7] Despite the fact that Pinel devotes considerable space to his own observations of the skull, his attitude toward such pursuits is less than sanguine. To Pinel's sensibilities, such theorizing is reminiscent of the arrogance of the *ancien régime*:

> In the present enlightened age, it is to be hoped, that something more effectual may be done towards the improvement of the healing art, than to indulge it with the splenetic Montaigne, in contemptuous and ridiculous sarcasms upon the vanity of its pretensions. (6)

To the extent that philosophy, ideology, and method cannot be separated, Pinel's asylum mirrors the conceptual space of his *Traité médico-philosophique*. "To avoid false reasoning," Pinel warns, "it is necessary to conduct the investigation upon the principles of accurate analysis and abstraction" (115). Such statements suggest that Pinel's writing of the *Treatise* was motivated as much by his perception of intellectual flaws within the thinking of fellow positivists as by his compassion for the mentally ill.

If Pinel's ambivalence toward basic scientific investigation is ideologically bound to a distrust of theorizing, its corollary is a devotion to presuppositionless observation—the *receptive* clinical gaze:

> From systems of nosology, I had little assistance to expect; since the arbitrary distributions of Sauvages and Cullen were better calculated to impress the conviction of their insufficiency than to simplify my labour. I, therefore, resolved to adopt that method of investigation which has invariably succeeded in all the departments of natural history, viz. to notice successively every fact, without any other object than that of collecting materials for future use; and to endeavour, as far as possible, to divest myself of the influence, both of my own presuppositions and the authority of others. (2)

Citing his observations both at the autopsy table and on the wards of Bicêtre, Pinel concludes that "the anatomy and pathology of the brain are yet involved in extreme obscurity," and he calls for "circumspection and reserve in deciding upon the physical causes of mental alienation" (133). Pinel's doubt that additional post hoc reflection will reveal the hidden loci of insanity, along with his belief in "the advantage of obtaining an intimate acquaintance with the character of the patient" (191), amounts to the first functionalist challenge to biological reductionism. Significantly, Pinel's counterargument is not simply based on moral therapeutics, but also springs from a new and psychodynamically oriented empiricism. To be sure, a nascent tradition of logotherapy, or "talking cures," can be dated back to Greek antiquity, but Pinel's *Treatise on Insanity* was the first widely disseminated medical text to examine empirically "the value of consoling language and . . . attention to the state of the mind exclusively" in the context of a recognizable model of disease (Altschule 1977, 131).[8]

The psychological orientation of Pinel's quest for a more complete scientific knowledge of insanity is exemplified by the attention to detail with which he treats patient encounters. In the *Treatise*, for example, Pinel does not rely on secondhand histories and conjecture based on physical examination to form an understanding of his patients. Instead, he focuses on the role and form of the patient interview. Earlier in his career, at centers such as Edinburgh and Montpellier, Pinel had noted an aggressively interrogative style that tended to cast the descriptive labor of clinical observation into an act that shaped the individual patient into a case of disease. "How, in the midst of this profusion of questions," he asks in *Médicine Clinique* (1815), "can one grasp the essential, specific features of the disease?" (qtd. in Foucault 1963, 111). Pinel engaged his own patients in conversation rather than interrogation, not simply as an empathic gesture, but also as a powerful data-gathering tool—a tool, he asserts, whose power surpasses not only theory, but also rivals that of autopsy. "By these and other means," he writes, "I have been enabled to introduce a degree of method into the services of the hospital [Bicêtre], and to class my patients in a great measure according to the varieties and inveteracy of their complaints" (Pinel 1801, 6).

Through his often informal and open-ended engagements with patients, Pinel reveals concerns well beyond the quotidian duties of an asylum physician. For Pinel, the personal and pathognomonic meaning of patient narratives are equally valued, for both elements contribute to his diagnoses and therapies. In the case of one young sufferer, Pinel recounts that "he often and earnestly entreated me to rescue him from the arms of death. At those times I invited him to accompany me to the fields, and after walking for some time, and conversing upon subjects likely to console or amuse him, he appeared to recover the enjoyment of his existence" (57). Later, he describes a cure of delusional mania effected through "repeated . . . visits daily [with] . . . the tone of friendship and kindness," during which "[h]e endeavoured from time to time to convince [the patient] of the absurdity of his pretension" (192). Similar encounters with other patients are described throughout Pinel's work, often with reference to their instrumentality regarding the ultimate disposition of the case. Pinel's approach represents a real and lasting departure from nihilistic viewpoints—be they demonic or organic—that marginalize the story and agency of the sufferer:

> To arrive at a diagnosis, the physician must carefully observe a patient's behavior, interview him, listen carefully, and take notes. He must understand the natural history of the disease and the precipitating event and write an accurate case history. Diagnosis and prognosis can then be made. (Weiner 1992, 726)

In the generation of "alienists" that arose after Pinel assumed the directorship of the Salpêtrière—and especially in his student J. E. D. Esquirol—we see the fruition of this approach into a clinical method in many respects as sophisticated as anything since.

THE ENDURING GAZE: MEDICAL AUTHORITY
AND THE SCIENCE OF PSYCHOPATHOLOGY

Justifiably, historical distinction is accorded to Pinel as a humanitarian, liberator, and "father" of modern psychiatry. His biography reads like that of the quintessential postrevolutionary man: inquisitive, reform-minded, and intent upon the progressive reorganization of theory, method, and ideology. But within the halls of France's most visible hospital, the salons of Paris and across the pages of his *oeuvres*, Pinel was also instrumental in the formation of a nexus of medical power. The empiricism that became operative in medicine at the end of the eighteenth century now carries a long and distinguished pedigree. But the modern medical gaze is as much about power as it is about knowledge. It would thus be naive to accept the positivist reformation of medicine as simply progressive, the successive elaboration of better ideas. As a means of production of medical *savoir*, the methods born in Pinel's age have been generative of both truth and authority. Well before the advent of germ theory, anesthesia, or vaccines, physicians were broadly able to legitimate certain forms of medical practice and to take control of that subset of the population they defined as a therapeutic target. At a critical period in its history, figures such as Philippe Pinel and Benjamin Rush bore responsibility for both the intellectual and the institutional reformation of medicine. From Edinburgh to Paris to Philadelphia, the institutions of the clinic and the medical school did not reflect a sudden efficacy, but rather solidified the paradigmatic extension of medical focus from the cause of disease to the laws of disease. As a result, pathology, nosology, etiology—concepts unthinkable as such before this transformation—entered the lexicon of the newly potentiated medical professional.

Within this professional community, Pinel was the first physician with the ability to command broadly both the physical and discursive spaces of insanity. As such, he is among those responsible for both the theoretical and the institutional groundwork of psychiatric modernity. Before the nineteenth century, most mentally ill people were kept at home, while others became vagabonds. During the eighteenth century at sites such as London's notorious "Bedlam" Hospital, lay administrators assumed responsibility for the institutional disposition of the most severely afflicted or those without familial support. In this context, it is important to realize that Pinel's acts of liberation were in no way tantamount to deinstitutionalization. Pinel was a strong, if by no means the first, advocate of removing the patient from the community. The benevolence of humane yet unequivocally institutional treatment conceals a subtler form of control than chains—therapeutic privilege:

> It is pleasing to observe so great a conformity of opinion, founded as it appears upon the results of observation and experience, prevail . . . on so important a subject as the utility of public and private hospitals . . . insan-

ity is much more certainly and effectually cured in places adapted for their
reception and treatment, than at home under the various influences of family interests and intercourse. (Pinel 1801, 214)

On the question of institutionalization, Pinel is willing to suspend his critical apparatus and accept at face value English physician John Haslam's dic-
tum that "confinement is always necessary in cases of insanity" (Pinel 1801,
215).[9] This notion proved as portable as it was popular, as evidenced by the
wide inclusion of references to Pinel, Tuke, Rush, and others by asylum
keepers over the ensuing decades. By the 1830s asylums were rapidly being
erected in America to protect the vulnerable from the excessive ambition
and diminished prudence of the postrevolutionary social order. Europeans,
although in general less willing to embrace the social etiologies popular
among their American counterparts, were just as avid beneficently to
sequester the mentally ill.

The asylum for Pinel represented the embodiment of a humanistic ideal
of reform, an optimistic space in which to effect curative measures. But the
asylum has ideological dimensions as well. It is a critical site for the production of medical knowledge, and so it served to validate the intellectual
agenda of the French Revolution:

> The principles of free enquiry, which the revolution has incorporated with
> our national politics, have opened a wide field to the energies of medical
> philosophy. But, it is chiefly in great hospitals and asylums, that those
> advantages will be immediately felt, from the opportunities which are there
> afforded of making a great number of observations, experiments, and com-
> parisons. (Pinel 1801, 46)

During Pinel's lifetime, the mentally ill population emerged as a therapeutic
target deeply enmeshed with social policy, political power, and social commentary. This trend extended throughout the Continent and across the English Channel, even spanning the Atlantic to America, where the concept of
madness became deeply enmeshed with notions of social order. Sadly, while
the asylums thrived in this well-intentioned era, within a few decades their
primary role became custodial rather than curative, allowing many of the
abuses that so outraged Pinel's reformist sensibilities to creep back into common practice within their walls.

Pinel's aim, however, was not simply to reinforce the institutional exercise of statutory power over madness. Rather, in his attempt to reconstruct
the forms of medical knowledge in the new French republic, he was among
the first to medicalize madness in the novel clinical setting of the asylum. By
virtue of his directorship at Le Bicêtre and La Salpêtrière, Pinel asserted—
both in word and deed—the importance of medical supervision of institutional patients: "These are the duties, and highly important they are, which

peculiarly belong to the governor. There are others, however, and they are certainly of no less importance, which . . . are connected with the character and province of the physician" (45).

To be fair, Jean Baptiste Pussin, the governor with whom Pinel served at Bicêtre and Salpêtrière, was much esteemed by the great physician, and is treated with much deference throughout the text of the *Treatise*.[10] But unlike Pussin, Pinel's status and celebrity as a physician-reformer ensured wide dissemination of his clinical perspective on insanity. Moreover, having labored to establish the axiomatic nature of clinical observation, and having addressed nosology and moral therapy earlier in the volume, Pinel reserved the final chapter of A *Treatise on Insanity* for medical treatment. Pinel begins with what seems like an apologia:

> Wearisome treatises, useless compilations, a scholastic dialect . . . have characterized the progress of almost all the sciences. Modern physics, the ancient doctrines of Aristotle, and the fanciful theories of Descartes, are examples perhaps equally illustrative of this truth. [I]f medicine be . . . chargeable with similar incumberances . . . it would however appear that this science be more or less distinguished for its habits of observation and analysis. (220)

However, it is clear that along with empirical methodology, Pinel saw the production of medical knowledge as inexorably linked with the day-to-day treatment and management of the mentally ill. It is naturally the physician who is best suited to "discriminate accurately between the different species of the disease, . . . avoid fortuitous and ineffective treatment [and] . . . furnish precise rules for the internal police and government of . . . asylums" (221). The power of medical surveillance flows seamlessly into custodial authority for the physician, a knowledge-power nexus that forms the basis for the roles of psychiatrists and patients alike to this day. Given the benefit of historical perspective, it is easy to question the innocence of Pinel's apologia for "the importance of an enlightened system of police for the internal management of lunatic asylums" (174), a subject upon which medical superintendents opined voluminously well into the next century.

It is in this context that we now approach the true import of the seemingly anachronistic content of A *Treatise on Insanity*; for here the notion of mental "illness" begins its conceptual evolution and becomes the subject of a new science. Combining the rhetoric of authority with the power of theoretical parsimony, Pinel deploys the asylum as a means to generate and test provisional hypotheses of madness. Through this process, a reconfiguration of existing opinions regarding the role of science in medicine is achieved, the centrality of clinical observation is ensured, and the promise of dynamically oriented therapies is first explored. As an Enlightenment thinker, Pinel was keen to reject the unicausality of Galenic medicine and its attendant methodological weakness, choosing instead to class diseases as distinct and reproducible entities. But as an idealistic son of the French Revolution, he wished to avoid the perceived arrogance of the *ancien régime*. Pinel attempted to preserve the strength of Hippocratic medicine, its focus on the experience of the diseased individual, without compromising the benefits of the positivist gaze.[11] As a result, he poses himself in square opposition to both somatic reductionism and demonic thinking. In short, Pinel opposes any subtractive gaze—medical or otherwise—that a priori annihilates the meaning of the individual and his sufferings.

The importance of these developments can hardly be overstated, for they extend well beyond the political and historical context in which they first came into being. Pinel represents a central figure in the establishment of the clinical precondition upon which the dialectic between form and function in psychiatry at present rests. Moreover, Pinel was among the first to translate the naive compassion of the reformists and moral therapists into a new mode of inquiry. He transformed the question "What is madness?" into "What is it like to be mad?" and challenged the clinical gaze to penetrate the otherness of its subject. But insofar as he failed to address certain implications of his nosology, Pinel's thinking is also problematic. For example, the *Treatise* lacks any experimental or otherwise systematic means for verifying clinical insights. In addition, the political and ideological entanglements of his age limited Pinel's ability to move beyond his powerful investigation of mental/medical experience to construct a theory of mind. Because Pinel regarded the extensive pursuit of insight-oriented analysis as inappropriately theoretical, it has been left to subsequent generations to realize the full heuristic value of his method. Alongside the questions of method, one must also inquire about Pinel's role in the establishment of the tremendous power that psychiatry has since wielded over its subject. For despite his reformist intentions, Pinel managed his population through subtle forms of control and intimidation. Born of an age that promised certainty—the retreat of ignorance from the light of inquiry—Pinel's legacy is provisionality.

CONCLUSION: PINEL AND THE PENDULUM REVISITED

In retrospect, several enduring themes are interwoven through the last two centuries of medical psychiatry, the span of its putative modern age. The acknowledgment of the phenomenological opacity of psychiatry's subject and the introduction of the mind-brain problem have given rise to a dialectic between formal and functional analyses of mental illness. In Pinel's wake, the patient speech act has been subjected to psychoanalysis, behaviorism, and cultural interpretation; yet it still remains enigmatic, in spite of the most recent advances of neuroscience. The debate first took shape toward the end of the eighteenth century with the emergence of competing empirical models upon which to build the nascent science of psychopathology. The site of emergence for these two gazes was Pinel's empirical asylum, from which vantage he offered a critique of both the anatomo-pathologists and the moral-environmental therapies of his day.

The specific debate between clinical and anatomo-pathological perception waged in that era represents a watershed in the intellectual and institutional status of the notion of mental derangement. The central arguments of this dialectic regarding the nature of medical perception can, and should, be marshaled to challenge the epistemological assumptions of current diagnostic instruments such as the *Diagnostic and Statistical Manual* or to expose the inherent contradictions of conciliatory syntheses such as the biopsychosocial model. The basic challenge of what was to become psychiatry was defined in Pinel's lifetime, and still remains: how most profitably to deploy the positivist gaze against the impenetrable otherness of the patient. Through its historical struggles, psychiatry tacitly acknowledges the problematic nature of the patient narrative, even when there is disagreement on how to approach it. The current rift between biomedical and dynamic psychiatry is therefore not an argument over whether or not psychiatry is a science, but rather the most recent iteration of the functional/formal dialectic within that science.

Finally, with the advent of a medical science of mental illness, an accompanying institutional drive to speak authoritatively about—and to multiply—those subject to its gaze has arisen. It seems almost intuitive that a new way of looking at the mentally ill should give rise to new powers and institutions. However, there is perhaps equal validity to the assertion that it was an institution, the asylum, that gave rise to Pinel's novel psychiatric perception. In any case, it would be a mistake to assume that the rise of medical psychiatry proceeded in lockstep with its increasing efficacy. Notably, medical personnel were able to exert a tremendous amount of control over large populations well before the production of any significant or legitimate evidence that they could accurately diagnose, treat, or even care for the mentally ill patient. The exercise of power has much to do with the manner in which the patient speech act has historically been interpreted. This struggle for interpretive preeminence over narrative is at the heart of both the claims and crises of legitimacy in psychiatric medicine.

At or very near the birth of the modern conceptual arrangement of psychiatric medicine is the figure of Philippe Pinel. Le Bicêtre and Salpêtrière were among the first institutions in which the patient narrative was considered at all, much less outside a demonic or mechanistic context. Pinel unchained his patients, but more importantly he listened to them. In doing so, he introduced the patient utterance as a legitimate object of study, with all of its attendant epistemological quandaries. In addition, Pinel pioneered the use of clinical observation to build nosological categories from the ground up, a necessary precondition to liberate his subject from Galenic theory, Christian theology, and various homespun medical pseudo-philosophies. Finally, Pinel proclaimed a new authority for the emerging discipline of psychiatry over mere asylum keeping: morally as a reformist, intellectually as an empirical clinician, and institutionally as the head of one of France's largest and most visible medical institutions. Pinel was present at—and in part responsible for—the introduction of that dialectical pendulum that has for two centuries swung between formal and functional analyses of narratives of madness. In the details of his *Treatise on Insanity*, we may find the release of a now-familiar mass whose alternating dominances have undergone various periodic iterations, but whose fundamental physics have proven remarkably durable.

NOTES

1. My adoption of the terms *madness, maniac, insanity, mental alienation,* and *ideotism* reflects their common use in Pinel's era, and is not intended to imply their validity as diagnostic categories. In addition, for the sake of consistency, the modern term *psychiatry* will be applied throughout the text to the medical surveillance of the mentally ill, even though it was not recognized as a medical discipline as such at the turn of the nineteenth century.

2. Literally, "Medical-Philosophical Treatise on Mental Alienation, or Mania" but conventionally translated as "A Treatise on Insanity." For the remainder of the present chapter, it will be referred to as the latter.

3. See Kramer and Sprenger's *Malleus Maleficarum* (1487), Johannes Weyer's *De Praestigius Daemonicum* (1563), and Burton's *Anatomy of Melancholy* (1621) for representative treatments of human behavior in the three centuries prior.

4. Given the relative indifference of the incipient moral therapy movement to the taxonomic complexities of the medical establishment, it seems curious that Pinel should be so well known as both a nosographer and moral therapist. On a political level, his discussion of moral therapy in the *Treatise* may have been, in part at least, motivated by a perceived need "to rescue France from the imputation of neglecting . . . this system of practice . . . hitherto almost exclusively awarded to England" (Pinel 1801, 107).

5. Considerable political controversy, for example, even surrounded the appropriate social role of disease classification. Many of Pinel's peers viewed the natural historical observation of disease processes as an inherently more "democratic" pursuit than the interventionist activities of experimental science and clinical medicine.

6. In the early nineteenth century, for example, "alienists" of the Paris school built upon Pinel's natural historical approach further to define the functional phenomena of mental illness, while a new generation of anatomo-pathologists, most notably Antoine Bayle (1799–1858), continued to champion the search for organic causes.

7. Curiously, in a much-publicized debate with Jean-Marc Itard over the prognosis of Victor, the celebrated "wild boy of Aveyron," Pinel deemed the youth uneducable.

8. In a remarkable example of consilience, Immanuel Kant's essay, "The Power of the Mind, Through Simple Determination, to Become Master Over Morbid Ideas," was published in 1798, three years before *A Treatise on Insanity*. And while both texts became influential sources for early-nineteenth-century logotherapists, only Pinel is routinely mentioned in discussions regarding the pedigree of modern psychoanalysis.

9. Haslam's *Observations on Madness* (1798) and Benjamin Rush's *Medical Inquiries and Observations Upon the Diseases of the Mind* (1812) were the two most widely read Anglo-American texts on mental illness during Pinel's career.

10. Pussin's wife Marguerite, in fact, is pictured alongside Pinel in Tony Robert-Fleury's 1878 painting, *Pinel Unchaining the Insane at the Hospital of Salpêtrière*.

11. Walther Riese argues compellingly that "Pinel's approach to the mentally ill is a logical result of his Hippocratic view of disease as an historical chapter in an individual's life" (1969, 3).

REFERENCES

Altschule, Mark D. 1977. *Origins of concepts in human behavior: Social and cultural factors*. Washington, DC: Hemisphere.

Foucault, Michel. 1961. *Madness and civilization: A history of insanity in the age of reason*. Trans. Richard Howard. New York: Vintage Books, 1988.

———. 1963. *The birth of the clinic: An archaeology of medical perception*. Trans. A. M. Sheridan Smith. New York: Vintage Books, 1994.

Grob, Gerald N. 1994. *The mad among us: A history of the care of America's mentally ill*. New York: Free Press.

McHugh, Paul, and Philip Slavney. 1986. *The perspectives of psychiatry*. Baltimore: Johns Hopkins University Press.

Morgan, William L., and George L. Engel. 1969. *The clinical approach to the patient*. Philadelphia: Saunders.

Pinel, Philippe. 1801. *A treatise on insanity*. Trans. Paul F. Cranefield. New York: Hafner, 1962.

Riese, Walther. 1969. *The legacy of Philippe Pinel; An inquiry into thought on mental alienation*. New York: Springer.

Weiner, Dora B. 1992. Philippe Pinel's "Memoir on madness" of December 11, 1754: A fundamental text of modern psychiatry. *American Journal of Psychiatry* 149, no. 6:725–32.

———. 1994. "Le geste de Pinel": The history of a psychiatric myth. In *Discovering the history of psychiatry*, ed. Mark S. Micale and Roy Porter, 218–40. New York: Oxford University Press.

FOUR

Narrative Medicine
and Negative Capability

TERRENCE E. HOLT

ONE

NOT LONG AGO, the critical, educational, and literary movement known as
"Narrative Medicine" received the definitive stamp of public recognition
when it was the subject of feature coverage both in *The New York Times*
(Smith 2003) and on National Public Radio (2003). Both pieces concen-
trated on the introduction of narrative writing and discussion groups into the
third-year clerkships at the College of Physicians and Surgeons at Columbia
University, featuring vignettes from students' autobiographical essays in
which they grapple with the ethical and existential crises they have faced in
their medical training. Both stories focused on this autobiographical element
as if it were remarkable. And yet the emphasis on autobiography in these features seems anything but surprising; indeed, when seen in cultural context, it
has an air of inevitability. Both the *Times* piece and the NPR broadcast situated their interest in the spectacle of doctors writing about themselves in the
broader context of the widespread attention that has been garnered recently
by doctors' autobiographical narratives. Atul Gawande's (2002) essays in *The
New Yorker*, for instance, are only the latest in a long series of narratives that

I would like to thank the Program on Aging at the University of North Carolina
School of Medicine, the R. J. Reynolds Foundation, and the Hartford Foundation for
support of this work. Thanks also to my colleagues in the Department of Social Medicine, UNC School of Medicine, for their helpful comments and advice.

have become a staple in its pages, reaching back to the days when Burton
Roueché's (1953; 1984) "Medical Detective" pieces spliced the disparate genres
of public health and the private eye into a literary form. Along the way, practitioners of the medical narrative, in the pages of magazines such as *The New
Yorker, Harpers,* and *Mademoiselle,* have included such well-known doctor-writers as Oliver Sacks (1974; 1985; 1997), Perri Klass (1987; 1992), and Richard
Selzer (1976; 1979), most of them writing in a style that owes far more to E. B.
White than to Sir William Osler, and in a mode not only autobiographical but
assertively personal. Considering the offerings before the public now, it would
seem that the dominant mode of medical discourse is the confessional.

On the one hand, then, we have mass publications holding up medical
autobiography as something remarkable; on the other, we have an established
tradition of confessional writing by doctors. What makes the element of autobiography in narrative medicine noteworthy, it would seem, is not the thing
itself, but a certain doubleness in our reception of it. It is something we regard
as a novelty even when it has become a commonplace. This now-you-see-me-
now-you-don't quality, as Michel Foucault (1975) has famously observed,
marks public-private boundaries generally. Here, however, this uncanniness
points to something important in the relationship between narrative and
medicine, between medicine and doctors, doctors and patients. There is
something here we do (not) want to see.

One way to trace that elusive something is by attending more closely to
the recent history of narrative medicine. At its inception, the narrative medicine movement was not exclusively, or even notably, linked to the autobiographical essay. It was, originally, a much more catholic undertaking, an
attempt to unite the long-sundered fields of medicine and the humanities.
The movement has grown into an initiative within medical education, one
that attempts to overcome the dehumanizing tendencies in medical training
by imbuing medical trainees and practitioners alike with, in Rita Charon's
words, "narrative competence," the ability "to recognize, interpret, and be
moved to action by the predicaments of others" (2001, 83). As such, narrative medicine has continued to emphasize interpretive skills far more than
actual narrative composition.

This emphasis on interpretation has still been regarded in some quarters as
revolutionary, and therefore unsavory: its practitioners have been accused by
one detractor of "advocating . . . the medical application of . . . deconstruc-
tionism, critical literary theory, or postmodernism." If we choose to ignore the
dangers of such "extreme relativism," he warns us, "we may do so at our own
and our patients' peril" (Poses 2001, 929). And it may be that this reaction is
correct, at least insofar is it identifies a tendency: for out of this relatively
innocuous attempt to articulate points of contact between the interpretive act
as practiced by doctors and by literary scholars has arisen what may well be the
most extreme relativism of all: autobiographical writing, an unseemly airing of

medical laundry, in which doctors, writing from a perspective that sets aside the impersonal plural of the journals and the labs, confess to having doubts, to making mistakes—sometimes even to doing harm. Our own and our patients' peril has in fact been the subject matter of the most widely noticed medical narratives, threatening (to such critics) to unleash a flood of revelation and self-regard that has already sparked a retrograde movement. Several recent essays in the medical literature (Charon 2001; Coulehan and Hawkins 2003) have issued cautionary statements warning practitioners of the potential harm they may do by revealing too much, undermining patient trust, even committing theft of narratives belonging properly to the patient, not the doctor.

This seems like a lot of history for such a small and youthful movement to have accumulated. But what I've sketched here is really only the tip of a much larger iceberg, a submerged mass whose actual outline is identified in the popular coverage the movement has recently received. The more sensational form of narrative medicine on display in the *Times* and on NPR shadows tendencies broadly disseminated in popular culture of the twentieth century, and exemplified in two highly influential sites of cultural production: *The New Yorker*, on one hand, and network television on the other. Given the measured restraint for which the former is famous, and the latter's uninhibited relish for spectacle, there might seem few points in common. But in their seeming opposition they represent two poles anchoring our culture's response to contemporary medicine. Between them, they articulate the same doubleness of blindness and recognition, a doubleness also inhabiting narrative medicine, medicine itself, and the educational process that makes doctors the strange creatures they are.

Read against the recent popular history of medical narrative, narrative medicine can be seen as offering a picture of the relationship between culture and medicine, doctor and patient, in which unity is deemed to be not only unattainable but undesirable, and where humane values are perceived as being more complicated than is sometimes assumed. Such a reading of the cultural representations of medicine offers, ultimately, a subject-position for doctors that may enable us to regain a portion of our humanity by taking the measure of its loss. By attending to this alternative history, where loss and division struggle with our desires for unity, I would like ultimately to come back to medical education, to suggest ways in which narrative can be incorporated in the medical curriculum not so much as a foreign body—tolerated, but effectively walled off in a kind of emotional abscess—but as something properly—indeed, already—a central part of medical education.

TWO

The New Yorker has been for the past generation the unchallenged arbiter of literary fashion in the United States (to the extent that the United States

can be imagined as having a single literary culture).[1] As such, it has imposed
a highly distinctive set of formal and substantive criteria on American literary production. On the one hand, there has been an extreme devotion to the
canons of literary realism, taking these conventions so literally that decades
of Ivy League graduates have made their entry into the world of letters in the
role of "fact checkers" for *The New Yorker*, verifying that the details not only
in nonfiction, but in pieces of fiction and even poems, conform to the reality
of the world as specified in their formidable reference library. One perverse
effect of this construction of realism has been a curious blurring of the lines
between fiction and fact: when both are expected to portray life with the
same fidelity to the world as construed by cartographers and encyclopedists,
it is natural to wonder where fiction ends and fact begins.

There has also been an understanding that, in short fiction at least, the
function of narrative personae should be as limited as possible, usually
through the formal mechanism of irony, by which any statements about the
world that might be deemed authoritative (beyond the location of certain
buildings on certain streetcorners) are rendered open to multiple and ultimately indefinite interpretations; in other words, the "meanings" of such stories should be apparently opaque, accessible primarily by reference to the
larger oeuvre of *New Yorker* stories. As a marketing technique, this has been
highly successful, allowing the creation of an audience larger than might otherwise have accrued to a literary magazine, because in its resistance to definition—fact or fiction, meaning this or meaning that—*The New Yorker* was
able to be many things to many people (a marketing technique that has been
explored in a variety of other ways by most of the successful mass media of the
past century).[2] But it has made the magazine a natural home for other cultural
trends that arise similarly from the exigencies of making a living in what the
Marxists hopefully call "late" monopoly capitalism: the decentering of the literary subject has been widely celebrated or condemned as chief among them.

The most familiar and influential instance of this tendency has followed
a trajectory of close to forty years, beginning with the first efforts identified
as the New Journalism in the 1960s, and continuing today in the flourishing
of the literary form known variously as creative nonfiction or more simply the
personal essay. The New Journalism, you may recall, was new because it was
a product of the sixties, and what marked it especially as a part of that era was
its skepticism about authority, which it expressed by reinserting the first-person singular point of view into journalism. Norman Mailer, Tom Wolfe, Gay
Talese, Joan Didion, and a host of others approached what had traditionally
been objects of journalistic interest—subjects approached, until then, with
an Olympian objectivity—with a perverse insistence on the reporter's identity as an individual, and by implication the limitations of the reporter's perspective. As such, the movement announced a principled rejection of what it
held to be an impossible and irresponsible claim to objectivity: in the com-

plex, highly charged political and social currents of the time, a claim to objectivity could only mask either self-delusion or a hidden agenda. Better to be up-front with one's position and prejudices, and thereby allow the reader to interpret the image in an avowedly flawed lens.

In their abdication of authority, the New Journalists tried to put into practice perhaps the most characteristic axiom of the time, "The personal is the political." But it also expressed a profound skepticism about the limits not only of knowledge but also of politics, an epicurean hand-washing of questions of truth and falsehood. As such, the New Journalism despaired of making sense of a society that had become too complex, too chaotic to see as a whole. But through its skepticism, the New Journalism also confessed to another wish: to hold itself, despite its pose of engagement, above the fray. By eschewing authority, by refusing responsibility for accuracy, the New Journalism also imagined itself managing somehow to escape the seemingly inevitable catastrophe toward which the times seemed a-heading. It is probably not an accident that the political dispute that brought the New Journalism into being was the war in Vietnam, where a protest against global entanglements reflected a profound skepticism about what had been verities of geopolitics, a refusal of the Manichean divisions of the world into categories of right and wrong that seemed doomed to reduce both sides to indistinguishable ash. Better not to be involved: at least then one could have the consolation of feeling oneself the innocent victim of others' mischief—about the only consolation one could imagine at the time. As a counterphobic response to the claustrophobically close perspective on the war offered by television coverage, the New Journalism offered cake both eaten and whole: the voyeuristic pleasures of participation without any of the guilt. The autobiographical impulse paradoxically emptied the subject position.

There is a problem with this originally principled position, of course, one of the several pitfalls into which irony by its nature threatens to tumble. It is a question of what might be termed the secondary gain that accrues from letting the observer off the hook: once above the fray, we're freed from taking sides and all the consequences such choices entail. Rather than leading to connection, saying "I" merely gestures toward engagement while actually refusing it. But rather than observe this from a safe distance and accuse the New Journalists of bad faith, we might more profitably observe that in doing so we merely repeat what we condemn, deploring from afar the unavoidable consequence of any attempt at social critique. We are never above the fray. Journalists, doctors, even literary critics are all part of what they examine. And our involvement extends even to the mixed motives and shameful pleasures that accompany the most virtuous acts. By the end of this chapter, I hope to show that this contradictory fragmentation of impulse is not necessarily a trap; indeed, if recognized as an inevitable part of ethical discourse, it offers a ground that actually enables a practical ethics of care.

THREE

If the elements of the story just told seem familiar, it may be because the key terms are essentially the same as those that mark the metamorphosis of narrative medicine from the academic purity that seeks to renew the unity of literature and medicine to the more spectacular autobiographies that chart disastrous complications. As we track the New Journalism forward through the seventies to the eighties, it morphs, as the rest of the culture did, from an intense interest in the political to a quietist concentration on the personal, emerging in the nineties in the form of creative nonfiction or the personal essay.[3]

And it is over precisely this period that the popular medical essay, which at its start was essentially the province of the traditionally reportorial Burton Rouché or the magisterially professional Lewis Thomas, gives over to the Carlylean excesses of Richard Selzer, the engaging confessional of Perri Klass, Oliver Sacks's quirky neuroethnographies, and ultimately the disturbing complications of Atul Gawande. It is an evolution marked by precisely the same reinsertion of the "I," the narrator-doctor, into what is revealed not as the pristine marble halls of Aesclepius but a charnel house of uncertainty, doubt, and error. In doing so, the doctor regains a personal contact with the audience, and ultimately with himself, but at a price: the surrender of the illusion of an identity somehow free of contradiction, pure of motive—the ideal provider.

As several commentators (Charon 2001; Coulehan and Hawkins 2003) have observed, the doctor who writes personally and honestly about the uncertainties and conflicts in medicine runs a number of real (and some I think imaginary) risks: from violation of patient privacy to undermining the confidence of the laity in the canons of medical professionalism to theft of literary property properly belonging to the patient to exploitation of suffering for personal gain. In abandoning the traditional prerogatives of the doctor— among them secrecy, detachment, and authority—doctor-writers risk alienating the very patients with whom they want to get personal. Who would trust a doctor who blabs the secrets of the examining room? Who would bare his belly to a surgeon who confesses his mistakes? Who would trust the prescriptions of a doctor who doubts? In trying to step down from his singular eminence, the doctor-writer may fall too far. The move to personalize, they say, may alienate instead.

But these attempts to discipline a popular form such as personal writing in general, or medical autobiography in particular, not only fail to achieve any reform, they also miss the point. Rather than condemn this tendency to expose, we might do better to ask what is driving it: What would move otherwise respectable doctors to open up the secrets of the sausage factory? And what patients would want to take the tour? When we consider the weight of professional tradition and prejudice, as well as legitimate ethical questions that arise when doctors stoop to storytelling, not to mention the reasonable revulsion such stories must elicit from readers (potential patients all), it is hard to escape the conclusion that there must be some powerful need driving not only the tellers but also the audience.

This question of audience seems to me centrally important. First, because the tendency in criticism of medical autobiography is almost universally to forget about audience altogether. Almost without exception, discussions of the attractions and pitfalls of medical autobiography turn on the doctor-patient relationship, or occasionally the doctor-doctor relationship (but even there the other doctor figures usually not as the reader, but an innocent bystander in the story, dragged in unwittingly as an extra in the storyteller's sensational tale). But second, and more important, because it is the existence (or creation) of an audience that has made—as the attention in the *Times* and NPR suggests—narrative medicine what it is. These narratives would not exist (not publicly, at least) without people willing—in fact, eager—to pay good money to read them. The question is, why? Where did this audience come from? What is motivating them to read things that most readers readily admit they find disturbing? And what is the relationship between that audience and the doctors doing the writing?

I think an understanding of this part of the history hinges on a recognition of one of the most important aspects of audience reception of these pieces. It is not unambivalent. The medical profession itself, in its distinct uneasiness about its own narratives, is acting (as it must) as a part of the larger culture, shocked, a little scared, a little titillated to find the secrets of the examining room and the operating room, the consulting room and the emergency room—all these rooms once closed off—now so readily accessible. This aspect of the trend was most clearly announced several years ago, with the possibly surprising success on niche cable channels of "documentary" programming devoted essentially to close-up images of gory surgery. The shows found a following, but it was clear that the appeal was essentially one of the frisson, of a voyeuristic entry into what should properly be concealed—our own insides, our bloody fragility—a spectacular relationship that has been best explained from the psychoanalytic perspective by Julia Kristeva (1980) and from a historico-political perspective by Michel Foucault (1975).

It is in the form of these recent, pseudodocumentary television essays that we find a suggestion that what draws people to such narratives is precisely what we have been warned against: a reveling in what one might call the medical sublime, a front-row seat at a display of mortal danger, where the boundaries of professional competence define as well the mortal boundaries of the self. Without this element of danger, danger constructed especially in terms of medical fallibility, it is doubtful that this audience would exist in the form that it does. But however crude or peculiar such attractions might seem, they underscore a more general appeal of medical narrative that has persisted for several generations in that hardy (seemingly immortal) subgenre of popular drama: the doctor show, where fallibility takes on a more personal form.

From its origins in radio soap opera through its manifestations among the most popular prime-time television programs in every decade since 1960 (*Dr. Kildare, Ben Casey, Marcus Welby, St. Elsewhere, ER*) as well as its persistence as a staple of afternoon programming, the doctor show has followed a very simple formula. In high-concept terms, it reduces to this: "personal medicine." Or, better, "romantic medicine." Perhaps even "family medicine."[4] No matter how it is inflected, the fundamental gesture is to take a remote institution—frightening because it insinuates itself into the most personal recesses of our lives while at the same time remaining impersonally aloof—and domesticate it. Once again, we find that troubling paradox: the personal points us to an impersonality it nervously dodges or covers over.

In these dramas, medicine can be domesticated in a number of ways. Sometimes the gesture is literal, as in the domiciliary architecture of the office in which Robert Young impersonated Dr. Marcus Welby (when we all knew he was really Father Knows Best). Similarly, we got the cozy home offices where Carl Betz went so Donna Reed could clean the house, or Bill Cosby disappeared while Phyllicia Rashad managed the children a generation later. Or it is figurative, as in the family romance enacted by Ben Casey and Dr. Zorba, Drs. Kildare and Gillespie. Or it appears as the most direct shorthand of all, the way sex just keeps happening all over these hospitals—something that (to the best of my knowledge, anyway) is not common at the institution where I practice. But I think the most telling way in which television domesticates the medical is also perhaps the subtlest, a matter of style more than substance. For the few minutes I last tuned into (I think it was) *Chicago Hope* a few years ago, I just felt bemused. Something wasn't right. It wasn't that they had the facts wrong (they had clearly hired the right consultants). It was something their medical fact-checkers had no power to correct: in every scene, doctors and nurses talked passionately about their work, their jobs, but especially their patients, as intensely as only actors on seasonal contracts can. They talked about them as if they deeply, *personally* cared.

Let me be clear. I am not at all suggesting here that doctors and nurses do not deeply, passionately, and in some sense personally care about the work they do. We do. But just what the personal means is the central issue in this essay. What we have to offer our patients isn't (ideally) *eros*, or even *agape*. At best, it rises to *caritas*, which may be the least personal (in the traditional sense), the most institutional form love can take. It is also, I think, the most powerful. It is certainly the most effective.

In understanding how the institutional reinflects the personal, we have the crux of the matter. For the audiences of the doctor shows—and, to the extent that they follow the logic of personalizing medicine, of all medical narratives—such stories address both a deeply held wish and an abiding fear: that doctors might (not) care for them; that anybody, in the enormous machine that is a hospital, might be personally concerned with their mortality; that somehow in the encounter with our utter helplessness that is the fundamental truth and shock of hospitalization, someone might intervene to make it all go away. Which, of course, we as doctors cannot. People come into the hospital, increasingly in this era of economically rationalized medicine, to suffer and to die. And no matter how deeply I may feel my commitment to ease that suffering, to forestall that death (if such forestalling be in fact humane), I know just as deeply that my powers in that regard are, to put it mildly, limited.

This is the problem that I think narrative medicine has come into being to address. I have been writing as if the confessional form were something new, as the entire discourse of the field has tended to assume. But *is* narrative medicine really a new form, a response to pressures on medicine in the postindustrial era? I actually doubt this. One persistent theme of contemporary critical theory would have it that writing happens all the time, that it is the base condition of existence: we live a narrative that inscribes itself in the world around us, and on ourselves. Perceiving the world through narrative because that is how we are made, we grasp the world only indirectly, and (believing too well the story we whisper in our ears) feel that indirectness as a flaw. It is a tale not of original and ultimate unity, but of originary, irremediable division, an alienation of the self within the self, the insurmountable gap between the self as idealized and the self as experienced, that language in its endless significations endlessly repeats.[5] Narrative medicine, it seems to me, is just a particularly revealing example of the fissures and paradoxes that necessarily result when we tell ourselves any story of the "I."

The particular version of this story that narrative medicine offers is a *Bildungsroman*, founded (as so many of them are) on an originary loss. It goes like this: out of a complex and poorly understood motivation, articulated (usually) idealistically and innocently in the AMCAS application essay, every year some thousands of young people go to medical school and start becoming doctors. The first thing that happens to them is that they dissect a cadaver. This is a nasty process, of dubious educational value, but we all know why it is such an essential introduction to medicine: it drives a wedge between the learned and perhaps instinctive taboos that inhabit most of us quite deeply, on the one hand, and the socially necessary instrumentality of the doctor, on the other. It is meant also (for good or ill) to erect a barrier between us and all the rest of the world for whom cutting up dead bodies would be criminally pathological. In fact, it is a symbol for this, an initiation that provides a key by which the initiate learns to understand a new relation to the world. Between the human being who feels a proper loathing and horror of the corpse and all it means and the doctor who will diagnose prostate

cancer by a rectal exam or deliberately rebreak a screaming child's arm so that
it will heal straight, there must be some division, some lasting estrangement,
or else the work will not get done: the cancer will be missed, the arm grow
twisted. So in order to create human beings who are able to do these things
day after day, we start by assaulting their fundamental emotional responses to
mortality.

I am not suggesting pity for the doctor—we are not the victims here. The
victims are the patients who find themselves under the care of people who
have had their capacity to connect with or care for others deliberately
altered. Not destroyed or incapacitated, but definitely changed, distanced,
disconnected from the way it works in most of us. The inscription left by this
process that matters most is not marked only on the doctor who cannot adequately respond to a patient's experience (although that is certainly a part of
the story). The larger story is made up of silences, of gestures not made, connections failed, of meanings misunderstood: it is in the entire institution of
medicine, with which nobody nowadays, at least in public statements, seems
all that happy. What is the story that the form taken by narrative medicine is
trying to tell us? How *can* narrative make us better doctors?

FOUR

I would like you to imagine me a few years ago, a resident in the cardiac ICU,
leaning against the wall of a patient's room. It is about eleven in the morning, and I have been up since six the morning of the day before. The patient
has been under my care eleven days, one of twenty or so I have taken care of
in that time. About five minutes earlier, in response to her request and after
several days of discussion, I had asked the nurse to turn off the pump that had
been keeping her alive. The family is gathered around the bedside. She is
awake, talking quietly. She will be dead within the hour.

As I lean against the wall, tears are coursing down my face. I am being
very quiet about it, but I am sobbing as freely as I know how. And meanwhile
I am thinking: if this is over by 12:30, I have got a chance of getting lunch
before I replace the art line in twenty-four. The tears are streaming down my
face, and I am utterly sad, haunted by memories of my father's nearly identical death ten years before. But somewhere a voice is also thinking: maybe
today I can sign out by three.

I am reluctant to offer myself here as an example of anything but a tired
man on the periphery of someone else's sad situation. Most doctors I know
can tell similar stories. Maybe with not so much weeping, but with the essential two-track mental process intact. The difference between my story and
other doctors'—the individual particularity that makes it worth casting as
narrative—has to do with my relationship to that process. When I was holding up that wall in the ICU, reviewing my to-do list and crying my eyes red,

I knew exactly what was going on. Psychiatrists call it "splitting," and it is a well-known defense mechanism. I was splitting. Even when my own father lay dying and my heart was broken, I remember noticing irrelevancies that made it somehow worse: the cramp in my neck, an itch on my nose, a bill coming due next Tuesday. Disloyal, shameful, and mine. Splitting. But what struck me most about it ten years later, when I was there again as a resident in the ICU, was not that I was splitting: it was that it did not bother me that I was doing so. In fact, in splitting, to myself at least, I was experiencing a truth about my presence in that room. And that, I think, was important. It set me free to do what mattered. As a resident, I had to think about other cases, my own duties, the burden of them I wished to have lifted for that day. As a human being, I also had to cry because of the shared human tragedy of mortality in that room. Or whatever it is that makes us cry. For the family in that room, the woman dying on that bed, I was there, both personally and impersonally, as doctor and fellow creature. She was not dying alone.

I do not mean by this digression to assign myself any particular virtue: I do not think anything about this story qualifies me as the historically necessary weeping doctor. But having gained this *aperçu*, I found myself wondering: what was it that enabled me to function comfortably within that split, to attend equally to both halves of my experience? Because I should emphasize that both halves were necessary, easing the suffering of that patient and her family in the only way I could, and, along that other track, still performing my obligations to the others who were depending on me that day: my remaining patients, who needed that art line, who needed a reliable handoff to the on-call team; and to my family, who unaccountably wanted me home. And to myself, who needed desperately to get some sleep. But I needed more than that, of course: I needed both of those tracks to function and function equally well. I needed to mourn that patient, to change that art line, to grieve my father, to sign out my patients, to feel *something* in the midst of so much institutional anomie, and to go home. I needed to think I was doing justice to everyone involved—in a situation where a single-minded response would have left many people uncared for. All of them, in fact.

If there was anything particular about my performance at that moment, it was simply that I was demonstrating the benefit of my training. Not as a doctor, but as a reader. As that celebrated doctor John Keats observed long ago, what constitutes the literary sensibility is precisely the capacity to entertain a schism within one's identity, a quality he called "negative capability."[6] If I was able to do my job fully that day, and also still somehow try to stay human and connected, I have to thank Keats as much as Hippocrates, and the people who taught me how to read Keats, probably, more than the ones who taught me to read an EKG. In entertaining two seemingly opposed responses—to pity and to duty, to death and to lunch—I was experiencing a fragmentation of the self. It is precisely this experience that bridges the worlds of medicine and art—or could, if medicine were to recognize it through the terms Keats made available two centuries ago. If we could recover a familiarity with, an acceptance of, the essentially fractured nature of our selves and our hearts, we might regain an insight that the empiricist disposition of contemporary medicine, for all its explanatory power, in its emphasis on the unifying hypothesis has lost the power to see, to express, or to accept. And that popular culture, for all that it revels in the frisson of the personal, shows us again and again (in the splitting of the New Journalists, for instance), but also fails consciously to assert, so long as it insists that the personal be something other than what it is: a realm not of unity but of division, where personal selfishness and humane care exist side by side. Because those are the only terms on which they can exist at all.

A reader reading well is simultaneously *experiencing* the text, responding to it emotionally, and *analyzing* that response, tracking it to its sources in narrative convention, in language, in culture and psychology and economics and all the other disciplines critics poach on these days. Doing one without the other is not reading. And it is not doctoring either. This is the story that the fractured history of narrative medicine has been trying to tell. Rather than ignoring or decrying our negative capability—the gap we pry open between our emotions and our function as doctors—rather than hiding it as a dirty secret of medical initiation, scotomizing it or pretending it is something other than it is, we need to address it, encourage it, cultivate it, learn it, and teach it. Make it not a loss but a gift, an instrument as important to medical care as any other technique at our disposal. And in literature we have ready-made the tool our culture has developed for this task. Both reading and writing are, as numerous exponents of narrative medicine have observed, performative acts, requiring just this capacity to think and to feel simultaneously, to experience and observe oneself in the act, and to know this disjunction not as a weakness or a wrong but as precisely what gives us the strength, the right, and the obligation to promise people care.

NOTES

1. Our wish to imagine a single literary culture helps generate organs such as the *Times* and NPR; the similar desire to believe in singleness of purpose and purity of motive informs much of the fantasy of what doctors and medicine might be.

2. Most trenchantly critiqued in that episode of *The Simpsons* where Homer appears as a freak act with a touring rock festival: "Dude! Are you being ironic?" "Dude! I don't even know anymore!" Or words to that effect.

3. For those who aren't sure what I'm talking about, the career of John McPhee, from *The Curve of Binding Energy* (1974) through *Coming into the Country* (1977) to *Basin and Plain* (1981) marks just this tandem process of personal engagement and public disengagement.

4. The identification of family medicine with television doctors was made explicit when *Marcus Welby, M.D.* attracted the College of Family Physicians as one of its prime-time sponsors, the logo of the organization succeeding the closing shot of Welby's home office in the show's final moments. Similarly, in its origins in the 1960s as a holistic alternative to a fragmentary medical establishment, family medicine offers a reassuring, totalizing response to the fragmentation both Kristeva and Foucault (as well as, originally, Freud) identify as the central horror of our mortality.

5. There have been numerous discussions in poststructuralist criticism of this aspect of writing, which Derrida (1967) seminally describes as *différance*. For an eminently readable introduction to the central themes of Derrida's work, see Barbara Johnson's (1981) introduction to her translation of *Dissemination*.

6. "Negative capability" is, as Keats himself recognized, a protean idea, one that, like most abstractions in his letters, resists determination. Although Keats criticism long received it as a univocal celebration of transcendence, more recent poststructuralists have tended to emphasize the ambivalence inherent in the formulation, and it is from this perspective that I approach the term. Keats's initial articulation of the concept on December 21, 1817, defines it as the "quality [that] went to form a Man of Achievement, especially in Literature, and which Shakespeare possessed so enormously . . . that is when a man is capable of being in uncertainties, mysteries, doubts, without any irritable reaching after fact and reason" (Forman 1952, 71). Ten months later, on October 27, 1818, returning to Shakespeare as an exemplar of this "poetical Character," Keats writes of that character that "it is not itself—it has no self—it is every thing and nothing—It has no character" (226–27). For Keats, this "negative capability" signifies a capacity to suspend especially the foundational certainty of identity: "A poet is the most unpoetical of any thing in existence; because he has no Identity" (215). "Identity" is a charged term in Keats's lexicon at this time, signifying especially the suffering of his brother Tom in his final illness (see his letter of September 21, 1818), and through that association becoming one of those peculiar words that suggests its own undoing. The association suggests also that Keats's career in medicine (which he abandoned only in 1816) formed an important basis for his formulation of questions of identity. For additional exploration of the multiple sites of uncertainty in Keats, especially in relation to poststructural theories of language and subjectivity, see the essays in Bloom (1985), which exhibit some of the range of interpretations to which this crux in Keats studies has played host over the past generation.

REFERENCES

Bloom, Harold, ed. 1985. *Keats, modern critical views*. New York: Chelsea House.

Charon, Rita. 2001. Narrative medicine: Form, function, and ethics. *Annals of Internal Medicine* 134:83–87.

Coulehan, Jack, and Anne Hunsaker Hawkins. 2003. Keeping faith: Ethics and the physician writer. *Annals of Internal Medicine* 139:307–11.

Derrida, Jacques. 1967. *L'Écriture et la différence*. Paris, Éditions du Seuil.

Forman, Maurice, ed. 1952. *The letters of John Keats*. Fourth ed. London: Oxford University Press.

Foucault, Michel. 1975. *Discipline and punish: The birth of the prison*. Trans. Alan Sheridan. New York: Pantheon Books, 1977.

Gwanade, Atal. 2002. *Complications: A surgeon's notes on an imperfect science*. New York: Holt.

Johnson, Barbara. 1981. Introduction to *Dissemination*, by Jacques Derrida, trans. Johnson, i–xxxiii. Chicago: University of Chicago Press.

Klass, Perri. 1987. *A not entirely blind procedure: Four years as a medical student*. New York: Putnam.

———. 1992. *Baby doctor*. New York: Random House.

Kristeva, Julia. 1980. *Powers of horror: An essay on abjection*. Trans. Leon S. Roudiez. New York: Columbia University Press, 1982.

McPhee, John A. 1974. *The curve of binding energy*. New York: Farrar, Straus, and Giroux.

———. 1977. *Coming into the country*. New York: Farrar, Straus, and Giroux.

———. 1981. *Basin and plain*. New York: Farrar, Straus, and Giroux.

National Public Radio. 2003. Stories in Medicine. October 28. Available via the link at narrativemedicine.org.

Poses, Roy. 2001. Narrative medicine. *Annals of Internal Medicine* 135:929–30.

Roueché, Berton. 1953. *Eleven blue men, and other narratives of medical detection*. Boston: Little, Brown.

———. 1984. *The medical detectives*. New York: Times Books.

Sacks, Oliver. 1974. *Awakenings*. Garden City: Doubleday.

———. 1985. *The man who mistook his wife for a hat and other clinical tales*. New York: Summit Books.

———. 1997. *The island of the colorblind and Cycad Island*. New York: Knopf.

Selzer, Richard. 1976. *Mortal lessons: Notes on the art of surgery*. New York: Simon and Schuster.

———. 1979. *Confessions of a knife*. New York: Simon and Schuster.

Smith, Dinitia. 2003. Diagnosis goes low-tech. *The New York Times*, October 11. Available via the link at narrativemedicine.org.

PART II

Psychoanalytic Interventions

FIVE

"The Past Is a Foreign Country"

Some Uses of Literature
in the Psychoanalytic Dialogue

VERA J. CAMDEN

THE USES OF psychoanalysis in the study of literature are familiar to us all, grounded as they are in Freud's own writings on art, literature, history, and religion. But the counterpoint to this, the uses of literature in the psychoanalytic process, is less familiar and less apparent in American psychoanalysis, which, practically speaking, reflects little of Freud's regard for the capacity of literature to instruct the analyst. As Pierre Bayard (1999) has put it, "As it is often practiced, *the psychoanalytical approach to texts places knowledge on the side of psychoanalysis and not on that of literature*. In doing so, it risks diminishing literature and underestimating literature's own ability to produce knowledge" (207–208). Too often in American psychoanalytic practice, Freud's indebtedness to the poets and philosophers is offered with sage reverence as a nod to the creative genius that Freud shared with those writers he credited with discovering the unconscious before him; but, as with most sage and reverential history, this regard has little practical impact.

The veneration of the artist as an agent of knowledge is ornamental in most psychoanalytic institutes. Indeed, it often seems that the trends in psychoanalytic training today reflect more regard for schools of business than

I would like to thank Murray Goldstone, MD, for his invaluable insight and support during my work on this analysis.

schools of the humanities. And yet as historian and psychoanalyst Peter Loewenberg remarked in 1999 to a class of psychoanalytic candidates in Cleveland on the topic of "applied psychoanalysis": "All of the practice of psychoanalysis is 'applied.'" To suggest otherwise, he continued, is to idealize a notion of a pure and scientifically repeatable psychoanalytic process. A psychoanalysis, however, like a work of literature, is unique. It is not typical; it is not in that sense "repeatable." For while we might not share Freud's erudition any more than we share his genius, we are heirs to his psychology of the mind and to his technique of treatment: that psychology and that technique were shaped by an intellectual legacy imbued with a humanistic as well as a scientific view of human experience. We do not practice psychoanalysis as well as we might if we do not keep that legacy in mind.

APPLIED LITERATURE:
THE HISTORY OF THE PRACTICE

On October 15, 1897, Freud wrote to Wilhelm Fliess of his discovery of what would later become known as the Oedipus complex: "I have found, in my own case too, [the phenomenon of] being in love with my mother and jealous of my father, and I now consider it a universal event in early childhood." He elaborates: "If this is so, we can understand the gripping power of *Oedipus Rex*," since "the Greek legend seizes upon a compulsion of which everyone recognizes because he senses its existence within himself. Everyone in the audience was once a budding Oedipus in fantasy and each recoils in horror from the dream fulfillment here transplanted into reality, with the full quantity of repression which separates his infantile state from his present one" (Masson 1985, 272). He goes on to explain that "the thought passed through my head that the same thing might be at the bottom of *Hamlet* as well. . . . [A] real event stimulated the poet to his representation, in that his unconscious understood the unconscious of his hero." Thus, what Frederick Wyatt (1989) terms the "extensive and auspicious" connection between literature and psychoanalysis marks Freud's dependence upon literature for the defining "paradigm" of this "prototypical event" in the psychic life of the individual (27). In this record of the process by which literature produces knowledge, Freud holds that literature operates cathartically—the audience sees its desire displayed full-blown upon the stage and responds with excitement, recognition, and (inevitably) a shrinking back from just such recognition.

Invoking another example of the stake of the literary in the origins of psychoanalysis, Shoshana Felman (1992) opines that it is on the testimonial aspect of Freud's dream-work that the foundations of psychoanalysis rest. In 1908, in the midst of his most fruitful research and clinical discoveries, Freud returned to the narratives and the interpretation of his own dream life that undergird his findings. He wrote in the preface to the second edition of *The*

Interpretation of Dreams: "During the long years in which I have been working at the problems of the neuroses I have often been in doubt and sometimes been shaken in my convictions. At such times it has always been *The Interpretation of Dreams* that has given me back my certainty" (1900, xxvi). Building on Freud's reflections, Felman highlights the "birth of knowledge through the testimonial process" and the literary event of Freud's record of the Irma dream, which results "not merely in the actual interpretation and elucidation of the dream, but in the transformation of this one particular event and of this one particular interpretation into a paradigmatic model not just of interpretation but of the very principle of psychoanalytic discovery" (1992, 16). Here is modeled "the very birth of knowledge through the testimonial process." It is this process of testimonial or narrative that will become, in the clinical setting, "the *psychoanalytic dialogue*" (15).

But for all Freud's indebtedness to literary paradigms and literary processes, psychoanalysis has always had an uneasy and ambivalent relationship to its literary origins. While on the one hand Freud parts company with those physicians who do not discern the relation between the psyche and the soma, he on the other hand exhibits considerable anxiety and ambivalence about the narrative appeal of his case studies, which often read like Victorian melodramas. He struggled with his audience, accusing some physicians of reading his case studies the wrong way, as novels or short stories, and for the wrong reasons. In his preface to the Dora case, he writes: "I am aware that—in this city, at least—there are many physicians who (revolting though it may seem) choose to read a case history of this kind not as a contribution to the psychopathology of neuroses, but as a *roman à clef* designed for their private delectation" (1905, 9).

The ambivalence that Freud reveals in his accusation of the prurient reader persists in the debates surrounding psychoanalytic reporting today: How does one convey the psychoanalytic process "scientifically" and yet retain the necessarily narrative form of the psychoanalytic dialogue, the record of a life disclosed in language? Psychoanalysis is haunted by literature: narrative functions like the repressed core that will ineluctably return, however disguised, to haunt the science of psychoanalysis.[1]

To embrace rather than resist the power of narrative as a clinical as well as a creative process, I should like to propose the usefulness of an argument recently offered by Peter Rudnytsky in his book, *Reading Psychoanalysis* (2002). Rudnytsky posits that a division needs to be made between our understanding of the metapsychology of psychoanalysis—or the theories of psychoanalysis as a science of the mind—and the clinical situation, the practice of psychoanalysis as it is applied in the psychoanalytic situation. He argues, "on the one hand, that a natural science model is not appropriate to understanding the existential dynamics of the analytic situation and, on the other, that metapsychologies are not mere metaphors but potentially testable theories" (230). Quoting John Bowlby, Rudnytsky remarks that there are "'two very different aspects of our discipline—the art of psychoanalytic therapy and the science of psychoanalytic psychology'" (238).[2] The confusion between these two aspects of the discipline has led to the neglect of the rich literary and hermeneutic tradition in psychoanalysis as it is practiced: "[I]n the always unique and never repeatable meetings between two human beings who call themselves analyst and patient, the ground rules are not those of scientific hypothesis-testing but rather of literary hermeneutics" (Rudnytsky 2002, 229). To paraphrase the remarks of Newell Fischer (2002), President of the American Psychoanalytic Association, psychoanalytic treatment is all too often popularly perceived as being aloof, overly intellectual, and ineffectual. Some of this negative perception can be attributed to the neglect of the ground rules of the hermeneutic tradition. The repression of the literary in psychoanalytic practice has contributed to the decline in interest in the actual experience of psychoanalysis.

A CLINICAL DISCUSSION

As literary critic Shoshana Felman and psychoanalyst Dori Laub claim in their work (1992) on Holocaust narratives, psychoanalysis and literature contaminate and enrich each other inasmuch as they both occur as events of *speech* and *writing*. Truth is begotten in the narrative act, a truth unavailable prior to the therapeutic dialogue. Psychoanalysis and the narrative that it unfolds construct a life testimony, a structure built in the space between analyst and analysand. In the following case material, I show one way in which the therapeutic process may utilize the competencies of literature to help achieve its purpose. By drawing comparisons between a clinical instance of a patient who recovered her memory of a childhood trauma and the narrative trope of a literary character's recovered memory in L. P. Hartley's novel, *The Go-Between* (1953), it becomes apparent how the resonance of a literary text in a clinical setting facilitated both analytic insight into the patient's inner life early in the treatment and helped intensify and inform my own countertransference response to her previously repressed childhood memory. This example dramatizes how a third voice, both hermeneutically and culturally inflected, may intersect and enhance the analytical dyad.

MRS. F.

When she first came to see me, Mrs. F. was fifty-nine years old and working in a health care field. She had been suffering from a chronic, life-long depression. She described herself as never having been happy; even in her childhood she contemplated throwing herself before cars and longed for death. As she portrayed herself to me in the first phases of the treatment, there was never any place to go back to psychologically; there was no nostalgia, no moments of joy. The psychiatrist who referred Mrs. F. to me for psychoanalysis had despaired of her ever getting better. After one year of trying various medications, he suggested to her that, as she seemed to want to talk with him about both her own childhood and her many regrets as a mother, she might want to try psychoanalysis as a last resort. I felt that this referral was a way of dispensing with Mrs. F. but also a test: Could I make any difference in this woman's life?

It is worth noting that Mrs. F. had in fact never reported any effect one way or another from medications for her depression. She had been on various medications for diabetes, hypothyroid condition, and high blood pressure. She had a lifetime of suicidal ideation but had only made one serious attempt in her twenties, which was followed by two weeks in the hospital. She remembered this time as being mixed: on the one hand, she enjoyed the time to rest and be away from family pressure; on the other, she felt that the psychiatrist whom she met with while in the hospital was worse off than she was. He seemed indifferent to her suffering; she recalled him routinely taking telephone calls during their sessions. My own fantasy was that, whatever this man's faults may have been, some of his readiness to interrupt the sessions may have reflected a need to erect barriers against Mrs. F.'s presence in the consulting room; my experience of Mrs. F. was that there was something about her that was draining and even deadening. I often fought the pull to doze off while she spoke. Her experience with the hospital therapist served the function of turning her off therapy for good: she received no treatment for her depression for some thirty-five years until she went to Dr. H., who then referred her to me. Mrs. F. knew full well that I am not an MD but rather a PhD in literature who is also a psychoanalyst. She was impressed that I have all of this learning while she enjoyed, it seemed to me, instructing me in medical matters. My relative ignorance of the technical details of her conditions gave her control over how her symptoms were understood between us.

Mrs. F.'s background was replete with trauma. It is this aspect of her case that I will highlight in the following discussion to illustrate the use of a literary text in my understanding of Mrs. F.'s suffering. Mrs. F. had been married to another health care worker for some forty years and had three grown children. When she met her future husband he was a lonely soldier who told her about his molestation by a priest and his own suicide attempt the preceding year while in the navy. She became pregnant with their first son while out of wedlock; however, she maintained that the real reason she married her husband was because she was afraid that if she did not respond to his importunity in courting her, he would repeat his suicide attempt. Much of their relationship over the years had been spent in keeping her depression at bay. She regarded her children as disappointments in various ways and often wished she had never had children and transmitted so much of her suffering to them.

Her contact with Dr. H. was the result of her despair over the hospitalization of her then-teenage son, who had been made a ward of the state after allegedly being involved in a satanic cult.

Mrs. F.'s own mother, the offspring of a rape, was raised by her (the mother's) grandparents, who blamed her for their daughter's death in childbirth. Mrs. F. was the last of six children and was told by her mother that she and her father had very seriously considered aborting her early in the mother's difficult pregnancy. Mrs. F. took this information as confirmation of her unwanted, unloved, and unworthy life. She had always despised her femininity and internalized her mother's attitude that childbearing is a curse. Affectively, she described herself as feeling enraged, numb, or dead. She longed for death as a kind of quietude, a cessation of suffering, consciousness, and choice. The history was not promising, and the prognosis perhaps even less so. Nevertheless, after having worked with this woman in psychotherapy for about a year, I felt that there was something in her determination to seek treatment and in her early attachment to and idealization of me in the transference which convinced me that an analysis might well help her come to grips with her own painful history and perhaps shape a more promising future for her and her family. This was what I could offer her, that she might have a chance to tell her story to someone who would listen to her and help her come to listen, with increased insight, to herself. And I still think now that that was enough.

One of my major challenges with this woman was to enable her to recognize that her traumatized history, the details of which she initially recounted with a kind of rote recitation, might meaningfully bear on her current suffering. Mrs. F. repeatedly resisted actively remembering or reconstructing any sort of sequence in her life. She had, for instance, moved very often (every year or two for the past thirty-five years), and before that at least half a dozen times with her parents. As if in response to this uprooted existence, she claimed that she could not remember much of her recent past any more than she could her childhood. While certain events stuck out in her mind, any attempt I would make to place them in a chronological sequence or in a geographical context was met with the complaint that I always asked her to remember things she could not put together. This incapacity to remember the facts of time and place—how old she was at any given time in her memories; where she was living—made piecing together a history nearly impossible at first and had the impact of thrusting our work into an intense contemporaneousness. It seemed to me as though Mrs. F. was enacting in her "not knowing" a truth about her life, which she wanted me to feel: that she had never really lived. All of my questions were really beside the point. Similarly, her account of her daily life at work, with her husband and children and grandchildren, had a deadpan, vacant quality to it. Her account of her life outside the analysis was "just the facts."

While the narrative of her life outside of the analysis was emptied of memory and meaning, Mrs. F.'s narrative of her dream life was, comparatively speaking, a flood. Her dreams, which she would frequently write down and then read to me, so as not to forget the details, were Byzantine. They were filled with what I would call "plot" complications—grotesque, vivid, and often violent imagery; diverse characterizations of her family, neighbors, and childhood friends; film stars and politicians. I was struck by the length and complexity of these dreams, which often would portray primitive and frightening scenes of murder, literal floods of feces, insects, maggots, and the like. I often felt as though I was witness to an uncensored Hieronymus Bosch–like world of raw humanity with none of the mediation of the artist's humanism. Mrs. F. would faithfully bring these productions to the hours we shared, recount them in scrupulous detail, and then after her rendition—which was never at all dramatic in the delivery but rather rote, as was her manner—wait for a response. It was as if the dream had been for her a thing that bore no particular relation to herself as she was lying there on the analytic couch. The dreams had the quality of stories. They were experienced, as she put it, as if they were movies, events that she saw, that happened to her, but were cut off from her own life, which was so abject, so dead. The work of interpretation therefore was mine because for her to provide associations to the dreams would have meant that she bore some relation to this bewildering, exciting, and libidinal material. I often felt as though I was drowning in the waves of these dreams.

In tandem with the expression of her flood of dream material, Mrs. F. began to discuss and actively experience in the analysis painful and unpredictable bouts with diarrhea. When I began to make inquiries into this condition, she described suffering from this explosive malady since childhood, when, to recall one event, she soiled herself in church and was forced to change into an uncle's clothes as his house was nearby. She remembered that the men's clothes were too big, and how humiliating this was for her. This pattern of interrupting outings and family activities with her self-soiling persisted into adulthood: she often had to rush home in the middle of shopping, movies, or hikes, and would end up in a gas station or McDonald's when she did not make it in time. She would make do with wet clothes or makeshift outfits pieced together in the car. Her diarrhea often interrupted the sessions. It was as if her body, like her mind, could not contain itself within its enclosure. She was a "mess" and continually fearful of messing up my couch.

Beneath this fear, however, was a thinly veiled wish to do just that. This wish came to an odd and to me infuriating climax in a series of sessions in which she announced to me that she had been diagnosed with scabies and had been infected, though untreated, for months. I was forced to clean the couch and other furniture in the office as well as to warn other patients of the possibility of infection. The breakthrough quality of Mrs. F.'s scabies incident helped us both to confront the pressure of her passive aggression toward me and everyone else whom she "touched." She was forced by this incident, and by the indignation it stirred up in me, to appreciate how her self-neglect in letting the scabies go untreated had had the effect of "contaminating" everyone she came into contact with. This "crisis" of soiling brought very close to the surface her passive expression of "jubilatory anality," as Julia Kristeva (1987, 15) has phrased the depressive patient's merger with her own waste. The anal preoccupation in these episodes suggested to me an archaic fusion not with me as a significant object so much as a fusion with disintegration itself. Kristeva has pointed out how for some depressives anality does not signal separation but rather an archaic fusion with waste as with death itself.[3]

In our work together we came to connect the explosive and riveting quality of these episodes of both diarrhea and scabies contamination with her dream productions. This metaphor of the mind and body began to take shape for us both when it became clear that, in her transference to me, my job was to do the work of interpreting Mrs. F.'s dreams; the dreams functioned between us like the diarrhea—impressive, overwhelming, excessive, and needing attention. Above all, I was to be the one to clean things up in these dreams. The challenge, then, was to help Mrs. F. recognize that the dreams were *her* productions. Our work together clustered around the construction of a narrative of her life through which we might integrate this unconscious material into a more contained and conscious expression of her daily existence. It sometimes seemed to me that Thanatos and Eros were at war within the analytic hour. Mrs. F. had developed in her daily life a "false self" that complied with the demands of the world and marched through the motions: in this life Mrs. F. felt no connection to time or place and reported only longing for death. My gamble in the analysis was that Mrs. F.'s dreams were at once an assault upon me and the analysis and yet were the only signs of life we had to work with. It often felt that she meant me to be as overwhelmed by this rehearsal as she was, but that she also expected me to interpret, to sift through her productions, looking for meaning. But perhaps most of all I was to come to understand that these dreams were the places where she felt alive; they seemed at times to take the place of memory.

TRAUMA AND RECOGNITION

Mrs. F. described to me a dream that both alarmed and intrigued me for its raw and uncensored description of aggression toward her mother. Images and themes emerged that came to dominate the visceral preoccupations of the analysis. I will only provide the outline of the dream and its highlights; the actual narrative was more extensive.

> I am standing in the kitchen cutting up a chicken with a butcher knife. The kitchen is from the house on X. St. where Mom actually had a yard and a

clothesline to hang up clothes. It was the only time I recall that we had a yard. The kitchen is larger than the one we really had and has a door, which opens up to a stairway going out of the house, into the yard. I am severing the bones of the chicken, and it turns into a bunch of small kittens which I can hold in my hand. Then I am no longer cutting but changing the diapers on a baby who looks like Billy [her grandson], who then somehow turns into a worm as I am holding his legs. There is a pounding on the door as if some-one wants to get in and I can't seem to finish what I am doing in time to open the door. The room becomes filled with dirt and maggots; I feel like I am swimming in filth and maggots and I can't get out or answer the door. My mother pushes her way into the room and I begin stabbing her and cut-ting her apart, like the chicken. The blood is everywhere and I can't even see. She is dead and I am drowning in all of this shit and blood.

Mrs. F. brought this dream with tears and distress. After some moments of tearful silence, I asked what this dream might be telling us about what she was going through; she replied that she had no idea what any of this "mess" meant. She could not stand looking at all of this or thinking about it. I had to help her get over these dreams. When I asked her what in particular she found most difficult, she said that the worst of it was that she felt bad telling me about this now, but that in the dream she only felt numb, as if she did not care about any of it at all. She too was dead and drowning. Mrs. F. was horri-fied at the images she had divulged in this dream and wanted me to know that she could not stand to go to sleep anymore with such horrible dreams waking her up to feel more tired and depressed than when she went to sleep.

How could I help her? At this point in the treatment, again, my approach to Mrs. F.'s flood of dream narrative was to talk about her wish and her fantasy that I would take these dreams from her and make sense of them for her. At the time she brought this dream, her ability to associate to it was minimal. Most of the work we did together was around how she felt telling me all of these wretched things that filled her sleep. I did not try to interpret the dream's various instinctual and flooding feelings and images, but rather kept with the feeling of the flood itself: the mess she had made of herself. She asked me tearfully what I thought was making her have these terrible dreams that haunted her life. She felt especially bad that I had to see all of this; she worried that I would find her too disgusting. I added that I thought she was also afraid that I would not be able to tolerate all the frightening and violent things that she was bringing for us both to look at. I wondered aloud with her if she felt as though I too would drown in the "shit" that she was filling the sessions with in these dreams. Here Mrs. F. did make an important association to an early concrete memory, the place if not the time of which she was able to recall. This was one of the first memories Mrs. F. was able to recount and that emerged, as it were, from the imagistic context of her dream narrative.

Mrs. F. picked up on the sensation of drowning, which this dream had captured, to recall an incident she remembered from a childhood visit to an aunt's house in the country. Aunt Marge, as she called her, was much feared and hated by Mrs. F. and her brother (who was two years older than she was). The young Mrs. F. was visiting this aunt over the summer holidays as a kind of last resort, really a booby prize in the distribution of vacation time among the children in the family. Her older sister (whom she was sure her mother favored in every way over her) always had had the enviable privilege of visiting a favorite paternal aunt in the summers and invariably came back with tales of all of the fun she had enjoyed. Mrs. F., meanwhile, was normally stuck at home. This summer, however, in response to Mrs. F.'s coaxing, her mother agreed to send her away, but not to the "good" aunt's house. She was stuck going to stay with Aunt Marge who was notorious for, among other things, keeping her cats locked in the outhouse. The memory of this summer, which Mrs. F. recalled with guilt, shame, and horror, was of being forced by Aunt Marge to take the kittens, which had recently been born to one of the outhouse cats, and to drown them in a bucket of water. Mrs. F. could not recall how old she was at the time but could only remember doing as she was told while her aunt watched and egged her on. It seemed to take forever for her to hold them down, and she cried hysterically as she was forced to do this. She saw their shit in the water. And she seemed to recall that she was given one to take home following this agony, but could only see herself sitting numb in the back seat of the car while her uncle, silently, drove her back to her home at the end of the week. She had no memory of whatever happened to the kitten she brought home.

I felt as struck by the horror of the event as by her telling me of it. I remarked to Mrs. F. that I believed this was one of the first sustained, narrated memories she had ever brought me. She said she was not sure if she had forgotten this incident or simply had not wanted to remember it. But one thing was for sure: she had never told anyone, for she could not bear for anyone to know what she had done. I pointed out that her aunt's sadism seemed psychotic, and Mrs. F. admitted to never really thinking about any of this before.

DISCUSSION: THE GO-BETWEEN

This particular moment in the work with Mrs. F. provides a context for an examination of how my own literary association enabled my affective response to this patient in a treatment context and illuminated my understanding of her affective deadness. I began to think of the brilliant Joseph Losey/Harold Pinter film adaptation (1971) of L. P. Hartley's novel *The Go-Between* (1953), which I had seen years ago; I reread the book to locate and revive the resonance with my impressions of Mrs. F.[4] I recalled, as I listened to Mrs. F.'s constrained and inhibited account of her daily life, the narrative voice of Hartley's Leo (in advanced middle age when we first meet him) introducing the story of his deeply traumatized early adolescence and subsequent constricted, eviscerated, and sexless adult life: "The past is a foreign country," Hartley famously writes in the opening line of the novel, "they do things differently there" (1953, 5). Hartley's evocation of the "sixty-odd" year-old Leo's alienation from his traumatic past, a past that is, like the victims of Felman's and Laub's testimonies, not verbalized and thus foreign and not fully known, would, I felt, teach me something about Mrs. F.'s affective deadness. The narrative voice of the middle-aged Leo, whose boyhood trauma had left him resolved that "the life of facts proved no bad substitute for the facts of life" (247), captured the paradoxical presentation of my patient whose teeming libido emerged only in dream narratives from behind the screen of facts that otherwise filled our sessions.

This discovery was to become enormously helpful to me in my own work with this woman as I reflected upon trauma and the repression of both sexuality and aggression in the context of Leo's narrative of his youthful confrontation with a violent, primal scene encounter. In the novel, Leo's encounter propels him into a nervous breakdown, a disavowal of the "facts" of life, and perhaps most of all into a complete repression of the sexual fantasies that had led him in the first place into being a "go-between" for the illicit love affair between the aristocratic Marian and her earthy, agrarian lover, Ted. Young Leo's primal scene encounter is forced upon him by a traumatizing parental imago, Marian's redoubtable mother, Mrs. Maudsley, who blames him for his part in the illicit coupling of the young woman he has been serving. Leo's own "Aunt Marge" figure, Mrs. Maudsley drags him across the fields to the outhouse nearby where the lovers, whose trysts he had arranged, are in the midst of flagrant and desperate intercourse. The scene is riveting:

> I cried, "Not this way, Mrs. Maudsley." But she paid no heed to me and plunged blindly on, until we came to the outhouse where the deadly night-shade had been. . . . I could not bear to aid her in her search, and shrank back, crying. "No, you *shall* come," she said, and seized my hand, and it was then we saw them, together on the ground, . . . two bodies moving like one. I think I was more mystified than horrified; it was Mrs. Maudsley's repeated screams that frightened me, and a shadow on the wall that opened and closed like an umbrella.
>
> I remember very little more, but somehow it got through to me . . . that Ted Burgess [the lover] had gone home and shot himself. (Hartley 1953, 244)

Critical to this scene is Leo's recognition that the horror of the encounter is not, as some critics have mistakenly implied (Blum 1995, 99), so much the "primal scene" of witnessing intercourse itself as it is in Mrs. Maudsley's "screams" and the "shadow . . . that opened and closed like an umbrella." Forced into a brutal confrontation with her hysteria, Leo displaces

his own fantasies of the poisonous nightshade plant, which figures promi-
nently in his exploits, onto the mysterious "shadow." Like Lear's yawning
hell, this sexual bloom opens and shuts "like an umbrella." The whole scene
creates in Leo "a loathing for the very idea of [human] coupling" (Tóibín
2002, vii). This theme of sexual repression is constant in Hartley's fiction; in
his first major work, *Simonetta Perkins* (1925), a young woman confronts even
the thought of sexual fulfillment with "a wall of darkness, thought-proof and
rigid like a fire-curtain, [rattling] down upon her consciousness. She was cut
off from herself; a kind of fizzing, a ghastly mental effervescence, started in
her head" (qtd. in Tóibín 2002, vii). So too Leo emerges from saturation in
adult sexuality and hysteria, incapable of feeling at all: "A foreigner in the
world of the emotions, ignorant of their language but compelled to listen to
it" (Hartley 1953, 261). "The past is a foreign country"; Leo's past is the place
of emotion and a place from which he is forever cut off.

Now, I believe my turn to Hartley and the literary realm both prepared
me for and protected me from my subsequent work with Mrs. F., who, like Leo,
was confronting memory and the foreign language of emotions that emerged
from that memory. The murderous fantasies replete in the dreams of Mrs. F.,
including her knowledge of the plan for her own "murder" as an unborn child,
were in various ways projected and displaced upon her memory of her "murder" of the kittens: like the kittens she had been unwanted and slated for
extinction. She had visited upon these kittens, barely able to resist and yet surprisingly vigorous, the drowning death she now relived in her dreams with all
their images of flooding. And in the kittens' feeble rebellion against her plung-
ing them to extinction, she was able to trace how, in the dream, which pre-
cipitated this memory, her rage became redirected at her mother whom she
meets with a bloody revenge and joins in an appalling mayhem. Our subsequent work in the analysis revealed how the objects of her rage were as multiple as the dreams themselves and how the images populating those dreams
were as overdetermined as her bodily symptoms. But the point I am making
here is that Mrs. F.'s capacity to connect those dreams with a very real and
traumatic memory signaled for her, as for Leo, a testimony, a witness to an
event the trauma of which, while only one thread in a tapestry of tragic and
repeated insults and agonies, provided us with the start of her story.

What Hartley evokes in this intense novel of sexuality and memory—a
novel in which, as Colm Tóibín puts it, Hartley "was writing to save his life"
(2002, v)—is familiar as a psychological response to trauma. The impact of
trauma is not fully registered at the moment of its occurrence but is, rather,
dissociated, met with a distancing of the self from the overwhelming event
and even with a denial or a forgetting. Having no categories with which to
register the overwhelming experience, memory does not serve: the past
becomes another country. What brings back the past, as Hartley so powerfully
dramatizes in the remembering of the sixty-year-old Leo as he rereads his boy-

hood diary, is the telling. In the telling the experience becomes real, and perhaps one saves one's life. "I . . . felt the sides of the lock relax and draw apart; and at the same moment, as if by some sympathetic loosening in my mind, the secret of the diary flashed upon me" (Hartley 1953, 6). As Cathy Caruth has recognized, in trauma "the greatest confrontation with reality may also occur as an absolute numbing to it," and "immediacy, paradoxically enough, may take the form of belatedness. . . . [T]he impact of the traumatic event lies precisely in its belatedness, in its refusal to be simply located, in its insistent appearance outside the boundaries of any single place or time" (1995, 6–9).

Hartley's Leo engages the reader as witness to his discovery of his boyhood diary, a testimony to the gauzy, sensuous summer of his youth that comes suddenly to an end with the discovery of raw adult sexuality, the violent storm of maternal rage, and the shock of Ted's suicide. Some knowledge cannot be borne without a witness. It is only with the discovery of his diary—a record that ends as suddenly as his summer, his youth, and any hope of a "normal" life—that Leo can remember himself as a boy and document for the reader the new record of recovered memory. It seemed to me then, in comparison, that what Mrs. F. was asking of me in her renditions of her overwhelming and impossibly intricate dreams was to experience the flood of knowledge that could not be contained, controlled, or interpreted in daily discourse. The analysis was reviving this knowledge by providing her with a witness to her history of trauma. Within these dreams were contained the disjointed fragments of her life. From them we were, over the years, able to construct not exactly a chronology but more like a tapestry of her history filled with repeated experiences any one of which might be expected to overwhelm normal development.

One thread in this tapestry, in particular, her first sustained childhood memory recounted in the analysis, seemed virtually to be borrowed from Hartley's chronicle and drew me deeper into the novel and into her memory as both witness and, eventually, in the transference, perpetrator. I was the figure of Aunt Marge forcing her to confront her "shit" in her dreams. Like the revenant of Leo's boyhood diary, I was the occasion of Mrs. F.'s remembering and the instigator of her reviving the narrative of her life. But I was also the reincarnation of her childhood self who was forced to endure and to carry the blame for traumatic encounters. In an aggressive identification, she was like her aunt, making me do the dirty work, both flooding me with her "shit" and making me clean it up with my interpretations and my attempt to contain its onslaught.

In the intervening years of our work together we wondered over the scene of the drowning kittens and thought about its many meanings both as a recovered, or at least revived, memory and as a shared encounter between ourselves. It frequently came up in the analysis after we had been talking about Mrs. F.'s masochistic sense that she both deserved to be punished and did not deserve the joys of life. "What have I done that makes me so dirty and worthless?" Other memories and desires erupted rather like the eels of the Fool's fishwife in *King Lear* who mutters "Down wantons" (II.iv.122–23) as they writhe out of her boiling pot. Lear recognizes in this metaphor of suppression the wantonness of his irrepressible hysteria; so too, Mrs. F. came to recognize in her recurrent memory of the struggling kittens a metaphoric locus for her sadistic and masochistic character. The memory became emblematic of her life's struggle: on the one side, she wondered why she complied with her aunt's demand and feared for her own safety—signs of animal suffering were everywhere. On the other side, she came to identify her excitement in the kittens' struggle and her haunting memory of the tenacity of their fight for life. She came to acknowledge in this scene and the related fantasies it evoked that she was still stirred by her aunt's brutality, and she realized why this memory erupted following the dream of her mother's murder. The intractability of her masochism was linked to her deep desire that her mother, who blatantly told her of her foiled plan to abort Mrs. F., should die herself. Her aunt's brutality evoked, at a deeper level, a traitor within the gates: her sense of herself as murderer. The death instinct of "the unwelcome child" was consonant with Mrs. F.'s lifelong wish for death. As Sándor Ferenczi observes, "children who are received in a harsh and unloving way die easily and willingly. . . . [T]hey retain a streak of pessimism and an aversion to life" (1929, 105). Whether Mrs. F. would in fact die any more "easily" than her unfortunate kittens is in the end beside the point: what is powerfully called up by Ferenczi's discussion is the traumatic fate of the unwanted child whose life is rife with the erotics of suffering and death from the outset.

Hartley's Leo is not an unwanted child: we are to believe that his mother dotes upon him, especially after the death of his father. But we might hazard that his extreme reaction to the primal scene—in which, as Hartley observes in a later introduction to the novel, he turns "into a misanthrope . . . cut . . . off from human fellowship" (1962, 13)—is overdetermined. Ted's suicide, an oedipal victory of sorts for Leo the "vanquisher" (1953, 246), whose own father had suddenly died the previous year, is an intolerable, terrifying triumph. In Leo's own words, "Ted hadn't told me what it [spooning] was, but he had shown me, he had paid with his life for showing me, and after that I never felt like it" (247). Mrs. Maudsley's displaced rage at Leo contributes to his utter dissociation—her "screams . . . were the last sounds heard by my conscious ear" (245). He represses his memory of the scene and retreats into an automaton-like existence for the rest of his life, until, that is, he finds his diary and begins within this narrative to write again. This is not, as Virginia Blum has argued, a regression to "latency" (1995, 97). Latency is not a time of numbness or dead factuality. The adult Leo's flight from sexuality is his post-traumatic retreat from feelings of all sorts.[5] He makes quite clear that he retreats from the realm of the senses. He lives a dissociated state, far from the "love affair with the world" characteristic of the latency child, far even from those who, neurotically arrested in a latency phase resistance to adult sexuality, may nevertheless draw upon a Peter Pan–like energy in their own worlds. Leo's response to the world is dissociation and a disavowal of the memories and the feelings of that hot summer of his adolescence.

Hartley's evocation of these hot days and the humiliation as well as the excitement of young Leo's drive to know and see the mysteries of "spooning" (Hartley 1953, 247) are framed by his narrative of the adult Leo's reluctant recovery of memory and desire in this text. His Epilogue to the narrative of the "unrelieved disaster" of "the whole episode" depicts the adult Leo's reunion with Marian in which he acts as a "go-between" one last time between her and her alienated grandson, the second-generation offspring of her affair with Ted; in this act and in his "talk" with the two of them, says the narrator, "he re-enters the world of the Feelings" (Hartley 1962, 13).

Hartley has been criticized for his Epilogue and his framing of Leo's narrative of his disastrous summer with the glimpse of his hero's final vanquishing of the traumatic past with a restored and hopeful future, even if in his late middle age. The voice of Leo in the Epilogue is a voice of the narrator who, having put down his pen after having recorded the traumatic summer memory, picks it up again one last time; his rationale is important for what it tells us about the curative effect of narrative: "When I put down my pen I meant to put away my memories with it. They had had days, weeks, months to settle, but in the end they didn't, and that is how I came to write this epilogue" (245). Leo's Epilogue records not his trauma but rather his adult reflections upon it and upon his eventual recovery in his return to Brandham Hall, the locus of his primal scene encounter. Hartley insists on giving Leo a future, secured by his having reentered "the world of the Feelings" through remembering and bearing witness through narrative to the pain of his youth. "Leo's self-rescue," according to Brooke-Davies, is Hartley's "attempt to demonstrate that our moral redemption resides in losing the numbness born of our saturation in suffering" (1997, xxix). This, I believe, is what I offered Mrs. F. in her analysis, the narration and the epilogue of a life's story, saturated in suffering.

I turned to Hartley to help me mediate my own sense of being flooded early in the analysis of this "hopeless" and deadened woman. I did not share my reading of this book with Mrs. F. as I saw no clinical benefit in that, but what I did share was my sense of how her numbed affective life seemed to belie a terrifying inner world, the substance of which was perhaps symbolically contained in her guilty, excited, and brutal memory of being forced to drown a litter of kittens. I mark a watershed moment of the analysis with the recovery of this memory in much the same way that Hartley's narrator marks Leo's "new" beginnings with his discovery of his boyhood diary and the flood of memory that flows therefrom.

EPILOGUE

I conclude this discussion with the description of a dream that Mrs. F. brought to me in the last year of her six-year analysis; this dream captures, I hope, some of the progress of our work together. Like Hartley, "I am not altogether a pessimist" (1962, 13), and I want to convey to my readers a sense of the progress in this treatment in which Mrs. F. enlisted me as a witness and even as a guide in her dream life. She became more equipped to interpret for herself her dreams along with her days, and her memories of both.

Mrs. F. had told me about a cat she had seen outside her apartment window that was caught in a tree. She and her husband and son had been worried about this cat because of the freezing weather. They had tried unsuccessfully to coax it down. Mrs. F. put out food for the cat overnight and was relieved when she saw the next morning that it was out of the tree. Unfortunately, as I heard the following week, the cat ended up back in the tree. Mrs. F. reported this to me in some distress and could not understand why the cat went back up in the tree again, especially in such weather. In the next session Mrs. F. reported the following dream:

> I am in the car with my own cat, Sam, and I drive around to the garage where I see the stray cat stuck in the tree. I safely stow my own cat in the apartment and try to bat something else down from the tree. I am not sure what it is, but I cannot do it. As I am reaching into the tree, I see that the cat is frozen—rigid and dead at the top of the tree. Next to it is a bloody squirrel. Along comes my husband and the dead cat falls on his head: he asks me to knock it off him. I refuse. I do not want to touch it. He is forced to pull it off on his own. In the meantime, I see a cougar come around the corner. It is not exactly threatening but not exactly friendly either. At some level, in the dream, I blame the cougar for the bloody squirrel, but I think that this is just its nature. I am drawn to this massive and beautiful cougar.

Mrs. F. recounted this dream to me, which she had first written down—as was her custom. She said she felt this was an important dream because it connected to her feelings about her analysis with me, and her life in general. She was like this cat in the tree: at first she had her hopes up that she was really better, that the analysis had taken away her rage and her deadness, but then, like the cat, she was back up in the tree: frozen and dead, unable or unwilling to come down. She had seen herself chased back up the tree by her failures of her life, which she could not change, and her despair over her children and her grandchildren. But she also had another feeling about the dream; and that was that she was not just the dead cat. She could be like that cougar: fierce and friendly. Displaying this aggressive side of herself at the hospital where she worked, she had been leading a campaign to get the shifts that she and colleagues worked reduced and more equitably distributed. Mrs.

F. was very pleased with her associations to this dream and felt a kind of relief that her thoughts about it seemed to have such resonance with what she was feeling as she and her husband were preparing to retire. They were both so overwhelmed by what appeared to be the inevitability of adopting the young grandson, Bill (who had appeared in the earlier dream as the worm), who was now older and in foster care.

I agreed with Mrs. F. that she seemed to be using this dream to understand the real dilemmas in her life; and I pressed her for more associations to other elements in the dream such as the bloody squirrel, the safe stowing of her own cat, and the image of the cougar. I felt curious and at the same time anxious about the "signs of life" in this dream. I wanted her to see everything I saw in this dream and to be able to take this analytic "tool" with her when she left. She was now less of a foreigner in her land of emotions and was thus able to react quite immediately to my series of questions with a kind of mock hurt and indignation, as if what she had done was not enough and that I was implying that I wanted her to do more. This really was right, and I told her so.

> *Patient:* Here I thought I had done so much, and now you bring up all of these other questions.
>
> *Analyst:* Questions which are hard to look at. It may be, as you say, that I have gotten carried away with my questions and all they might suggest about where you are in your life now. I think you feel that I am not giving you enough credit for what you have seen or that I am not looking at that carefully enough in my eagerness to do more, to see it all.

Here we reflected on my wish, which I had already expressed, that she could do "more" analysis and not retire so early and leave the area.

> *Patient:* But I want to talk about the cougar. I really want to tell you where I think that comes from.

Mrs. F. explained that one of her favorite mystery series is about a young woman, an American Indian who works as a Park Ranger who is always solving mysteries in the West. She recently read a book in which this ranger saved a population of wild cougars from environmental hazards caused by certain unethical developers who were indifferent to their habitat. She thought that this is where she got the idea of the wild cougars. I remarked, "In your dream you are somehow hovering between being the clueless cat who hopelessly returns to the tree top and finally falls from it, frozen and dead, and this other cat, the wild cougar who is able to be both fierce and friendly and who is given the chance to live, rescued really, by the good offices of a conscientious Park Ranger." At this we both smiled as we recognized together whom this Park Ranger might represent. And this is the note that she wanted to stress above all things: that I was like this Park Ranger to her. I had helped her recognize that behind the dead cats of her "factuality" there lingered the prospect of memory "long hidden" from view (Hartley 1953, 261)—fiercely energetic, blindingly destructive, but capable of power and even beauty.

NOTES

1. As Roy Schafer (1997) remarks of the connection between narrative and Freud's case histories: "Self-consciously, Freud had declared early that he drew back from writing only stories. I would say that he did so once he recognized that, inevitably, case histories . . . are narratives. That is to say, they are *tellings* of human events, not measurements or simple records of process and materials in the physical universe" (338).

2. This passage from Bowlby is taken from his "Psychoanalysis as Art and Science" (1979).

3. In my thinking about the intractability of Mrs. F.'s depression, I have found useful Kristeva's (1987) depiction of "another form of depression" from the classically neurotic, that is, a "narcissistic" depression that distinguishes itself as being more primitive. Her description of this state clarifies the cherishing of sadness itself as a libidinally charged object: the substitution of depressed affect for the object itself. These depressives believe themselves afflicted with "a congenital deficiency" and find that "sadness is really the sole object; more precisely it is a substitute object they become attached to, an object they tame and cherish for lack of another" (12).

4. L. P. Hartley (1895–1972) was described by Lord David Cecil as "one of the most distinguished of modern novelists; and one of the most original." He is quoted in the current Penguin edition as praising Hartley's "keen and accurate" observations "of human thought and feeling," while noting that Hartley "is also a sharp-eyed chronicler of the social scene." Both aspects of Hartley's gift inform *The Go-Between*, in which a lament for a childhood destroyed by trauma is orchestrated by a longing for a Victorian social order, gone forever. Though beyond the purview of the present chapter, it is worth noting that Leo's personal trauma robs him of his memory and any hope of a fulfilled future corresponding, according to Hartley, to England's own vanquished condition in the modern age.

5. In an observation regarding the social context of Hartley's fiction, Brooke-Davies reinforces this sense of the "post-traumatic" quality of Leo's experience. The breakdown to which Leo refers in his Epilogue is "explained more specifically in the holograph: 'Nervous prostration and loss of memory following shock was the diagnosis of my illness.'" "It recalls," notes Brooke-Davies, "the young Osbert Sitwell's meeting in 1914 with his idol Debussy which left him no recollection of the encounter: 'The intensity of the emotion killed memory'" (Hartley 1953, 291–92). Brooke-Davies further emphasizes the pressing and traumatic realities of the Boer War and World War I that frame *The Go-Between*, equating the "screams" of Mrs. Maudsley and the screams of gun shells: "Shell and scream testify to the same thing: that the world which would follow would never be the same as the one that had been lost" (1997, xxviii).

REFERENCES

Bayard, Pierre. 1999. Is it possible to apply literature to psychoanalysis? Trans. Rachel Bourgeois. *American Imago* 56:207–19.

Blum, Virginia L. 1995. *The child between psychoanalysis and fiction*. Urbana: University of Illinois Press.

Brooke-Davies, Douglass. 1997. Introduction. In Hartley 1953, xi–xxiv.

Caruth, Cathy. 1995. Introduction: Trauma and experience. In *Trauma: Explorations in memory*, ed. Caruth, 3–12. Baltimore: Johns Hopkins University Press.

Felman, Shoshana. 1992. Education and crises, or the vicissitudes of teaching. In Felman and Laub 1992, 1–56.

Felman, Shoshana, and Dori Laub. 1992. *Testimony: Crises of witnessing in literature, psychoanalysis, and history*. New York: Routledge.

Ferenczi, Sándor. 1929. The unwelcome child and his death instinct. In *Final contributions to the problems and methods of psychoanalysis*, ed. Michael Balint, trans. Eric Mosbacher et al., 102–107. London: Karnac, 1980.

Fischer, Newell. 2002. We have a date. *The American Psychoanalyst* 36, no. 3:3–4.

Freud, Sigmund. 1900. *The interpretation of dreams*. In *Standard edition of the complete psychological works*, ed. and trans. James Strackey et al., vols. 4 and 5. London: Hogarth Press, 1953–1974.

———. 1905. *Fragment of an analysis of a case of hysteria*. S.E., 7:7–122.

Hartley, L. P. 1953. *The go-between*. Ed. Douglass Brooke-Davies. London: Penguin, 1997.

———. 1962. Author's introduction to *The go-between*. New York: New York Review Books, 2002, 7–15.

Kristeva, Julia. 1987. *Black sun: Depression and melancholia*. Trans. Leon S. Roudiez. New York: Columbia University Press, 1989.

Masson, Jeffrey M., ed. and trans. 1985. *The complete letters of Sigmund Freud to Wilhelm Fliess, 1887–1902*. Cambridge: Harvard University Press.

Rudnytsky, Peter L. 2002. *Reading psychoanalysis: Freud, Rank, Ferenczi, Groddeck*. Ithaca: Cornell University Press.

Schafer, Roy. 1997. Conversations with Elisabeth von R. In *Storms in her head: Freud and the construction of hysteria*, ed. Muriel Dimen and Adrienne Harris, 323–40. New York: Other Press, 2001.

Tóibín, Colm. 2002. Introduction. *The go-between*. By L. P. Hartley. New York: New York Review Books, 2002, v–xiii.

Wyatt, Frederick. 1989. The uses of literature in the psychoanalytic process. In *Compromise formations: Current directions in psychoanalytic criticism*, ed. Vera J. Camden, 26–43. Kent: Kent State University Press.

SIX

It's Really More Complicated than You Imagine

Narratives of Real and Imagined Trauma

BENNETT SIMON

INTRODUCTION

IT IS BY NOW commonplace that the clinician working with individuals or groups that have been subject to severe trauma may find that the people involved have difficulty telling the story of their trauma, remembering all of what happened, or integrating the story and the import of the trauma into their ongoing lives. The press to tell, whether coming from within or without, is associated with fear of great pain in the telling and retelling. At times, especially outside the clinical setting, the person could be discounted as a confabulator, or a liar, or someone with just a very poor and unreliable memory. This clinical observation, and the distress experienced both by the person trying to tell and by the person eliciting the telling, is the motor driving the present chapter.

I shall attempt to weave a narrative about narrative, trauma, and memory. The threads are strands of my own career and interests, and, undoubtedly, pieces of my internal world, some known to me, others not so clearly known. I am a psychoanalyst and psychiatrist, very much interested in issues of trauma. As a clinician, I did not always know how interested I was in trauma. I am also a student of literature and of ancient cultures, and have written and taught on various aspects of the interpenetration of psychoanalysis and literature. My more explicit interest in trauma was first actualized in my writings

(1988) about tragic drama, where I suggested that tragic drama could be usefully conceptualized as telling stories about the transmission of trauma within families or societies, from one generation to the next. In a way, literature first raised my awareness of life and influenced my clinical concerns. I have also studied how political trauma, especially the trauma of violence and persecution, affects people, both children and adults. Here too, the issue of how trauma is transmitted, how trauma may be transmuted, across the generations is salient in my own thinking and writing. Like many others, I am intensely interested in the controversy that can be labeled "the memory wars"—the polarized battle between "recovered memory specialists" and groups such as the False Memory Foundation.[1] I am drawn to this question not only as a clinician but also as a member of our society, curious as to how and why this issue has become so political and so polarized.

I will, then, be weaving with these different threads, hoping for a more or less pleasing design, but not to produce a "crazy quilt" of my interests. So, I will be addressing: (1) the dynamic interrelationship of trauma and narrative; (2) narratives of trauma within the clinical setting, including the ways a traumatic history is presented and represented in affects, sensory experience, and at times dramatic reenactments; (3) how the memory of trauma differs from less charged autobiographical memory, and how memory accompanied by post-traumatic stress syndrome (PTSD) is still more different; (4) developmental perspectives on how trauma can interfere with the capacity to develop a fluent narrative and meaningful narrative; and (5) considerations about the nature of narrative, especially verbal narrative, and the relation of narrative to veridical truth. The question is not whether or not the narrative tells exactly what happened—by its nature, narrative cannot—but whether and how much historical actuality and what aspects of historical actuality are registered and represented.

By trauma, I mean events that are threatening and overwhelming, that shake the very fabric of your being, that "shatter assumptions," that make the ground beneath you give way. They at once demand to be made meaningful yet also resist understanding. Events such as the birth of a sibling in an ordinary family I categorize as troubling, possibly painful, but more amenable to integration, explanation, and even pleasure.

THE DYNAMIC INTERRELATIONSHIP
OF TRAUMA AND NARRATIVE

Trauma requires and generates narrative. Narrative is a sequence of "begettings"—this happened, which led to that happening, which in turn led to something else happening. In ordinary life, too much that is problematic interferes with, interrupts, limits, aborts, and leads to stillborn narrative. But too little trauma results in flat narrative or the absence of narrative. Ideally, you need "trouble," not trauma, and certainly not overwhelming trauma, to stimulate narrative. Narrative helps make meaning out of puzzling or disturbing events. Events that are too disturbing may overtax the meaning-making capacity of the child. The place, ideally, where "trouble" but not overwhelming trauma takes place is the family. The expectable problems of the child growing up in family life generate stories, and the stories in turn help the child make meaning, make sense of the problems.

The writer Grace Paley once advised a student that the next step in his development as a writer should be to study the Book of Genesis, wherein, she said, all the basic plots can be found. I would qualify her advice by saying, "Begin with chapters two and three—the second account of creation." The first account, Genesis 1–2:4, tells how God created and ordered the world in six days, proclaimed it all as good, man as very good, and rested on the seventh day. It's beautiful, but it's the end of the story. Not too good to be true, but too neat to be interesting and generative. You need a Garden, a man, a lonely man, a God who makes a woman for him, a snake who is deceptive, forbidden fruit, disobedience, discovery, shaming, expelling, intercourse, procreation, brothers, murder—now you have the makings of a story! And notice how replete the early chapters of the Book of Genesis are with "begats"—with generations, and lists interspersed with allusions to trouble. "Generations" and "stories" overlap, intertwine, and one without the other just doesn't work.

What happens when there are events in the life of an individual or group that threaten the end of the existence, the extinction of that person, or group? How do you tell the story of something that might end all stories, destroy all who tell and all to whom the story might be told? Here I refer to my studies (1978; 1988) on the transition in classical Greece from epic poetry to tragedy. Epic poetry represents continuous telling of heroic tales, with virtually no interruption. Characters are in dialogue in their dreams, Achilles is talking with his horses on his way to battle, people cannot go to sleep because they want to hear the story. There is an implicit expectation that there will always be ongoing narrative, ongoing generations to hear the stories, and that a reason to be heroic is to generate stories that will lead to a kind of "narrative immortality." Characters in Homer say, "What we are doing today will be a subject for stories for men in time to come."

Greek tragedy introduces a world in which things might come to an end, certainly within a particular family. The house of Atreus, the house of Oedipus, the house of Medea and Jason can be extinguished. Concomitant with this threat, we see the appearance of interruptions in narrative, specifically silences. Silences signal the presence of the unspeakable or the not-to-be-recalled; interruptions in the dialogue of the play signal a story of interruption in generational continuity, or in the sanctity of intergenerational boundaries within the family. Murder, incest, infanticide, betrayal of marital bonds—these are represented as too terrible to be told, and the telling is skewed, erratic, not linear, and interrupted. Shakespeare introduces other ways of representing deeds that threaten extinction, along with silences— elaborated madness, frenetic humor, and nonsense. These characterize the worlds of *Hamlet* and *King Lear*, where the houses are threatened with extinction by the nefarious deeds of their members.

CLINICAL NARRATIVES OF TRAUMA

I now highlight the nature of the narratives of trauma in the clinical psychotherapeutic and psychoanalytic setting. There is always a tension between telling and not telling. Past trauma shapes the present relationship and the entailed narrative, and the present relationship shapes the narrative of the past. There is "telling" that is primarily in symbolic form, or enacted in the patient-therapist relationship. That which is not symbolizable may be known mainly by the uncanny or despairing affects in the patient or those induced in the therapist or both (see Laub and Auerhahn 1993).

Early in my psychiatry training, a young African American man was admitted to our psychiatric ward with a complete amnesia for personal identity and any personal history. Hypnosis, with a sodium amytal interview, was tried, and information progressively emerged over several hypnotic sessions about his parents, especially his father, who was a Caucasian and a psychiatrist. We soon realized that the description of his father was the description of the psychiatrist doing the hypnosis! Other information eventually led to the verifiable story that he suffered from sickle-cell anemia (a potentially crippling and at times fatal disease that in the United States is mostly found in African Americans), and had been told that he would be dead by age thirty. His amnesia set in a few days before his thirtieth birthday! As the true history emerged through investigation (e.g., tracing him through fingerprints and missing-person bulletins), not hypnosis, the young man became progressively more depressed and suicidal, and it emerged how many other issues in his life were contributing to the onset of an amnesiac state. In this instance, a false narrative arose to encode an otherwise difficult-to-articulate true and complex story. The false narrative probably also encoded a wish to have different parents, and perhaps also a wish to have different parents in order to have different genes, to be free of the burden of the genetic illness.

An intergenerational transmission of trauma and the accompanying interruption of the narrative, transmitted only in unexplained and unconnected images and obsessions, is exemplified by a man in his thirties who came for analysis seeking help with the problem of his incredible silence. He noted that his father was even more silent. He also placed a stringent limit on the length of the analysis, and at various junctures revealed that there were important issues he had with me about which he remained silent. In the course of analysis he mentioned that he had in his head an image that made no sense—an image of a gas pipe or lead pipe. He also mentioned an obsessive thought he had had since his teenage years. Did he or did he not sexually molest an infant girl when he was babysitting for her? (There was no reason to think he actually did do it.) Several years after the end of treatment, he returned to tell me that after the death of his mother and decline of his father from Alzheimer's, he discovered in a drawer newspaper clippings from the father's teenage years. They detail how the father's father—a respectable citizen in a small town—had been accused of sexually molesting young girls, and on the day he was to go to court, he was found hanging in his basement from a gas pipe. We pieced together that the father's extreme silence communicated something unspeakable to the son, my patient, and that perhaps he had some years earlier come across these articles and repressed the memory. The discovery helped further elucidate and reduce his proclivity to silence. We were left with some mystery as to how this transmission had occurred.

A third vignette illustrates reenactment involving both patient and therapist, leading to the recollection and integration of a traumatic event and climate. A thirty-five-year-old woman sought treatment for repeated conflicts and disappointments with her sexual partners, about having children, and her work. One day in the third year of her analysis (perhaps following a brief interruption or a change in our schedule) she was irritable and demanding, and nothing I said or didn't say was right. I sensed, helplessly, her mounting frustration and anger; suddenly she got up, denounced me, and stormed out of the room, slamming the door. I was caught by surprise—nothing like this had ever happened with her—and said to myself, "She'll never come back." In distress, I called a colleague with whom I had previously discussed the case, and she was quite surprised to hear my conviction that the patient would not return. She tactfully reminded me of all the evidence that the patient and I had a good working relationship, and suggested that there was something off-kilter about my feeling. The patient did return, and in the subsequent sessions it emerged that one day when she was about eight years old, she and her sisters huddled behind the couch in the living room as they heard the parents engage in violent, screaming recriminations and threats behind their closed bedroom door. They heard a gunshot, and were of course terrified that one of the parents had killed the other. The door burst open, the father ran out, the mother stood there holding the gun, with plaster coming down from the ceiling. The father left the house, slammed the door, and the little girl had the horrible thought, "He's never coming back!" Actually, he did come back to fight with the mother many more times until they were divorced when the patient was a teenager. Over the next few weeks in analysis what emerged was a much more elaborate history of parental fights, always mutually humiliating, often violent and terrifying to the children. The patient's storming out and my conviction that she would never return were thus part of a reenactment of perhaps the most terrifying of the chronic parental fights, with one or the other parent dis-appearing and leaving the children feeling helpless and fearful with the other parent. This was a memory (actually series of memories) that had not been totally out of awareness—she was not amnesic for the event—but neither had it been in her consciousness for many years. It was simply not "recallable" until something triggered off this strong visceral reaction, a memory that "recruited," as it were, all the bystanders in the terror of death and abandon-ment. I surmised that in our relationship she was afraid to speak of a disagree-ment with me, lest it would lead to an argument with terrible consequences.

My reaction clamored for some self-analysis. I revisited a difficult part of my own childhood history, though not nearly as dramatic or dangerous as this incident in her childhood. But somehow she touched a part of me that was afraid of irreconcilable argument and one or the other parent leaving. Subse-quent to the revelation of this violent scene, I found myself recurrently imag-ing a scene from Frank Conroy's popular novel *Prince of Tides*, which involves a doctor and patient and where the family had kept a tiger as pet! A violent intruder came into the house to rob and rape and possibly kill, and somehow one of the family members managed to let loose the tiger, who mauled the intruder. My fantasizing about this scene from the novel led me to the hypothesis that the patient was not only a victim and helpless onlooker, but possibly also an aggressive tiger, who might maul me, the intruder. Part of her integrating the traumatic scene involved acknowledging her "identification with the aggressor." Over time, she became much more skilled at knowing when she needed to be a bit of "a bull in a china shop" in personal and work relationships, and when quieter and subtler forms of interaction were needed.

Such dramatic reenactments, while not the everyday stuff of analysis and therapy, are not rare either. They are especially liable to happen when some-thing triggers off a traumatic memory, and the affects associated with that memory are activated and somehow enacted. Accordingly, in working ana-lytically with a patient one knows has been traumatized or with a patient where only as treatment proceeds does this awareness dawn, the analyst must be prepared to experience some powerful emotional jolts and onslaughts. One day, one session, the analyst says or does something that seems perfectly ordi-nary and reasonable, whether an act of omission or commission, and the patient explodes. The analyst has stepped into a minefield without knowing it. Such moments are of extreme importance therapeutically and I, along with many others, believe that often only through such an encounter can the analyst begin to comprehend the depth of feeling and pain in the patient's traumatic past.

My fourth and last vignette is of a case where both "true" and "false" memories appear, and where adjunctive therapies other than talking made a major difference. A married woman in her late fifties, the mother of two grown sons, came for psychotherapy, seeking a male therapist, after a number of years of working with a woman therapist, with some success, but still living with serious limitations. She was professionally extremely competent, a very caring person, and had a wide circle of devoted friends. She felt she had made great gains in terms of basic self-esteem, in learning how to deal with a loving but demanding husband, and in coming to terms with the pain of her older son being quite alienated from the two of them. This son was not responding to any efforts from the parents or from his brother to come to even a limited reconciliation.

Her main complaint was that she remained extremely anxious in regard to any and all medical situations, especially if she had to wait for the results of a test for several days or weeks. Each visit to a doctor's office was a severe trial, often leading her to delay getting necessary consultations or tests. She and a psychiatrist friend of hers had concluded that, given her history, she should have some time with a male therapist. The history relevant to that decision was of a physician father who was extremely tyrannical, took exclusive medical care of his family members, and often interfered with or outright forbade any consultation with physicians other than himself or those few of his own choosing that he might allow. He and the patient's mother together demanded no display of weakness, no tears, no complaining, no admitting of pain. He had died about two months before her coming to see me, and the patient and he had had some sort of deathbed reconciliation of their differences.

She later related to me that "my anxiety really grew out of a sense that I was riddled deep inside with a cancer that would be discovered. I feared that I would not be able to maintain my outward appearance of being a 'trooper,' and tears, fear, dependence, lack of courage, inability to keep my life together would ensue. Because my anxiety had no other outlet, it was reflected in my body. Constant medical situations therefore were created and played out."

The patient curiously evinced no particular apprehension about seeing me, a male physician. She felt that this was a purely professional relationship, that I was rather aloof, remote, and unresponsive, probably not caring too much about her. It also gradually emerged that she would not tell me very important things on her mind—whether about a feeling, a memory, a comment about me, or, at times, a painful physical symptom she was having even while in my office (e.g., that she had fallen earlier in the day and severely bruised her leg, which was quite painful and clearly needed medical attention).

In recounting her story to me, she rather matter-of-factly alluded to quite a few incidents of totally outrageous behavior on the part of her father with her, her older brother, and various relatives and friends. These often involved abuse of his position as a doctor to examine and treat her and her body quite inappropriately, as if she were his personal property. I would say to her very clearly that these actions were totally unacceptable, and that it was awful that her mother condoned, and at times encouraged, the father in them. The behaviors included massive parental indifference to, or even joking about, serious childhood physical and emotional symptoms (e.g., severe rocking behavior, even in public). She gradually began to say that she knew I was right, but it was still very hard for her to condemn her father.

We discussed some outrageous fathers and their daughters' relationships with them. Through her reading about the case of Stalin's daughter, and later, reading (at my suggestion) more broadly about trauma, she began to realize the power of her own denial and minimization, her need to defend not only her father but also her mother. These discussions had nothing to do with "recovering" buried memories of trauma, but rather with owning up to the implications of what the father had done.

We came to understand why she could not tell me everything on her mind—sometimes a week or two later she would admit to me that she had not told me something very important going on in the session. In fact, my clarity was a threat to her need to maintain an illusion about her parents. As a result, her defense of dissociation, including during the sessions, gradually emerged into view, and she could see how much she had dissociated all through her growing up with her father. Her anxiety symptoms began to be less severe and crippling, but they remained very disturbing and problematic. I referred her to a female colleague for concomitant EMDR (Eye Movement Desensitization Reprocessing) therapy, which was extremely helpful. Something in that process facilitated a profound and inescapable experience of the affects associated with the memories of the father's behavior. It also included a good deal of discussion, especially of how she withheld from me and how, with the encouragement of this woman therapist, she could develop a sense of a "two-parent family," of a man and a woman as a parental couple with whom she could safely see and acknowledge the truth.

Gradually, even more outrageous stories emerged, including some she had not totally repressed, but had somehow lodged way at the edge of consciousness. These involved much franker sexual invasions by the father in the course of his alleged "medical" examinations. The reproduction of these scenes was accompanied by a good deal of painful affect, at times leading her to a state of near-terror (which was treated with some medication), but resulting eventually in a decided alleviation of her medical anxiety symptoms.

The striking thing was that as she began to acknowledge the awfulness of the way she was treated in growing up, she began to get (or to register) comments from relatives and friends that substantiated a number of her memories and perceptions. She then produced her adolescent diaries and, with great reluctance, shared them with me. In these diaries she recorded a number of events and feelings that she had in fact nearly forgotten. She also expressed her outrage at her father during those years—something that she had given no hint of as an adult. These revelations facilitated the work that the patient was doing both with me and with the EMDR therapist, and led to a clarity about her past and its consequences that was extremely salutary.

The overall outcome was a quite wondrous improvement in her general well-being and relief of the medical anxiety symptoms. As it happened, both she and her husband developed serious cancers. These were fortunately quite treatable, and she managed both their treatments with focus, concern, and appropriate apprehension about the outcome, but no crippling anxiety. To date, she has maintained and built upon these very substantial gains, recognizing that she is still somewhat vulnerable to alarming medical news and having some setbacks, but now equipped with many more tools for coping.

In general, neither I nor the EMDR therapist suggested to her that she had buried memories that had to be retrieved. Rather, it was mostly affective appreciation of what she did remember that was so problematic. She had to uncover and eventually master the pattern of dissociation in both the past and the present. The remembered record of abuse and neglect was quite impressive, even without the scarcely remembered incidents that emerged later in the therapy.[2]

Now, the son who was alienated from her and her husband had been a problematic child since early in his development. He had had therapy as a child and adolescent, and there had been much family therapy around him. He had severed relations with his family and then minimally resumed them several times. As an adult, he entered treatment with a "recovered memory" specialist, and "recovered" memories of being taken by his grandfather, the patient's father, to Satanic worship in the basement of a local house of worship, where there was sexual abuse of children, child sacrifice, and the drinking of blood from skulls. He blamed his mother for not knowing that her father was doing this to him, and further blamed her for refusing to acknowledge that it was true. Until she did so, he would not have contact with her.

Needless to say, this topic occupied a good deal of attention in the course of our work together. The accusations were the standard fare for Satanic cults that investigators (e.g., Ganaway 1989) have argued are inherently quite unlikely, and the format of the accusations had itself become almost ritualized. We both felt that the accusations of the Satanic abuse were most implausible, but we were being hoisted on our own petard! We were accepting her account of the abuse she had suffered, but not accepting her son's account of *his* abuse. The patient and I came to a necessarily tentative conclusion that there was a kernel of truth in the son's allegations. It had to do with the patient's preoccupation with defending her father—and with the father more generally—during the years of the son's development. She was painfully aware, however, that her own capacity to minimize, indeed overlook, terrible things involving her father, and the implausibility of the son's accusations, did not relieve her of the responsibility for not having stood up more to her father, especially when she was a grown woman, wife, and mother. At the time of termination, it was clear that the integration of this sense of responsibility, placing it in perspective, would be an ongoing task.

Coincidentally, over much of the course of our therapeutic work, I was working with colleagues on a psychoanalytic case record from 1912, which we published with commentaries (Lunbeck and Simon 2003). That case involved sexual abuse, incest, and a mixture of plausibly true memories and probably fantasied or hallucinated memories. We saw, as had Freud in the 1890s (see Blass and Simon 1994), that the problem of sorting out true memories from fantasies was enough to drive the clinician *meshuge*.

TRAUMATIC MEMORY DIFFERS FROM OTHER AUTOBIOGRAPHICAL MEMORIES

In the next two sections, I address some research that helps illuminate why the verbal telling of a person's traumatic history is often so problematic, including why the veridical nature of the story can easily be questioned. First, I summarize some research on adult traumatic memory, and then some research on the development of the capacity to narrate in children, and how trauma can interfere with that development.

There is much evidence to suggest that events in the life of a person are encoded in several different channels and circuits of the brain. Thus, we may speak of memories residing in the mind, the soul, and the body. The nature of traumatic memories—their encoding, their recalling, their retelling—and even more the nature of traumatic memories in people who have PTSD (which should, rather, be called "complex traumatic stress syndrome" because the trauma is ongoing and the person is not "post-"), is different from that of less charged autobiographical memories. Memories of trauma are much more prone to be encoded in bodily form—sensations, affects, images—and to be less successfully registered as communicable narratives. Research summarized by Grolier, Yehuda et al. (1997) and Van der Kolk (1997) finds, broadly speaking, that traumatic experiences are initially imprinted as sensations or feeling-states that are not immediately transcribed into personal narratives; and that personal narrative does develop, but later than the sensory-motor-imagistic-affective record. The two levels can therefore coexist, but are more walled off from each other than in ordinary autobiographical memory. Thus, there are memories of trauma that the patient chooses not to tell, but also memories that are not easily accessible in verbal form. Talking therapy may help enormously, but it feels at times like swimming against the tide of bodily "right-brain-encoded" experience.[3] Socially communicable symbolic representation is more difficult with traumatic memories, but particularly during recovery more communication does open up between the verbal and nonverbal representations of the memory.[4]

A further research finding is that flashbacks, which are part of PTSD, are different from memories; they cannot be evoked at will, though they may be readily triggered by any number of stimuli that may not make sense to an outside observer. The flashbacks are not necessarily veridical representations of an event, though they often are, but they may reflect the charged affective states at the moment of assault (e.g., terror, rage, disbelief), augmented by subsequent brain processes in the amygdala nuclei. It appears that more neutral memory retrieval and recall engages different sections of the brain from traumatic memories, especially memories returning as flashbacks (Solms and Turnbull 2002). As a general rule, traumatic memory is more likely to be activated in the right brain, and ordinary episodic memory in the left brain (Lanius, Williamson et al. 2004).

Research on post-traumatic dreams and nightmares suggests that the person may report he has the same nightmare night after night, but careful inquiry often reveals a fair bit of variation, and that it is not always or only a veridical representation of the event (Lansky and Bley 1995). The nightmare may incorporate symbolic representations of overwhelming affective states. A traumatic event that took place on land, for example, might become a nightmare with overwhelming waves and fear of drowning representing the affective state, not necessarily the literal event (Hartmann 1998).

Finally, as with all important memories, different facets of an event may be the starting point (or stimulus) for recall, so that the same event takes on different meanings and emotional aspects in different contexts. Traumatic memories are subject to this kind of variation, which may give the impression of inconsistency and inaccuracy, especially in legal settings.

DEVELOPMENTAL PERSPECTIVES ON NARRATIVE AND TRAUMA

A number of lines of research converge to paint a broad picture that children need narrative to help contain, make meaningful, and come to terms with important events in their lives. But severe trauma, especially in very early childhood, may impair the ability to form coherent and fluent narratives. As Bruner and Lucariello (1989) have shown, during the second year of life the child's narratives represent efforts to express and integrate the earlier seeds of agency, sequencing, intentionality, perspective, and "canonicity"—that is, the way things are supposed to be. Trauma at this stage of development can impair the development of these skills, especially the knowledge of "canonicity"—what's right and wrong, expectable and not expectable in the world.

By three, the child may be capable of rather complex moral judgments and acts of empathy, and have a corresponding ability to put these into verbal and verbal-play narratives. Trauma at this age may interfere with the child's freedom imaginatively to try out different moral scenarios (Buchsbaum and Emde 1990). It may also interfere with the child's growing ability—detectable as early as two years—to spin out an imaginary world and a real world and to know the difference between them. This leads to constrictions in storytelling and play (Emde et al. 1997). In other words, trauma interferes with development of the capacity to symbolize (Cicchetti and Beeghly 1987). Later, threats around specific or repeated episodes of abuse that the child "better not tell anyone," especially if accompanied by violent threats, may lead to significant amnesias and related varieties of difficulties in recalling and telling (Briere and Conte 1993). From recent research on attachment, we have learned how extensively negative internal representations of difficult childhood attachment-separation issues with the parent (mostly the mother) are associated in adulthood with problems in fluency and coherence of narrative (Lyons-Ruth and Jacobovitz 1999; Fonagy et al. 2002; Waldinger et al. 2001). In some of the research there is reliable prospective or retrospective information on the problematic nature of the earlier attachment patterns. In broad sweep, one can say that "bad internal objects" make for bad narrative, not just in terms of content, but of form.

The narratives of a traumatic event by somewhat older children may contain significant defensive distortions to deal with the helplessness and impotency of their plight. A now-classic study by Pynoos and Nadir (1997) of a schoolyard shooting reveals how important are distortions that involve "intervention fantasies"—what the child might have done or wished he or she could have done. Also involved are spatial relocation fantasies. Children closer to the represented shooting tend to place themselves farther away, while those farther away tend to place themselves closer (as part of their "intervention" fantasies).

At the same time, the children in this study had a very accurate "motor" memory of exactly where they were if someone walked the grounds with them. Thus, memories of a trauma are encoded in several different channels that may be differentially tapped to produce an account of the event.

Young children's narratives are indeed susceptible to influence and shaping by adults or other children or both. While this potential "co-construction" is utilized by some primarily to insist on the unreliability and suggestibility of children's memory, it is also the pathway for helpful adult interventions that can mitigate effects of a trauma. There are ways of enhancing the memories of school-age children for traumatic events without "leading the witness" and suggesting what "must have been."

Most early memories are clearly "interpretations" of what happened, as signified by the fact that they are typically recalled as containing the rememberer. That is, our early memories resemble looking at photos of the scene. Research (Schacter 1996) shows how memories are altered in the course of development and affected by the adult situation in which they are being elicited. Interpretation enters again in terms of "memory markers"—that is, which aspect of the story the child begins with or attends to at a particular time. This is important to understand, as shifts related to "markers" can give the (misleading) impression of great inconsistency in the story. The child may need to tell about the blood, leading to one narrative sequence, or about the reactions of other children, leading to a different narrative sequence.

CONSIDERATIONS ON
NARRATIVE AND VERIDICAL TRUTH

The extremes of the "memory wars," in which "recovered memory therapists" battle the False Memory Foundation, leave most of us in a middle position. Numerous publications (and Web sites) have taken a partisan stand on accusations of sexual abuse, especially when adult children bring charges against their parents about events that allegedly took place years before.[5] The most convincing review and deepest analysis of this controversy that I have found is Janice Haaken's *Pillar of Salt: Gender, Memory, and the Perils of Looking Back* (1998). Haaken brings together a clinical psychoanalytic perspective, a feminist perspective, and a detailed sociohistorical exploration of issues such as narratives of Satanic Ritual Abuse, multiple personality, and the founding of the False Memory Syndrome Foundation.[6]

Given the complexities of memory and narrative revealed by the clinical situation and more systematic research on adults and children, it is not surprising that there is often great confusion around "true" and "false" traumatic events. Absent external verification, there is no consistently reliable method of "recovering" memories of trauma. Relatively well documented (Haaken 1998, ch. 6, 291n40, 291n68, 293) is how much various methods such as hypnosis, police interviewing of young children, and the techniques employed by "recovered memory" therapists can influence the process of recollection. Problems of ascertaining truth or falsehood of abuse memories can be very complex, and at times insurmountable. Did the school principal fondle you, at age seven, in his office? Sometimes there are indirect means of verification. Everyone knew the principal was an alcoholic, he was seen stumbling in public places after school, he always had problems with the school board, but no one did anything about it because he was well connected.

Sometimes verification is not sought until a certain threshold of salience has been crossed by the person, such as becoming a parent. "Now that I am experiencing frustration with my young child, I must know what happened to me. How did my parents handle their anger and frustration with me?" Sometimes indisputable verification does appear. A man seeking political asylum from the former Yugoslavia claimed that "the Serbian government wants to arrest me and maybe kill me because I told secrets of their abuses." He was obviously psychotic, and hence his claim could easily have been dismissed. Fortunately, a humanitarian relief organization turned out to have documentation of his heroic efforts to blow the whistle on Serbian atrocities. Contrariwise, there are false accusations, both by individuals and groups. Physicians for

Human Rights, for instance, is frequently asked to ascertain the truth or falsity (or partial truth and partial falsity) of allegations of brutality and atrocities by one side or another of a conflict. That difficult task takes a major effort to be objective. Sometimes there is nakedly self-serving lying or propaganda. A sadistic attempt to settle a grudge over real or imagined slights, or simply to distract attention from other issues, can also be operative. Repeatedly, one must ask, "What goes into these false or even totally fabricated claims?" and not ignore the conditions facilitating these claims.[7]

Given the evidence that traumatic memories are subject to even more problems of recall and placing in a consistent and coherent frame than ordinary memories, one can easily slip into a position of either dismissing an incoherent memory or too readily accepting every detail and every version. My brief review has suggested that it is in the very nature of memory, and even more of traumatic memory, to select, "editorialize," revise, recontextualize, and reinterpret. This does not mean that the trauma did not happen but, rather, shifts the question to how the traumatic event is registered and recalled in the narrative version or versions we receive.

But let us return to my earlier clinical vignette of the son who broke off relations with his parents for their alleged failure to acknowledge that his grandfather had taken him to participate in horrible Satanic rituals. It seems to me from my experience with this and a few other cases, and hearing and reading of other people's experience, that what turns out to be a false accusation, or a severe doubting of "did it or did it not happen," may reflect an attempt by the child (now an adult) to concretize a difficult-to-name problem with the parents. In one instance, it became clear that a patient's recurrent obsessive question about whether or not the parish priest had abused her at the age of seven was used to screen off the more painful awareness of extreme neglect by her middle-class professional parents, who had severe alcohol problems. Her pain at acknowledging the actuality of neglect by these parents she loved led her to reach for an "exterior" explanation that could be endlessly questioned. What was repressed were memories too shameful to discuss even as an adult, which led back to experiences that as a child had to be rationalized and hidden from adults outside the family (e.g., school). (It was ultimately not possible to determine whether or not she had been sexually abused, but the patient ended up with a very different perspective on her initial question.) I cite this as one possible line of explanation for some cases where an accusation turns out to be false, but there is nevertheless a serious ignored or repressed problem. My first vignette also illustrates the interweaving of fantasy and fact, and the crucial need to understand why and how this came about. Haaken provides several of her own compelling examples of this complex interweaving, especially in chapter 11, "Sex, Lies and Therapy." Most therapists can readily provide examples of these complex situations from their own practices, as I have from mine.[8]

But why have the "memory wars" taken on such a prominent place in contemporary society? Haaken attempts to define several culturally widespread "narratives" that have developed sequentially over the last decades: "In the 1980s, there was a decisive shift from rape to incest as paradigmatic of women's sexual oppression" (1998, 126). These narratives of victimization have served, in her view, both to articulate previously suppressed women's suffering in the culture and, at the same time, to cover over some of the complexity of women's psychological issues, especially those around sexual desire.[9] Again, the pervasiveness of such narratives does not mean that real traumas do not take place, but rather that it may be difficult to know whose narrative means that she or he has indeed been a victim of incest, and who uses the narrative to name a more amorphous, or repressed, developmental problem within the family.

The controversy over "true" and "false" memories has certainly become politicized in contemporary American culture. At the extremes, the polarization has to do with whether you are on the side of the child or the parent. If on the side of the child, you are liberal and open (or too liberal, too permissive, and hence dangerous to societal stability); and if on that of the parent, you are a conservative, believing in the virtues of authority and discipline (or authoritarian, rigid, and child-hating, and hence dangerous to societal decency). But consider the statistic that fewer than one-quarter of American children are being brought up in households with their two biological parents. This suggests that we may be in a period of confusion about what exactly parents and children ought to expect of each other. We may well be uncertain about whether our own memories of childhood provide sufficient guidance as to how to raise our children. Hence, we have trouble knowing what really happened, and who really did what to whom. We can be traumatized and overwhelmed by the uncertainties, and fail to develop adequate narratives of what it is to be a parent or a child. Not being able to tolerate the ambiguities and complexities, we then reach for simplistic solutions. Or we can be creatively troubled by these realities, recognize that we stand on shifting and uncertain ground, and seek new ways or renew old ways of coping. As suggested by my title, I vote for the latter: it can be much more interesting and creative to imagine how complex are the realities in which we are living and will doubtless continue to live.

NOTES

1. My own Department of Psychiatry at Harvard Medical School in recent years has encompassed national leaders on both sides of the debate, with Judith Herman stating that "false memory" accusations are rare compared to the incidence of actual abuse, and Fred Frankel, a consultant to the False Memory Syndrome Foundation, speaking to what he considers the very weak evidence for valid "recovered memories."

2. See Harvey and Herman (1997) for an account of the treatment of three members of a family with sexual abuse of the children.

3. A woman in her twenties with major psychiatric illness, refractory to treatment, had been a hidden child in Poland during World War II. It emerged that she could access memories of sexual abuse on the farm where she was hidden but only in Polish, and not in English. Fortuitously landing with a Polish-speaking therapist brought this to light. The two languages had vastly different emotional and interpersonal valences.

4. There is considerable controversy, often needlessly polarized, on the treatment of traumatic stress syndromes. Many indictments of "talking therapy" seem to presume a rather abstract, nonaffectively charged set of interactions between patient and therapist. See the critique of nonverbal therapies assembled by Varvin (2003) and reviewed by Leuzinger-Bohleber (2004), as well as Applebaum et al. (1997) for more detailed discussion.

5. For scholarly, but still partisan, treatment, see two books, both published by Harvard University Press: Freyd (1996) and, in some disagreement with Freyd, McNally (2003), as well as the critical review of McNally's work by Putnam (2003). See also Prager (1998).

6. For critiques of her work, see Roundtable (2004).

7. See Volkan (1979) on the Greek-Turkish conflict over Cyprus for examples of such claims, and an effort to make sense of them.

8. See Davies and Frawley (1994), and Good's (2004) symposium on the "seduction hypothesis." My therapeutic approach, though different from case to case, errs on the side of tending to affirm the validity of the patient's history. I do try to establish a "truth-seeking alliance" with the patient that, ideally, allows us to explore all the possibilities and ramifications of the memories. However, there is room for disagreement as to the stance of the therapist in handling the discussion of the veracity of the memories. See, for example, Grand's (2004) critique of Haaken's approach, and Haaken's (2004) reply. It is clear no stance is immune to countertransference issues on the part of the therapist or free of risk either to the therapeutic alliance (perhaps by repeating the parental denial of abuse in childhood) or of a *folie-à-deux* between patient and therapist that prematurely affirms the veracity of the memories and precludes further analysis.

9. I might add orphanhood as another example of a cultural narrative that serves to "explain" a whole host of problems. Nineteenth-century novels are replete with characters who have lost a parent early in life. For example, in *Moby Dick* Ahab has lost his mother to psychosis and death before he was one, while Ishmael has lost his parents by age four.

REFERENCES

Appelbaum, Paul S., Lisa A. Uyehara, and Mark R. Elin, eds. 1997. *Trauma and memory: Clinical and legal controversies.* New York: Oxford University Press.

Blass, Rachel B., and Bennett Simon. 1994. The value of the historical perspective to contemporary psychoanalysis: Freud's "seduction hypothesis." *International Journal of Psychoanalysis* 75:677–94.

Briere, John R., and Jon R. Conte. 1993. Self-reported amnesia for abuse in adults molested as children. *Journal of Traumatic Stress* 6:21–31.

Bruner, Jerome, and Joan Lucariello. 1989. Monologue as narrative recreation of the world. In *Narratives from the crib*, ed. K. Nelson, 73–97. Cambridge: Harvard University Press.

Buchsbaum, Harriet K., and Robert N. Emde. 1990. Play narratives in 36-month-old children: Early moral development and family relationships. *Psychoanalytic Study of the Child* 45:129–56.

Cicchetti, Dante, and M. Beeghly. 1987. Symbolic development in maltreated youngsters: An organizational perspective. In *New directions for child development. Vol. 36: Atypical symbolic development*, ed. Cichetti and Beeghly, 5–29. San Francisco: Jossey-Bass.

Davies, Jody M., and Mary-Gail Frawley. 1994. *Treating the adult survivors of sexual abuse: A psychoanalytic perspective*. New York: Basic Books.

Emde, Robert N., Lorraine F. Kubicek, and D. Oppenheim. 1997. Imaginative reality observed during early language development. *International Journal of Psychoanalysis* 78:115–34.

Fonagy, Peter, Gyory Gergely, Elliott Jurist, and Mary Target. 2002. *Affect regulation, mentalization, and the development of the self*. New York: Other Press.

Freyd, Jennifer J. 1996. *Betrayal trauma: The logic of forgetting child abuse*. Cambridge: Harvard University Press.

Ganaway, George K. 1989. Narrative truth: Clarifying the role of exogenous trauma in the etiology of MPD and its variants. *Dissociation* 2:205–20.

Good, Michael, ed. 2004. *The seduction theory in its second century*. New York: International Universities Press.

Grand, Sue. 2004. Uncertainty and incest—Beyond true and false: Commentary on Janice Haaken's *Pillar of salt. Studies in Gender and Sexuality* 4:178–85.

Grolier, Julia A., Rachel Yehuda, and Stephen M. Southwick. 1997. Memory and post-traumatic stress disorder. In Appelbaum et al. 1997, 225–42.

Haaken, Janice. 1998. *Pillar of salt: Gender, memory, and the perils of looking back*. New Brunswick: Rutgers University Press.

———. 2004. Pleasures and perils in looking back: Responses to Fogel, Grand, Kahane, and Namir. *Studies in Gender and Sexuality* 4:208–25.

Hartmann, Ernest. 1998. *Dreams and nightmares: The new theory of the origin and meaning of dreams*. New York: Plenum.

Harvey, Mary R., and Judith L. Herman. 1997. Continuous memory, amnesia, and delayed recall of childhood trauma: A clinical typology. In Appelbaum et al. 1997, 261–71.

Lanius, Ruth A., Peter C. Williamson et al. 2004. The nature of traumatic memories: A 4-T fMRI functional connecting analysis. *American Journal of Psychiatry* 161:36–44.

Lansky, Melvin R., and Carol R. Bley. 1995. *Post-traumatic nightmares: Psychoanalytic explorations.* Hillsdale, NJ: Analytic Press.

Laub, Dori, and Nanette C. Auerhahn. 1993. Knowing and not knowing massive psychic trauma: Forms of traumatic memory. *International Journal of Psychoanalysis* 74:287–302.

Leuzinger-Bohleber, Marianne. 2004. Review of *Mental survival strategies after extreme traumatization,* by Sverre Varvin. *International Journal of Psychoanalysis* 85:236–42.

Lunbeck, Elizabeth, and Bennett Simon. 2003. *Family romance, family secrets: Case notes of an American psychoanalysis, 1912.* New Haven: Yale University Press.

Lyons-Ruth, Karlen, and D. Jacobovitz. 1999. Attachment disorganization: Unresolved loss, relational violence, and lapses in behavioral and attentional strategies. In *Handbook of attachment,* ed. Jude Cassidy and Phillip R. Shaver, 520–55. New York: Guilford Press.

McNally, Richard J. 2003. *Remembering trauma.* Cambridge: Harvard University Press.

Prager, Jeffrey. 1998. *Presenting the past: Psychoanalysis and the sociology of misremembering.* Cambridge: Harvard University Press.

Putnam, Frank. 2003. Memory wars featured in trauma book. *Traumatic Stress Points. Bulletin of the International Society for Traumatic Stress Studies* 17(Fall):8–9.

Pynoos, Robert S., and Katherine Nader. 1989. Children's memory and proximity to violence. *Journal of the American Academy of Child and Adolescent Psychiatry* 28:236–41.

Roundtable on *Pillar of salt.* 2004. *Studies in Gender and Sexuality* 4:150–225.

Schacter, Daniel L. 1996. *Searching for memory: The brain, the mind, and the past.* New York: Basic Books.

Simon, Bennett. 1978. *Mind and madness in ancient Greece: The classical roots of modern psychiatry.* Ithaca: Cornell University Press.

———. 1988. *Tragic drama and the family: Psychoanalytic studies from Aeschylus to Beckett.* New Haven: Yale University Press.

Solms, Mark, and Oliver Turnbull. 2002. *The brain and the inner world: An introduction to the neuroscience of subjective experience.* New York: Other Press.

Van der Kolk, Bessel A. 1997. Traumatic memories. In Appelbaum et al. 1997, 243–60.

Varvin, Sverre. 2003. *Mental survival strategies after extreme traumatization.* Copenhagen: Multipress.

Volkan, Vamik D. 1979. *Cyprus—war and adaptation: A psychoanalytic history of two ethnic groups in conflict.* Charlottesville: University Press of Virginia.

Waldinger, Robert J., Sheree L. Toth, and Andrew Gerber. 2001. Maltreatment and internal representations of relationships: Core relationship themes in the narratives of abused and neglected preschoolers. *Social Development* 10:41–58.

SEVEN

Narrative and Feminine Empathy

James to Kristeva

JANET SAYERS

INTRODUCTION

"I CAN FEEL HIM. I can smell him. I can hear him. It's *too* real." A woman complains of the abuse she has suffered. It eludes straightforward telling. Neuropsychology tells us that in trauma "the high level of emotional arousal impairs memory and the hippocampus can atrophy from high levels of the stress hormone cortisol" (Emanuel 2004, 75). This causes "the memory difficulties of trauma victims who are able to retain the physical and emotional aspects of the experience, the encoded body changes of emotional memory, but cannot recall the actual details of the event."

Trauma evades narrative memory; according to Roland Barthes, it "is a suspension of language, a blocking of meaning" (1961, 209). Paradoxically, this impediment makes trauma akin to the ineffability or transcendence of mystical experience. One of the founding fathers of academic psychology, William James (1902), regarded just such experience as a cure for the ills of "the divided self." Today, by contrast, thanks to developments in psychoanalysis associated in England with the work of D. W. Winnicott and Wilfred Bion, the healing of trauma is seen to take place through the narration made

---

I am grateful to the British Academy for making possible my trip to Gainesville to attend the conference on Psychoanalysis and Narrative Medicine at which this paper was originally presented.

possible by the intersubjectivity associated with what could be called feminine *receptive* empathy. In her recent trilogy, *Feminine Genius* (1999; 2000;
2002), Julia Kristeva modifies this tradition derived from Melanie Klein by
stressing the *projective* empathy of women as daughters and mothers as integral to transubstantiating the dislocations of trauma into a linguistically
expressible form.

WILLIAM JAMES

In his abbreviated textbook *Psychology* (1892), James affirmed: "It is, in
short, the reinstatement of the vague and inarticulate to its proper place
in mental life which I am so anxious to press on the attention" (165). Having adopted this as a maxim in the epigraph to his book *The Psychoanalysis of Artistic Vision and Hearing* (1953), Anton Ehrenzweig argued in his
later book, *The Hidden Order of Art* (1967), that "chaos" is the starting
point of all that is best in music and art, just as James had held vagueness
to be the fount of religion. More crucially, as regards narrative medicine,
James maintained that the evanescent, fleeting oneness with what is godlike or divine in mystical experience often marks the turning point in healing those suffering from a crippling self-division between love and hate,
good and bad.

James described how an ecstatic oneness with God is mediated by the
subliminal self. It is accessed by a lowering of the usual barrier between the
subconscious and wide-awake consciousness. He allied this lowering with the
experience of women cured of hysteria through surrendering to the injunc-
tions put to them under hypnosis by their doctors, and with the openness of
mediums (also usually women) to visitations from the dead. Ironically, James
himself was fearful of specters. Perhaps that was why he scarcely, if ever,
attained mystical states of mind. He nevertheless revered their ineffability as
"noetically" insightful and revelatory. In a vicious circle, the very fears that
caused these breakthroughs to elude him may have contributed to the ills for
which he sought soul-healing.

Freud, who was vehemently opposed to religion, tended to reject such
spiritualistic approaches to the psyche as unscientific. He disparaged mystical
experience as a regressive return to primary narcissism, that is, to the infantile illusion of oneness with the mother. Nevertheless, he acknowledged
(1923) that Havelock Ellis (1919), among others, had explicitly connected
his "fundamental rule" of free association with the methods adopted by a fol-
lower of the Swedish mystic Garth Wilkinson, after whom one of William
James's younger brothers had been named. Thus, despite his own protestations, both Freud's clinical practice and his preoccupation with dreams and
dream interpretation tie him at least indirectly to nineteenth-century spiritualism and to mystical traditions more generally.

WINNICOTT

Writing in the British tradition influenced as much by Klein as by Freud, Winnicott (1945) argued that the narratives we tell ourselves in dreams first come into being intersubjectively. He suggested that our ability to sustain the mystical states of mind (celebrated by James), which many then as now associated with dreaming, depends on early experiences of being held psychologically as well as physically by those who first mother us. If all goes well, we can learn to bear, and even enjoy, such states of "primary unintegration": "There are long stretches of time . . . in which a baby does not mind whether he is many bits or one whole being, or whether he lives in his mother's face or in his own body, provided that from time to time he comes together and feels something" (150). Through her identification with her baby, Winnicott went on, the mother anticipates and meets his or her proto-narrative illusions and fantasies. She enriches them with details of what is "actually available" (153), and thereby enables mother and child to *live an experience together* (152; italics in original).

At first, of course, the baby has no knowledge of its fantasies and dreams, or of their interrelation. Putting this in somewhat Kleinian terms, he pointed out that the baby initially does not know that "the mother he is building up through his quiet experiences is the same as the power behind the breasts that he has in mind to destroy" (151). Young children need the assistance of others to become aware of what they narrate to themselves as they sleep: "It is normal for small children to have anxiety dreams and terrors. At these times children need someone to help them remember what they dreamed."

A cornerstone of Winnicott's subsequent theory was that the discovery of external reality depends on our mothers' surviving our fantasies of destroying them, so that we can use them (and later others) as figures on whom to test our imaginative pictures and narratives about them. This is the means by which inner subjective and outer objective reality come together. When this does not happen, as Winnicott's close friend and colleague Marion Milner put it, "the world becomes grey, lacking in affective coloring, prosaic" (1952, 191).

BION

Although Bion remained more Kleinian in his thinking than either Milner or Winnicott, he agreed with them in allying this fusion of inner and outer reality with mysticism. He too argued, in effect, that the transformation of experience into narrative meaning brought about through a successful psychoanalysis is akin to what one could call the receptive empathy or identification of women with their lovers and babies. Shortly after falling in love with and marrying Francesca McCallum (his first wife, Betty Jardine, having died in 1945 just after giving birth to their daughter, Parthenope), Bion noted: "In group treatment many interpretations, and amongst them the most important, have to be made on the strength of the analyst's own emotional reactions" (1952, 149), reactions to the group's "proto-mental system in which physical and mental activity is undifferentiated" (154).

In another essay at about the same time, he explored how schizophrenic states of mind obstruct the transformation of such undifferentiated activity into what can be known and thought about through the narrative form of dreaming. As an illustration, he cited an analysand who said, with several minutes' silence between each utterance:

> "I have a problem I am trying to work out."
> "As a child I never had phantasies."
> "I knew they weren't facts so I stopped them."
> "I don't dream nowadays."
> "I don't know what to do now." (1955, 227)

Although the patient became distressed as he spoke, Bion commented: "About a year ago you told me you were no good at thinking. Just now you said you were working out a problem—obviously something you were thinking about." "Yes," said the patient. Bion accordingly concluded, "Without phantasies and without dreams you have not the means with which to think out your problem." Bion frequently mentioned analysands who treated sensations as things and ejected them by convulsively jerking their bodies, depositing what they took in visually onto walls and into corners of the consulting room. In their hallucinations, they would enviously attack any link between themselves and others that might make it possible for Bion to take in and render what they experienced bearable.

Armed with such clinical data, Bion cogitated on Henri Poincaré's notion of a "selected fact" in mathematics. Echoing the words of Apollinaire on Matisse, "To make order out of chaos—that is creation" (1907, 38), Bion said that such facts

> must unite elements long since known, but till then scattered and seemingly foreign to each other, and suddenly introduce order where the appearance of disorder reigned. Then it enables us to see at a glance each of those elements in the place it occupies as a whole. (1962, 72)

Bion attributed the lack in schizophrenic states of mind of any synthetic powers, such as are essential to narration, to an inability to tolerate the frustrations that come with forming ties with others, or with seeing others form ties with each other. The result, he argued, is that "in the psychotic we find no capacity for reverie, no α [alpha element], and so none of the capacities . . . which depend on α, namely attention, passing of judgment, memory, and dream-pictures, or pictorial imagery that is capable of yielding associations" (1992, 53).

In normal functioning, he argued, the α-activity of dream work is continuous night and day. Its narrative capacity operates on stimuli arising both within and beyond the psyche. In psychosis, however, there is neither any integrative nor any disintegrative function. Consequently, there is "a lack of associations . . . as if the word were a counterpart of the pure note in music, devoid of undertones or overtones" (1992, 63; see also Ogden 2003). In such cases, Bion maintained that the analysand needs the analyst to be like an artist or scientist:

> He [the artist] is someone who is able to digest facts, i.e. sense data, and then to present the digested facts, my α-elements, in a way that makes it possible for the weak assimilators to go on from there. Thus the artist helps the non-artist to digest, say, the Little Street in Delft by doing α-work on his sense impressions and "publishing" the result so that others who could not "dream" the Little Street itself can now digest the published α-work of someone who could digest it. (1992, 143–44)

Bion compared this process of transformation to a mother's metamorphosing her baby's inchoate sense data and self-sensations into the stuff of narrative thinking. He speculated that the baby's experience of frustration at the mother's not feeding it when it wants to be fed might become the beginning of the thought of "no breast." Alternatively, the baby might experience this frustration as a "β-element" or "bad object" that must be gotten rid of, which always carries the risk that what has been banished will return as a persecuting "bizarre object." The recourse, Bion further speculated, is for the mother neither to collapse nor to be indifferent. It resides in her "containing" the baby's projected β-elements and transforming them, through her "capacity for reverie," into the α-elements that allow experience to be registered, stored, known, and narrated. Bion (1967, 116) also conceptualized this process in terms of a man contained by a woman in sex. He accordingly schematized the analysand-analyst, contained-container relation as "♂♀."

Further sexualizing this coupling, Bion stressed the importance of treating its resulting interpretations as preconceptions open to revision by whatever their future "mating" with reality might reveal. He thus urged the same openness to what is vague or unknown advocated by William James many years before. He theorized this capacity for reverie in terms of a free movement between what Klein called paranoid-schizoid and depressive states of mind, which he schematically rendered as Ps↔D. He argued that it entails the analyst's being able to tolerate the anxieties aroused in both these states of mind—the same anxieties that, as previously indicated, James seemed to have found it hard to bear.

KRISTEVA

Bion's critics would argue, however, that he advocated too passively contemplative an analytic stance. Julia Kristeva, by contrast, has recently depicted psychoanalysis in much more active terms. In the past, she concurred with Winnicott and Bion that it essentially involved what one could call receptive empathy. In this earlier phase, she suggested that analysts should model themselves on Sonia in Dostoevsky's *Crime and Punishment* (1866). The nonjudgmental quality of this idealized female figure is exemplified by her response to Raskolnikov's confession that he had murdered her friend, Lisaveta:

> [S]he looked at him helplessly for some time, and with the same expression of terror on her face [as Lisaveta's] and thrusting out her left hand all of a sudden, she touched his chest lightly with her fingers and slowly began to get up from the bed, moving farther and farther away from him and staring more and more fixedly at him. Her feeling of horror suddenly communicated itself to him: exactly the same expression of terror appeared on his face; he, too, stared at her in the same way, and almost with the same *childlike* smile. (424; italics in original)

Later, as they sat side by side:

> He looked at Sonia and felt how great her love for him was, and, strange to say, he felt distressed and pained that he should be loved so much. Yes, it was a queer and dreadful sensation . . . and suddenly now, when all her heart was turned to him, he felt and knew that he was infinitely more unhappy than before. (435)

In Bion's terms, Sonia had transformed, through her receptive empathy, Raskolnikov's previous thing-like terror from a β-element into a consciously alive, albeit unhappy, α-element form.

Summarizing this transformation, Kristeva writes:

> According to Dostoevsky, forgiveness seems to say, through my love . . . I recognize the unconscious motivations of your crime. . . . It raises the unconscious from beneath the actions and has it meet a loving other—an other who does not judge but hears my truth in the availability of love, and for that very reason allows me to be reborn. (1987, 204–205)

More recently, Kristeva has extended this principle of forgiveness to the whole of psychoanalysis:

> Forgiveness—that is to say, the gift of meaning at the heart of the transference—is also at the heart of the talking cure of psychoanalysis. . . . From beneath action, it involves the encounter of the patient's unconscious with a loving other, who does not judge, but who understands the patient's truth without acting on the love that enables their rebirth. (1997, 32)

Having thus presented psychoanalysis as a process seeking to bring about the analysand's rebirth through the analyst's receptive feminine empathy, Kristeva has now (2000) come to view the work of the analyst more as a process of projection that transforms the analysand's thing-like, β-element experience into narrative form. She instances Klein's elaboration of her four-year-old son Erich's inhibited curiosity into fantasies by weaving his nascent images together with her own stories and ideas. In Klein's account of their interaction:

> He had spoken of his "kakis" as naughty children who did not want to come. . . . I ask him, "These are the children then that grow in the stomach?" As I notice this interests him I continue, "For the kakis are made from the food; real children are not made from food . . . they are made of something that papa makes and the egg that is inside mamma." (1921, 33)

Kristeva likewise adduces Klein's (1930) interweaving of her own ideas and narratives with those of another four-year-old, Dick, a patient who would today be diagnosed as autistic. Certainly, Dick seemed affectless at their first meeting. He ran aimlessly around the room and treated Klein as though she were a piece of furniture. In the absence of any expression of curiosity on the child's part, Klein intuited what he might be fantasying based on what she had been told about him and his obsessions, particularly with trains. Taking up two toy engines and calling the bigger one the "Daddy-train" and the smaller one the "Dick-train," she put them side by side. Dick then picked up the Dick-train and rolled it to the window, saying "station" (225). Construing the situation in light of her mother-centred version of the Oedipus complex, Klein hazarded: "The station is mummy; Dick is going into mummy." Dick responded by running in and out of the space between the double doors of her room and saying "dark." Klein interpreted, "It is dark inside mummy. Dick is inside dark mummy." Through the anxiety aroused by Klein's theory-based projections, Dick became more aware of what he felt. He became visibly upset and asked when his nurse was coming to collect him.

In subsequent sessions, Dick began incipiently to narrate his feelings. On one occasion, for instance, he pointed to a little toy coal-cart, saying "Cut," at which, wrote Klein, "Acting on a glance which he gave me, I cut the pieces of wood out of the cart, whereupon he threw the damaged cart and its contents into the drawer and said, 'Gone'" (1930, 225–26). Another time, "Dick lifted a little toy man to his mouth, gnashed his teeth and said 'Tea daddy,' by which he meant 'Eat daddy.'" Later he expressed concern for her, saying "Poor Mrs. Klein." He thereby put into words the "premature empathy" that had, in her view, been "a decisive factor in his warding-off of all his destructive impulses . . . [and] brought his phantasy-life to a standstill by taking refuge in the phantasy of the dark, empty mother's body" (227).

Kristeva (2000, 139) comments that, by putting Dick's fantasies into words, Klein transformed his mental universe from one "based on identities" (e.g., father = train) to one "based on similarities" (e.g., penis akin to father). In Lacan's terms, she propelled his mental universe from the register of the

Imaginary to that of the Symbolic. Kristeva argues that, drawing on her own experience as a mother, Klein developed a technique enabling mothers to bring their fantasies together with the pre-narrative (yet object-related) drives of their babies, thereby endowing these proto-fantasies with a form capable of linguistic representation and narrative meaning.

By analogy, analysts do something similar in projectively identifying or empathizing with their analysands, which aids in restoring life to formerly deadened psyches. In keeping with her biological essentialism, Kristeva believes that women analysts are likely to be particularly adept at projective empathy given their susceptibility to their mothers' "seductive osmosis" when they were babies. Although Kristeva emphasizes that the mother also has in mind her desire for her father or for her child's father, the receptivity of the girl's genitals, as well as of her mouth and anus, greets this seduction with bodily excitement. As infants, in Kristeva's view, women compensate for being the objects of their mothers' seduction by "the early elaboration of a relationship of introjection/identification with the loving-and-intrusive object" (2002, 411). The little girl thereby forms her first "internal representation." This launches her into the organization of her psyche—"psychization"—and, from here, eventually into narrative. Kristeva traces the novels of Colette to her seduction by her mother, Sido, and by her first husband, Willy.

Kristeva cautions that, from a clinical standpoint, the analyst's maternal seduction of, or projective identification with, his or her analysand raises the problem of treatment by suggestion. But Kristeva sidesteps this problem. Nancy Chodorow (1978), by contrast, has addressed the danger of intrusiveness in mother-daughter relations. She argues that women as infants are much more at risk than are men from their mothers' seductive projections. She cites Enid Balint's (1963) observation that, as a result of their mothers' "false empathy," women often grow up feeling they cannot "interpret the world in their own way" (Chodorow 1978, 100). Balint based her formulation on the case of a woman whose mother had responded to her as an infant with "her own preconceived ideas as to what a baby ought to feel" rather than by paying attention to "what her baby actually felt" (qtd. in Chodorow 1978, 101). Chodorow brings to bear further examples of women whom another researcher, Christine Olden (1958), describes as "unable to empathize with their children" except through the narcissistic "closeness" involved in projecting themselves onto the child (qtd. in Chodorow 1978, 102).

According to Chodorow, boys as well as girls go through an early "symbiotic phase of unity, primary identification, and mutual empathy with their mother and then go through a period of differentiation from her" (1978, 108n). But this process of differentiation is less marked in girls since, because of her shared sex with her daughter, the mother is liable "to experience a sense of oneness and continuity with her," leading her (the mother) to project "unconscious meanings, fantasies, and self-images about this gender" (109) as well as "her own internalized early relationships to *her* mother" (167; italics added). As a result, explains Chodorow, "girls emerge from this period with a basis for 'empathy' built into their primary definition of self in a way that boys do not." But this secondary gain, as Marilyn Lawrence (2002) has recently emphasized, derives from the same process of projective identification that often leads daughters to experience their mothers—and later their analysts—as overly intrusive.

CONCLUSION

Unlike Chodorow, many analysts celebrate the female-centered empathic oneness with another person involved in mothering, femininity, and "feminine genius," to borrow the term used by Kristeva as the subtitle of her trilogy celebrating Klein's achievements in child analysis, as well as those of Colette and Hannah Arendt in their respective domains of literature and political philosophy. But though it too arguably arises from a preverbal ground of being, psychoanalysis, unlike religious therapy, seeks to put into narrative form what William James celebrated as transcending language. The process of verbalization enables analytic hunches to be tested against reality, unlike the ineffable experience to which religion all too often appeals in refusing to open its dogmas to scientific investigation. The transformation of psychoanalysis from an impersonal (and implicitly male) surgical procedure, as Freud (1912) envisioned it, into one more closely linked with women's femininity and mothering also beneficially highlights the importance of analysts' attunement with their analysands.

Whether conceived, in the manner of Winnicott and Bion, as receptive empathy, or with Kristeva as projective empathy, this quintessentially feminine quality can be healing in bringing the shattering experiences of both mysticism and trauma into assimilable narrative form. But if this celebration of the ineffable becomes excessive, psychoanalysis can become as impervious to the truth as religion. Hence the need for narrative and its openness to what it evokes and reveals—an openness splendidly captured by Henry James's (1902) image of a doctor's "great empty cup of attention," to which Rita Charon refers in her essay in this volume when she asks, "Where does narrative medicine come from?"

REFERENCES

Apollinaire, Guillaume. 1907. Henri Matisse. In *Apollinaire on art*, trans. Susan Suleiman, 36–39. London: Thames and Hudson, 1972.

Balint, Enid. 1963. On being empty of oneself. *International Journal of Psychoanalysis* 44:470–80.

Barthes, Roland. 1961. The photographic image. In *Selected writings*, ed. Susan Sontag, 194–210. London: Fontana, 1983.

Bion, W. R. 1952. Group dynamics: A re-view. In *Experiences in groups*, 141–91. London: Tavistock, 1961.

———. 1955. Language and the schizophrenic. In *New directions in psychoanalysis*, ed. Melanie Klein, Paula Heimann, and Roger E. Money-Kyrle, 220–39. London: Tavistock.

———. 1962. *Learning from experience*. London: Heinemann.

———. 1967. *Second thoughts*. London: Heinemann.

———. 1992. *Cogitations*. London: Karnac.

Chodorow, Nancy. 1978. *The reproduction of mothering: Psychoanalysis and the sociology of gender*. Berkeley: University of California Press.

Dostoevsky, Fyodor. 1866. *Crime and punishment*. Trans. David Magarshack. Harmondsworth: Penguin Books, 1951.

Ehrenzweig, Anton. 1953. *The psycho-analysis of artistic vision and hearing*. London: Routledge and Kegan Paul.

———. 1967. *The hidden order of art*. London: Paladin, 1970.

Ellis, Havelock. 1919. *The philosophy of conflict and other essays in wartime*. Boston: Houghton Mifflin.

Emanuel, Ricky. 2004. Thalamic fear. *Journal of Child Psychotherapy* 30:71–87.

Freud, Sigmund. 1912. Recommendations to physicians practicing psychoanalysis. *Standard edition of the complete psychological works*, ed. and trans. James Strachey et al., 12:111–20. London: Hogarth Press, 1953–1974.

———. 1923. Two encyclopaedia articles. *S.E.*, 18:235–59.

James, Henry. 1902. *The wings of the dove*. London: Penguin, 1965.

James, William. 1890. *The principles of psychology*. New York: Holt.

———. 1902. *The varieties of religious experience*. London: Fontana, 1960.

Klein, Melanie. 1921. The development of a child. In Klein 1975, 1–53.

———. 1930. The importance of symbol-formation in the development of the ego. In Klein 1975, 219–32.

———. 1975. *Love, guilt, and reparation*. London: Hogarth.

Kristeva, Julia. 1987. *Black sun: Depression and melancholia*. Trans. Leon S. Roudiez. New York: Columbia University Press.

———. 1997. *La révolte intime*. Paris: Fayard.

———. 1999. *Hannah Arendt*. Trans. Ross Guberman. New York: Columbia University Press, 2001.

———. 2000. *Melanie Klein*. Trans. Ross Guberman. New York: Columbia University Press, 2001.

———. 2002. *Colette*. Trans. Jane Marie Todd. New York: Columbia University Press, 2004.

Lawrence, Marilyn. 2002. Body, mother, mind: Anorexia, femininity, and the intrusive object. *International Journal of Psychoanalysis* 83:837–50.

Milner, Marion. 1952. Aspects of symbolism in comprehension of the not-self. *International Journal of Psychoanalysis* 34:181–95.

Ogden, Thomas. 2003. On not being able to dream. *International Journal of Psychoanalysis* 84:17–30.

Olden, Christine. 1958. Notes on the development of empathy. *Psychoanalytic Study of the Child* 13:505–18.

Winnicott, D. W. 1945. Primitive emotional development. In Winnicott 1958, 145–56.

———. 1947. Hate in the counter-transference. In Winnicott 1958, 194–203.

———. 1958. *Collected papers: Through paediatrics to psychoanalysis*. London: Tavistock.

EIGHT

The Fortunate Physician

Learning from Our Patients

FRED L. GRIFFIN

INTRODUCTION

IN THE 1960s, the author John Berger and the photographer Jean Mohr spent six weeks with an English doctor, John Sassall, who lived and worked in an impoverished community in the west of England, near Monmouth. Berger and Sassall had met earlier, when Berger was living in a neighboring village and had consulted Sassall about abdominal pain. A friendship developed, and Berger eventually approached Sassall with the idea of writing a book that would chronicle the doctor's interactions with his patients as well as reflect on his personal and professional development. Near the end of the ensuing remarkable three-way collaboration, *A Fortunate Man* (1967), Berger observes that "Sassall, with the cunning intuition that any fortunate man requires today in order to go on working at what he believes in, has established the situation he needs" (158). The "situation" to which Berger refers is the set of circumstances that allowed Sassall to satisfy his desire simultaneously to learn more about the humanity of his patients and about himself as both a physician and as a man.

As a psychoanalyst in my thirtieth year as a physician, I have been reflecting on how fortunate I am to be engaged in a process that, while constantly challenging me to become a more effective clinician, provides the dual opportunity to try to grasp what is essential to the lives of my patients and to comprehend more about myself.[1] My training has taught me to focus closely on what is "written" intersubjectively in the two-person relationship between analyst and patient as a path to "reading" what my patients are trying to communicate about their lives. In order to do so, I must constantly confront my limited self-understanding and engage in self-inquiry; and this, to my mind, is a fortunate set of circumstances.

Like psychoanalysts, physicians on the front lines of patient care are continuously afforded moments where they can achieve a partnering of self-reflection with engaged, attuned clinical work. But because medical training has traditionally devalued subjective (and intersubjective) experience, it may not adequately prepare physicians to appreciate the unique experiences they are creating with their patients at particular moments of time.

Consequently, I have sought a way to communicate what I have gained from my clinical experience as a psychoanalyst that might be of value both to practicing physicians and to the growing body of literature on narrative medicine.[2] Recognizing that the terminology and frames of reference that psychoanalysts use to speak about their work often seem irrelevant, if not off-putting, to outsiders, I take it for granted that if I hope to enter into substantive conversations with physicians, I am obliged to find a language that is meaningful to them. I believe that A Fortunate Man offers a medium through which I can convey elements of my work as an analyst in a form that is accessible to my colleagues in various branches of medicine.

Several years ago, I inaugurated a series of evening classes titled "Conversations for Physicians" in which I took Berger's book as a stimulus for discussing the physician-patient relationship, the professional and personal development of the physician, and the practice of narrative medicine. Although there are obvious differences between the medical culture of an English country doctor in the mid-twentieth century and that of contemporary physicians in the United States, I believe that A Fortunate Man captures something that is universal and enduring about what it means to be a doctor. Furthermore, I found that Berger's book spoke to the doctor-with-patient experience in a manner that allowed me to bring a "psychoanalytic sensibility"[3] to the discussions and to introduce concepts such as unconscious motivation, transference, intersubjectivity, empathy, the therapeutic alliance, and the use of the self as a clinical tool without resorting to arcane terminology.

INTERNAL LANDSCAPES

Throughout A Fortunate Man, Berger's prose is complemented by Mohr's evocative photographs. The opening pages feature bucolic scenes: a winding road amid forest and field, two men in a boat fishing on a calm river. But as the book progresses, the photographs turn from crisp and sunny to dark, foggy, and barely discernable. The following words are found in the lower right-hand corners of the first two photographs:

Landscapes can be deceptive. Sometimes a landscape seems to be less a set-ting for the life of its inhabitants than a curtain behind which their strug-gles, achievements and accidents take place. For those who, with the inhab-itants, are behind the curtain, landmarks are no longer only geographic but also biographical and personal. (Berger 1967, 13–15)

Berger is an essayist of the highest order who most often writes about life from the perspective of the world of art. His collections—*Ways of Seeing* (1972), *The Look of Things* (1971), *The Sense of Sight* (1985), *Toward Reality* (1962), and *About Looking* (1980)—develop the reader's aesthetic sensibility by suggesting more encompassing ways of perceiving and understanding what—and more importantly *how*—he or she is viewing.[4] We know, there-fore, that when he speaks of "landscapes," Berger refers not only to external landscapes but also to the internal, psychological world.

The frontispiece of *A Fortunate Man* shows Sassall at the threshold of his office, his gaze directed inside (perhaps toward a patient to whom he is lis-tening) and his hand resting on the outside of the opened door. This liminal space between inside and outside is where the mature clinician knows that he or she must live: poised with binocular vision to perceive what originates within but is manifested in both the physical and psychological lives of the patient. As psychoanalysis reminds us, the physician likewise needs to be attuned to his or her own somatic and psychic worlds.

THE DEVELOPMENT OF THE PHYSICIAN

Sassall did not always possess the capacity to see beyond the external presen-tations of his patients. Early in his career, he held the simplistic belief that the physician was an active, objective agent who encountered a passive and subjective patient. Berger writes:

He had no patience with anything except emergencies or serious illness. . . . He dealt only with crises in which he was the central character . . . in which the patient was *simplified* by the degree of his physical dependence on the doctor. . . . [This] made it impossible and unnecessary for him to examine his own motives. (1967, 55; italics in original)

Berger informs us that as a boy, Sassall read Joseph Conrad's stories of the sea, through which he constructed a model of what a physician should be. Like the mariners who conquer the elements of the weather and sea, Sassall viewed himself as a heroic figure who vanquishes disease. He and the disease were locked in combat, while patients were relegated to the sidelines. He did not consider how the patient's entire personality shaped the manner in which the illness was expressed or how his own personality and approach may have impacted his diagnosis and the effectiveness of his treatment.

But Sassall brought something more from Conrad's vision of the hero to the practice of medicine. For Conrad's mariners, the dangers of the sea could be faced only by men who were outwardly controlled and devoid of emotional response. The physician whose life was to be patterned after these mariners likewise had to renounce his imagination:

> The quality which Conrad constantly warns against is at the same time the very quality to which he appeals: the quality of imagination. . . . It is to the imagination that the sea appeals; but to face the sea in its unimaginable fury, to meet its own challenge, imagination must be abandoned, for it leads to self-isolation and fear. . . . [Sassall] admired physical prowess. He enjoyed being practical and using his hands. He was inquisitive about things rather than feelings. (52)

Then something happened, a sudden revelation that showed Sassall that the truth of his patients' lives was not always what it seemed to be on the surface:

> They had lived in the Forest for thirty years. . . . The husband said that his wife "was bleeding from down below." . . . When he [Sassall] went back into the parlour, the wife was lying on the ottoman. Her stockings were rolled down and her dress up. "She" was a man. He examined her. The trouble was severe piles. Neither he nor the husband referred to the sexual organs which should not have been there. (56)

Shocked and then perplexed by this experience, Sassall was confronted with the fact that he had no way to go about understanding how these two males had sustained a life as man and wife. The recognition of the unreliability of appearances led Sassall to a new approach to his work, one that seeks to fathom what motivates people and makes them who they are. Sassall began to span the distance between the external "landscape" presented by his patient and the internal world of meanings that informed the patient's self-representation and relationship with others. He no longer aspired to emulate the mariners' denial of imagination in their confrontations with the sea:

> He had done just that—using illness and medical dangers as they used the sea. He began to realize that he must face his imagination, even explore it. It must no longer lead to the "unimaginable," as it had with the Master Mariners contemplating the possible fury of the elements—or, as in his case, to his contemplating only fights within the jaws of death itself. . . . He began to realize that imagination had to be lived with on every level: his own imagination first—because otherwise this could distort his observation—and then the imaginations of his patients. (56–57)

After Sassall's imagination came to life in his work, it became not only possible but necessary for him to explore his personal psychology and that of his patients in order to develop into a more complete physician. Allowing his imagination a clinical function, he became able to create personal narratives from what he observed of his patients. In Arnold Weinstein's phrase, Sassall now "*restories* the patient" (2003, 160; italics in original). Sassall likewise recognized that in order to understand his patients' stories and to differentiate them from his own, he had to learn more about himself—his character, motivations, personal history, and ways of comprehending the world. He read Freud and began a self-analysis that he initially found so disturbing that he became sexually impotent for a time.[5] He emerged from his six months of self-examination with the realization "that the patient should be treated as a total personality, that illness is frequently a form of expression rather than a surrender to natural hazards" (Berger 1967, 62).

Now a more mature clinician, Sassall no longer needed to create such emotional distance between himself and his patients, and his therapeutic relationships improved. He came to understand that illness deforms the patient's sense of who he or she is, and he imagined how he might help to restore to the patient a more coherent sense of self: "Illness separates and encourages a distorted, fragmented form of self-consciousness. The doctor, through his relationship with the invalid and by means of the special intimacy he is allowed, has to compensate for these broken connections" (69).

Sassall found that the physician-patient relationship was far more complex than he had formerly believed it to be. Not only do patients inevitably experience feelings about their encounters with diseases, their intimate contact with him evoked emotions in him as well. His subjective reactions to his patients and their diseases affected his diagnoses and how he proceeded with treatment. Worlds apart from the earlier model of the physician-patient relationship, this conception takes into account the subjectivity of both doctor and patient. Rather than denying the patient's emotional impact upon the physician, the more developed physician makes fuller use of his senses and imagination to apprehend the patient and the manner in which his or her *disease* may present itself in the form of an *illness*.[6]

It was here that Sassall's good fortune began, with his recognition that his earlier model of himself as the hero who exists to conquer disease limited his capacities to be a physician in the fullest sense. By listening to his patients' stories and understanding who they were as people, Sassall now grasped that disease expresses itself in unique ways that are shaped by the patient's personal psychology as well as by the social and interpersonal context, including the doctor-patient relationship. Sassall was also fortunate because his work fostered his own emotional development. He became a better man as he became a better doctor, achieving a stronger connection with his own emotional life as well as with his patients. Through his increasing capacity to discern his feelings and reflect upon personal meanings, he grew more competent in finding words to communicate his understanding of their experience to his patients:

Once he was putting a syringe deep into a man's chest; there was little question of pain but it made the man feel bad; the man tried to explain his revulsion: "That's where I live, where you're putting that needle in." "I know," Sassall said, "I know what it feels like. I can't bear anything done near my eyes, I can't bear to be touched there. I think that is where I live, just under and behind my eyes." (47–50)

The patient was telling Sassall what it *meant* to him to be penetrated by a needle in that part of his body. Because Sassall now had better access to his own feelings and to his own world of meanings, he was able to make a genuine connection with his patient. By cultivating his own human sensibility, he came to possess a clinical instrument that addressed what lay hidden in the patient's interior just as powerfully as the stethoscope and as effectively as medication.

A FAILED CONNECTION

Placed among the vignettes describing Sassall at his best is one that illustrates his experience with a case that "failed"—where he felt that his approach was inadequate to the problem that his patient presented. A cautionary tale, demonstrating that the physician—even when his intention to help is most operative—may not always connect with his patient, it serves as a reminder that powerful psychological and social forces may stand in the way of our best therapeutic efforts.

The vignette presents a thirty-seven-year-old unmarried woman, now living with her ill mother, who was first seen by Sassall ten years earlier when she consulted him for a cough and a sense of weakness. Her chest film at the time was normal. Sassall felt that she wanted to talk about something, yet she refused to look at him directly, "casting him quick anxious glances as though somehow by these to bring him closer. He questioned her but could not gain her confidence" (Berger 1967, 21). A few months later she returned, complaining of insomnia and asthmatic symptoms. Berger describes Sassall's observation of the change taking place in his patient in a way that also illustrates the change in the physician-patient relationship:

Now when he saw her, she smiled at him through her illness. Her eyes were round like a rabbit's. She was timid of anything outside the cage of her illness. If anybody approached too near, her eyes twitched like the skin round a rabbit's nose. . . . He was convinced that her condition was the result of extreme emotional stress. Both she and her mother insisted, however, that she had no worries. (21)

Two years later Sassall discovered the cause of her problems through a chance conversation with a woman who had worked with the patient at a dairy. The woman told Sassall that the manager of the dairy—a member of the Salvation Army—had had an affair with the patient and promised to marry her. Overcome with religious scruples, however, he abandoned her. On a house call to see her ailing mother, Sassall, armed with this information, again tried to reach his patient:

> The doctor once again questioned the girl's mother. Had her daughter been happy when she worked at that dairy? Yes, perfectly. He asked the girl if she had been happy there. She smiled in her cage and nodded her head. He then asked outright whether the manager had made a pass at her. She froze—like an animal who realizes that it is impossible to bolt. Her hands stopped moving. Her head remained averted. Her breathing became inaudible. She never answered him. (23)

Thereafter, the woman's asthma worsened, causing structural damage to her lungs. She survived by taking steroids, which left her face moon-shaped. Effectively giving up on life, she rarely left the cottage where she lived with her mother; her existence had devolved into the cage of her illness. Sassall recognized that the manner in which she resigned herself to the role of one-who-is-sick expressed how she felt about herself and what life she believed she deserved. Berger writes: "Before the water was deep. Then the torrent of God and the man. And afterwards the shallows, clear but constantly disturbed, endlessly irritated by their shallowness as though by an allergy. There is a bend in the river which often reminds the doctor of his failure" (23).

Clearly, Sassall was also "constantly disturbed" by the course his patient's life had taken, and he blamed himself for it. He did not fully accept that there are times when, even in the hands of the most experienced, determined, and humane practitioner, a patient may fall into his or her own angle of repose.[7] That is, there are elements of character and motivation that powerfully (even irrevocably) determine an individual's psychological response to trauma. These forces may not be overcome by the most seasoned of clinicians.

Beyond this woman's manner of coping with her painful experience, moreover, Sassall may himself have unknowingly contributed to this failed connection because he had not completely given up his fantasy of being the hero who could "conquer" disease, or had not accepted that all physicians face limitations in their attempts to treat illness. Frustrated and threatened by his lack of therapeutic potency with the patient, Sassall attempted to force her to "open up" about her experience, ignoring the extraordinary sense of shame and guilt she must have experienced (both in the original event of the affair and in her retelling of the story to her physician).[8] Her sense of humiliation must have been even more excruciating in her mother's presence. While Berger suggests that Sassall remained haunted by this missed connection—he never ceased looking for what it was within him that interfered with his effort to reach this patient—we never learn

whether he discovered how his own personal psychology may have contributed to the therapeutic impasse.

The physician, like the psychoanalyst, must seek to discern where the
patient is emotionally at every moment of an encounter in order to intuit
how his or her own words may be received. This kind of trust can only be
built up over time, and in some instances it may not develop at all. Although
it is not always possible to undo the harm that may have been done to our
patients, we are fortunate that they can teach us to be better doctors—and
more attuned human beings—even through our failures with them. Although
it is always painful and humbling for the physician, we are fortunate that
patients can remind us of our inevitable limitations.

RECOGNIZING THE PATIENT

As Sassall began to listen more carefully to his patients, he realized that the
forms in which disease are expressed are largely determined by the entire personality of the patient. He strove to engage in a physician-patient relationship that would facilitate a more comprehensive type of healing than he had
achieved when attempting to "conquer" disease. This kind of healing can still
take place even if the patient's disease cannot be cured; indeed, it may even
take place as the patient lies dying.

Berger also describes Sassall's experience with the mother of the afore-
mentioned traumatized female patient, a woman whose congestive heart failure had forced her to live in her bed. As Sassall entered the house, he found
that she had contracted pneumonia. He gave her an injection, after which
the old woman said, "It's not your fault" (Berger 1967, 26). Berger captures
who this woman was, who she had been, and what the doctor saw and
thought as he examined her:

> He listened to her chest. Her overworked brown arms, her deeply lined face,
> her creased, strained neck were suddenly denied by the soft whiteness of her
> breast. The grey-haired son down in the yard with the cows, the daughter at
> the foot of the bed in carpet slippers and with swollen ankles, had both once
> clambered and fed here, and yet the soft whiteness of her breast was like a
> young girl's. This she had preserved. (26)

This passage beautifully demonstrates how Sassall came to recognize his
patient by viewing her and her environment as a narrative to be "read." Her
story was "written" not only by the presence of the family members who
attested to her life as mother and wife. Sassall could also read what was written *on her body*—"overworked brown arms, her deeply lined face, her creased,
strained neck"—and this illustrated how her life had been lived. But the "soft
whiteness of her breast" reminded him of the young woman she had once

been, which was equally part of her narrative. Her past and her present were captured in a single moment.

Sassall spoke to the old woman's husband, promising that he would come back that evening. When he did so, what he saw disturbed him:

> The parlour was in darkness. . . . He called out and receiving no answer felt his way up the stairs. . . . The room smelt now of sickness. . . . The old woman was paler and a piece of damp rag was laid over her forehead. . . . The doctor listened once more to her chest. She lay back exhausted. "I'm sorry," she said, not as though it were an apology but simply a fact. He took her temperature and blood pressure. "I know," he said, "but you'll sleep soon and be rested." (27)

The old woman knew that she and Sassall had both done their best, but the end was near. "I'm sorry" may in part have been an apology, for she sensed that her physician had a personal need to heal and that he would be disappointed in himself for not saving her. Sassall's response, "I know," communicated many things at once: "I understand how you feel. I know the place, the inner and outer landscapes where you now live in your illness and where you used to live when you were young; I have been here many times before. I will not let you suffer unnecessarily. I am here with you."

Sassall told the husband and daughter that his patient had pneumonia and instructed them about the medication. The old man was silent, yet his hands—"clutching and unclutching the heavy material of the overcoat across his knees" (28)—communicated how he felt. As the doctor was leaving, the patient's husband began to cry. The tears welled up in his eyes. Sassall put his bag down, leaned back in the chair, and asked, "Can you make us a cup of tea?" (29). He spoke with the man about the apple orchard and with the daughter about her father's rheumatism.

The next morning the old woman died quickly, after a second attack. Berger reports the scene: "In the parlour the old man rocked on his feet. The doctor deliberately did not put out his hand to steady him. Instead he faced him . . . [and said], 'It would have been worse for her if she had lived. It would have been worse'" (29). Here Sassall was a fortunate man—the fortunate physician. Having learned from his patients that all the elements of their lives contribute to their larger biopsychosocial world—and to his own role in that world—he was attuned and responsive to the old woman, and he engaged the husband and daughter as a part of the totality of her "illness." His perceptions extended beyond the signs of congestive heart failure and the sounds of pneumonia and beyond his evaluation of the patient's color, pulse, respiration, and temperature. Because Sassall was able to register his own feelings, as this particular medical situation impacted him emotionally, he could empathize with the pain that her family members felt. And because he could do so, Sassall's treatment extended beyond caring for the dying woman to meeting the emotional needs of the other people with whom he came into contact. Through this holistic approach, he too found a modicum of comfort and actualized himself.

In *A Fortunate Man*, Berger demonstrates that Sassall achieved a narrative competence that allowed him to envision his patients' lives as coherent stories and thereby to help them restore a sense of wholeness that had been shattered by illness: "In illness many connections are severed. Illness separates and encourages a distorted form of self-consciousness. The doctor, through his relationship with the invalid and by means of the special intimacy he is allowed, has to compensate for these broken connections" (69). In striking agreement, Charon draws an explicit comparison between the work of the family physician and the clinical process that takes place in psychoanalysis: "As in psychoanalysis, in all of medical practice the narrating of the patient's story is a therapeutically central act, because to find words to contain the disorder and its attendant worries gives shape to and control over the chaos of illness" (2001a, 1898).

According to Berger, to be a physician requires above all the capacity for *recognition* and for creating authentic conditions that heal:

> What is required is that he should recognize his patient with the certainty of an ideal brother. The function of fraternity is recognition. This individual and closely intimate recognition is required on both a physical and psychological level. On the former it constitutes the art of diagnosis. Good general diagnosticians are rare, not because most doctors lack medical knowledge, but because most are incapable of taking in all the possible relevant facts—emotional, historical, environmental as well as physical. They are searching for specific *conditions* instead of the *truth* about a man which may then suggest various conditions. . . . On the psychological level recognition means support. As soon as we are ill we fear that our illness is unique. . . . The illness, as an undefined force, is a potential threat to our very being. (1967, 73; italics added)

Berger anticipates the central insights of both narrative medicine and contemporary psychoanalysis when he insists that the physician must recognize the patient as a *person*—one like himself or herself—in order to be effective. He writes:

> How is it that Sassall is acknowledged as a good doctor? By his cures? . . . I doubt it. . . . No, he is acknowledged as a good doctor because he meets the deep but unformulated expectation of the sick for a sense of fraternity. He recognizes them. Sometimes he fails—often because he has missed a critical opportunity and the patient's suppressed resentment becomes too hard to break through—but there is about him the constant will of a man trying to recognize. (76)

Berger's phrase, "the constant will of a man trying to recognize," captures what is asked of the physician when he enters into a relationship with the patient intent upon discovering the human being who is ill. Sassall's own words describe his entry into a patient's world:

> "The door opens," he says, "and sometimes I feel I'm in the valley of death. It's all right when once I am working. I try to overcome this shyness because for the patient the first contact is extremely important. If he's put off and doesn't feel welcome, it may take a long time to win his confidence back and perhaps never. All diffidence in my position is a fault. A form of negligence." (77)

The physician must have the courage to cross the threshold into the patient's universe—"the valley of death"—in order to imagine what it might be like *to be* the other person at the moment of their encounter. Berger expatiates on the kind of relationship Sassall creates through his *recognition* of his patients, his *intention* to understand and to be helpful, his capacity to *communicate* physically and emotionally: "It is as though when he talks or listens to a patient, he is also touching them with his hands so as to be less likely to misunderstand; and it is as though, when he is physically examining a patient, they were also conversing" (77).

What motivates a physician to engage in such relationships with patients? There is, of course, the wish for excellence as well as the need to be fully actualized as a practitioner of the art and science of medicine. There are love and respect for humankind and the desire to be helpful to others. But Berger hits upon other attributes of Sassall's character that he believes drive him to such excellence—his curiosity and imagination: "He has an appetite for experience which keeps pace with his imagination and which has not been suppressed. It is the impossibility of satisfying any such appetite for new experience which kills the imagination of most people in our society" (78). Berger continues:

> When patients are describing their conditions or worries to Sassall, instead of nodding his head or murmuring "yes," he says again and again "I know," "I know." He says it with genuine sympathy. Yet it is what he says whilst he is waiting to know more. He already knows what it is like to be this patient in a certain condition: but he does not yet know the full explanation of that condition, nor the extent of his own power. (81)

THE USE OF IMAGINATION

As Sassall reconceived his role with his patients and lessened the emotional distance between them, he used his imagination to envision who the patient *is* and where the patient "lives" in the unfolding narrative of his or her life.

Sassall was then able to employ his "imaginative 'proliferation' of himself in 'becoming' one patient after another" (Berger 1967, 143). This capacity is captured in the words of the physician and writer William Carlos Williams:

> I lost myself in the very properties of their minds; for the moment at least I actually *became* them, whoever they should be, so that when I detached myself from them at the end of a half-hour of intense concentration over some illness which was affecting them, it was as though I were reawakening from a sleep. For the moment I myself did not exist, nothing of myself affected me. As a consequence I came back to myself, as from any other sleep, rested. (1948, 356; italics in original)

Berger presents an encounter between Sassall and a sixteen-year-old girl who entered his office crying. She could not tell him what was the matter: "I just feel sort of miserable" (Berger 1967, 31). He gently but persistently ran down his list of possibilities:

> "What's getting you down?"
> No answer.
> "Sore throat?"
> "Not now."
> "Water-works all right?"
> She nodded.
> "Have you got a temperature?"
> She shook her head.
> "Periods regular?"
> "Yeah."
> "When was your last one?"
> "Last week."
> The doctor paused.
> "Do you remember that rash that you used to get on your tum? Has it ever come back?"
> "No."
> He leaned forward in his chair towards her.
> "You just feel weepy?" (31–32)

Sassall then inquired how she felt about her work. "It's a job," she replied. As he continued to probe her feelings about her job—determinedly, for he knew that he was now on the right track—she finally confessed, "It's terrible, that laundry. I hate it" (33). Sassall asked the young woman what she would like to do. She had always wanted to be a secretary. How much education did she have? It turned out that she left school early. He wrote a note to excuse her from work for a few days and asked her to come back to discuss her options.

> "You can come up again on Wednesday and I'll phone the Labour Exchange and we'll talk about what they say." "I'm sorry," she said, beginning to cry

again. "Don't be sorry. The fact that you're crying means that you've got imagination. If you didn't have imagination, you wouldn't feel so bad. Now go to bed and stay there tomorrow." (33)

In this dialogue with his patient, Sassall did not perceive her crying merely as a sign of disease or reduce this human expression of pain to a biological indicator of depression that would prompt the writing of a prescription. He neither ignored her tears nor ran from them. This young woman's crying had meaning to Sassall in the context of her illness. Her tears signified that she hated the way her life was going, that she wanted more. But she did not possess the capacity to imagine how she might find her way out, or the resources to do anything about it.

Although the patient was able to recognize that *something* was wrong with her life, she needed Sassall to help her identify *what* was wrong and *how* she could remedy it. Sassall recognized that if she was unable to imagine herself into a new place in her life and to change her circumstances accordingly, she would likely return to his office time and again with symptoms she could not explain. As with his other patients, he had to use *his* imagination to put into words "some of what they know but cannot think" (109). He moved beyond viewing the external "landscape"—that of an attractive young woman "with her whole life in front of her"—to exploring her internal world. He considered all of the circumstances impinging upon this young woman that contributed to her illness. By imagining what it would be like to *be* in her particular situation, he achieved a depth of understanding of her plight. Sassall then envisioned who she might *become* so that he could assist his patient in taking the first steps toward a new life.

DR. SASSALL'S PRACTICE OF NARRATIVE MEDICINE

In *A Fortunate Man*, Berger's commentary on Sassall's work captures the substance of narrative medicine: he creates stories out of Sassall's clinical experience. These are stories about the patient, about Sassall himself, and about the physician-patient relationship. Information is transformed into words and words into new knowledge—narrative knowledge. Narrative knowledge provides a way for physicians to gain a fuller grasp of their patients' illnesses beyond the bioscience of the disease with which they present. This in turn requires that the physician be attuned to his or her own emotional reactions to his or her patients. As Rita Charon explains:

As the physician listens to the patient, he or she follows the narrative thread of the story, *imagines* the situation of the teller (the biological, familial, cultural, and existential situation), *recognizes* the multiple and often contradictory meanings of the words used and the events described, and in

some ways *enters into and is moved by* the narrative world of the patient. . . .
[A]cts of diagnostic listening enlist the listener's *interior resources* . . . to
identify meaning. (2001a, 1898–99; italics added)

Much like a sonogram sending out sound waves that reach internal
structures, which then return echoes that can be fashioned into a three-
dimensional representation of the patient's interior, the physician uses his
feelings—as they resonate with those of his patient—as a means of creating
a picture of what is taking place inside the other person's psyche. In Berger's
words, "Sassall accepts his innermost feelings and intuitions as clues. His
own self is often the most promising starting point. His aim is to find what
may be hidden in others" (1967, 102). This way of working is what psychoanalysts mean when they speak of utilizing their own emotional responses in
the countertransference, and Berger evinces a psychoanalytic sensibility
when he adds of Sassall: "He confesses to fear without fear. He finds all
impulses natural—or understandable. He remembers what it is like to be a
child" (108).

Sassall achieved narrative competence only after he re-envisioned the
physician-patient relationship as one between two human beings—an intersubjective experience where each has his or her own distinct role. He came
to recognize his patient as a human being experiencing an illness, not an
object taken over by a disease. The physician who can develop such acute
diagnostic skills and who can refine his treatment procedure to fit the individual in need of help may indeed be described as fortunate.

TRANSFORMATIONS

Physicians who use themselves in this manner to explore the patient's inner
and outer worlds must engage in a disciplined process of self-inquiry that
leads to better self-understanding. It is physicians' good fortune to spend their
life's work engaged in a profession where—hand in hand with developing
proficiency in helping others—they may increase their own humanity and
learn to grapple with the dilemmas that they too must face in life. Charon
describes this as being granted "access to knowledge—about the *patient* and
about *myself*—that would otherwise have remained out of reach" (2001b, 84;
italics added). Such experiences may be transformative for physicians who
avail themselves of the opportunities for personal and professional growth
through relationships with their patients. As Berger says of Sassall, "He cures
others to cure himself" (1967, 77).

When physicians are willing to engage in this process, they are much
more likely to find their work meaningful; they are less likely to become
"burned out" by the daily impact of their patients' suffering and of the
emotional demands placed on them. This statement is only apparently

paradoxical. The conventional wisdom that doctors must achieve great emotional distance from patients in order to protect themselves has led to the creation of a therapeutic relationship that often proves to be emotionally deadening for the physician. Doctors who function predominantly as detached observers often feel more like human "doings" than human "beings."

Most physicians enter medicine because they wish to engage in helping relationships with patients. But years of clinical practice as "objective" participants in the physician-patient relationship may lead to robotic interactions and fewer opportunities for personal and professional growth. The physician who is emotionally present and sufficiently attuned—while at the same time maintaining his or her psychological separateness from the patient—is more likely to find clinical work satisfying over time (Horowitz et al. 2003).[9]

THE DOCTOR'S STORY AND THE PATIENT'S STORY

Though written nearly forty years ago, A Fortunate Man affords an extraordinary introduction to elements of both contemporary psychoanalytic practice and narrative medicine. This text demonstrates to today's physicians an approach that may assist them in creating situations in which clinical practice will be meaningful and self-sustaining. By listening to the patient from the perspective that a narrative can unfold through the doctor-patient relationship, the physician gains the capacity to create stories from what may appear to be the disparate elements of the patient's history and physical examination as they emerge in the clinical moment. The narrative act transforms an identified patient into a human being.

Undoubtedly, primary care physicians are constantly confronted by the *subjective experience* that is generated, in Berger's words, by "the anguish of dying, of loss, of fear, of loneliness, of being desperately beside oneself, of the sense of futility" (1967, 113). To witness the patient's suffering is itself "a hidden, subjective experience—the generalized impact on a doctor's imagination of the suffering which he meets almost daily and which cannot be settled by writing prescriptions" (126). In order to make creative use of such moments, the physician must identify his or her own subjective experience with that of the patient and have sufficient understanding of his or her own emotional life. Knowingly or unknowingly, the physician may feel that the patient's story too closely approaches his or her own life story—or the story that the doctor fears his or her life may become. As a consequence, the doctor may *react* (through withdrawal or overinvolvement) rather than *reflect* on the experience. But by the disciplined practices of self-reflection and self-inquiry that lead to self-understanding, difficult clinical moments may lead physicians to learn more about themselves.[10]

CONCLUSION

The story of Dr. John Sassall teaches us that medical practice characterized by the approach to the physician-patient relationship espoused by both narrative medicine and contemporary psychoanalysis creates a fortunate situation for both patient and doctor. It is certainly fortunate that the same process designed to create diagnostic and therapeutic stories from what the patient brings to the doctor—and one that fosters engagement with the patient as a fellow human being—may also teach the physician ways to be a more complete clinician. And it is fortunate that interacting with patients in this manner may lead to more meaningful and satisfying clinical work. It may even be true that this process can come to assist the physician in achieving better self-understanding and a richer grasp of his or her own life story.

NOTES

1. Henry Smith comments appositely on the process of psychoanalytic treatment: "In analysis we are continuously doing 'two things at once,' consciously or involuntarily, as we proceed with the analysis of the patient, which is our aim, and simultaneously extend our own self-understanding, which is our good fortune" (1997, 29).

2. See, for example, Charon (1986; 1993; 1994; 2001a; and 2001b) and Greenhalgh and Hurwitz (1998; 1999).

3. McWilliams (2004) organizes the elements of the psychoanalytic sensibility under the following rubrics: curiosity and awe, complexity, identification and empathy, subjectivity and attunement to affect, attachment, and faith.

4. When asked what attributes must be possessed by a good creative writer, Wallace Stegner (1988) replied: "Ultimately, what one looks for is sensibility . . . and sensibility is essentially *senses*. One looks for evidence that eyes and ears are acute and active, and that there is some capacity to find words for conveying what the senses perceive and what sense perceptions do to the mind that perceives them" (16).

5. It is likely that Sassall's systematic self-inquiry through reading Freud was of immense benefit to his understanding of his patients and, to a lesser degree, of himself. But such solitary introspection only rarely achieves results similar to what may be accomplished by engaging in a therapeutic process with a psychotherapist or psychoanalyst. The latter may not only lead to an expansion of self-understanding, it may also help one to learn ways of listening to oneself and to others that can be especially valuable to physicians in their work with patients.

6. For a probing commentary on the distinction between illness (the biological or physiological event) and disease (the social and existential dilemma in the context of the individual's personality and social network), see Weinstein (2003, xxvii).

7. The term *angle of repose* refers to "the greatest angle between two planes which is consistent with stability" (*Shorter Oxford English Dictionary*, fifth ed., s.v. "angle of repose"). It is an apt metaphor for the solutions patients may discover when encoun-

tering the forces of internal conflict (as when the wish for a fulfilling life is opposed by the need for punishment) and corresponding internal representations of the self and others. These are resolutions that may create psychic stability, but often lead to a degree of emotional deadening.

8. See William Carlos Williams's story, "The Use of Force" (1950), for a moving example of how—even in the context of a desperate wish to heal—a challenge to a physician's therapeutic potency may generate powerful emotional forces within him that compel him to overpower the patient.

9. This recent study reports that "nearly all the doctors" who engaged in narrative writing about their clinical encounters "described nontechnical, humanistic interaction with patients as experiences that fulfilled them and reaffirmed their commitment to medicine. Rather than recounting tales of diagnostic triumph, they uniformly told stories about crossing from the world of biomedicine into their patient's world. They described how relationships deepened through recognizing the common ground of each person's humanity" (Horowitz et al. 2003, 773–74).

10. In his introduction to *The Doctor Stories*, Robert Coles (1984) quotes Williams's eloquent remarks on what the physician may learn from such clinical experiences: "as William Carlos Williams appreciated, 'There's nothing like a difficult patient to show us ourselves. . . . I would learn so much on my rounds, or making home visits. . . . I was put off guard again and again and the result was—well, a descent into myself'" (xiii).

REFERENCES

Berger, John. 1962. *Toward reality: Essays in seeing*. New York: Knopf.

———. 1967. *A fortunate man: The story of a country doctor*. New York: Vintage Books, 1997.

———. 1971. *The look of things*. New York: Viking, 1974.

———. 1972. *Ways of seeing*. London: Penguin.

———. 1980. *About looking*. New York: Pantheon.

———. 1985. *The sense of sight*. New York: Pantheon.

Charon, Rita. 1986. To render the lives of patients. *Literature and Medicine* 5:58–74.

———. 1993. Medical interpretation: Implications of literary theory of narrative for clinical work. *Journal of Narrative and Life History* 3:79–97.

———. 1994. Narrative accuracy in the clinical setting. *Medical Encounter* 11:20–23.

———. 2001a. Narrative medicine: A model for empathy, reflection, profession, and trust. *Journal of the American Medical Association* 286:1897–1902.

———. 2001b. Narrative medicine: Form, function, and ethics. *Annals of Internal Medicine* 134:83–87.

Coles, Robert. 1984. Introduction to *William Carlos Williams: The doctor stories*. New York: New Directions, 1984. vii–xvi.

Greenhalgh, Trisha, and Brian Hurwitz. 1998. *Narrative based medicine*. London: BMJ Books.

———. 1999. Narrative based medicine: Why study narrative? *British Medical Journal* 318:48–50.

Horowitz, Carol, Anthony Suchman, William Branch, and Richard Frankel. 2003. What do doctors find meaningful about their work? *Annals of Internal Medicine* 138:772–75.

McWilliams, Nancy. 2004. The psychoanalytic sensibility. In *Psychoanalytic psychotherapy: A practitioner's guide*, 27–45. New York: Guilford Press.

Smith, Henry. 1997. Resistance, enactment, and interpretation: A self-analytic study. *Psychoanalytic Inquiry* 17:13–30.

Stegner, Wallace. 1988. *On the teaching of creative writing*. Ed. E. C. Lathem. Hanover, NH: University Press of New England.

Weinstein, Arnold. 2003. *A scream goes through the house: What literature teaches us about life*. New York: Random House.

Williams, William Carlos. 1948. The practice. In *The autobiography of William Carlos Williams*, 356–62. New York: New Directions, 1967.

———. 1950. The use of force. In *The doctor stories*, ed. Robert Coles, 56–60. New York: New Directions, 1984.

PART III

The Patient's Voice

NINE

Learning How to Tell

LISA J. SCHNELL

Perhaps the only way to overcome a traumatic severance of body
and mind is to come back to mind through the body. We recall
how voice dries up, and chokes its way out again.
                        —Geoffrey Hartman, "On Traumatic
                              Knowledge and Literary Studies"

IT IS MARCH 1997; my daughter Claire is four months old. My mother-in-law is
staying with us until May so that we can get through the semester. My husband,
Andrew, and I are working; our other daughter, Emma, who is three, is at day
care three days a week. We are all learning how to take care of Claire. We are
"going through the motions," hardly an original phrase but an apt one. Nothing
seems particularly motivated anymore. I know I need to take care of Claire and
Emma; I know I'm not doing a particularly good job of it. Oh, they are both fed,
and clean, and warm; they are held and kissed, played with, and read to. The
motions we are going through are the right ones. And yet there is a roaring blank
space just outside of our little sphere of motion that threatens to destroy me.

Two months previously, in mid-January, after almost eight weeks of my
insisting over and over again that something was horribly wrong with my

I am grateful to the Open Society Institute's Project on Death in America for the fellowship that first allowed me the time and space to begin to tell my story. This chapter also bears witness to some of the papers I heard and to many of the generous and
stimulating conversations I had with participants at the Psychoanalysis and Narrative
Medicine conference.

baby, after we'd seen at least four doctors, including a pediatric neurologist, and after I'd finally agreed to see a psychologist to talk about the possibility of postpartum depression, Claire had what was obviously a seizure and was finally admitted to the hospital for a battery of inpatient tests. The MRI showed that her brain was smooth and that some important-sounding things were missing: a corpus callosum, a septum pellucidim, words I'd never even heard before. The doctors told us that something had happened very early on, maybe as early as eight weeks into the pregnancy: a neuron didn't migrate from one developing hemisphere of her brain to the other. Like a smudge on a blueprint, someone said. It feels much worse than a smudge: she will never see, or walk, or talk, or even really recognize us. She will not necessarily even "think," at least not in the way we imagine thinking. She will have constant seizures, some tiny—the subtle twitching I have noticed since she was just hours old—but many of them big and bad, intractable, impervious to drug treatment. If we shun "heroic medical intervention"—tubes and vents and all that sort of thing—she will live perhaps a year or two, the doctors tell us. They have a name for this horror, a sibilant terror of a word: lissencephaly.

I don't sleep much anymore; I eat sporadically. Some days I am ravenous, but there are days in a row when all I can eat is a little breakfast. It's not quite that I'm not hungry; it's that I can't stand to have anything in my mouth, in my throat. I can't swallow. At one point I am struck by the fact that my problem with food, though quite clearly an emotional one, mirrors Claire's. She, too, cannot swallow properly; she is starting to aspirate, just as they said she would when those protective little fat pads start to recede from her cheeks and the musculature starts to change in her throat. And then my muscles start to twitch, subtly at first and then a little more insistently and much more frequently. What started as an occasional twitch in my left calf muscle has now become a twitching in both my legs and sometimes in my hands. There is a muscle on the left side of my face that thrums gently but persistently; the muscles around my right eye start to spasm when I am tired. It is not noticeable to anyone but me, and it doesn't interfere at all with any of the deliberate things I do with my muscles. But it bothers me, and it does begin to occur to me that my body is imitating Claire's in a very subtle but unmistakable way.

I imagine all the horrible things it could be. I've never been a hypochondriac, but I'm so steeped in the epistemology of diagnosis at this point that I spend almost all my time, when I'm not diagnosing Claire, diagnosing myself. It's MS, I think for a while. In fact, I'm pretty convinced of it. But then there's an article in the paper about Jacobs-Kreutzfeld syndrome (mad cow disease as it manifests itself in humans), and I'm sure that's it. Or maybe it's ALS (Lou Gehrig's disease). Or Parkinson's. A friend of my neighbor, a previously healthy man in his late forties, has just been diagnosed with Parkinson's. I ask after him in a way that I hope does not reveal the obsessive self-interest that

I am truly ashamed of but that I am in total thrall to: I ask only because I want to compare his symptoms to my own.

I call my doctor, whom I haven't seen since my last physical, about two years previous. I tell him about the twitches (not about any of my own speculative diagnoses) and he asks me if I've been taking any "funny drugs." The question is so completely absurd to me that it sits outside the range of my comprehension for a few seconds. "Oh good god, no!" I finally respond, laughing, trying to imagine what all this would feel like in an alternative reality. And so he asks me to come in for a visit.

My doctor is a very smart, very engaging man whom I've known for about four years and who is properly sympathetic about my situation, even truly compassionate. He takes a lot of time in this first visit just to listen. He then does a bunch of rudimentary neurological tests (close my eyes and touch my nose; close my eyes and hold my arms out to the side; balance on one leg and then the other), asks me how much I'm sleeping, how much I'm eating, and reassures me that I almost certainly don't have a degenerative neurological disease (I have, by this time, revealed to him some of my specific fears about my symptoms). "What you have," he tells me without a trace of condescension or dismissal, "is stress. What you need to do is go into a corner and cry for about a week, and you can't do that because you have people to take care of. Your body is behaving in a perfectly normal way—it's telling you that you need to take better care of *yourself*. You need to sleep more, eat more, and probably let yourself cry a little more." He tells me to try to get more exercise: endorphins will make me feel better emotionally, and the physical exertion should start paying off in better sleep patterns. He tells me that I am doing amazingly well given the circumstances, that I am brave and kind of inspiring. He tells me how much he admires me. I feel a little embarrassed about the last bit—I *feel* neither brave nor in any way inspiring; I certainly do not feel admirable. But for a second or two I am relieved of the pressure of myself. I enjoy the fact that even though he might be way off in his estimation of my courage—maybe *because* he is way off in his estimation of my courage—I get to be someone other than the grieving, self-obsessed person I've become, even if it's just for a moment. Perhaps owing to this momentary relief of the burden of my own self, but mainly owing to his compassionate reassurances about my health, I leave feeling a lot more hopeful than when I walked into the examination room.

But the twitching doesn't go away. And now I'm feeling light-headed a lot of the time, like my brain is not quite attached to the rest of my body. The only time I feel well is when I'm running—and I'm running a lot: about thirty miles per week. And yet, in spite of my now obvious physical fitness, I remain obsessed with my own health in a way that I know is not healthy. I can't help it: I am convinced that I am going to die. "Whatever got Claire has gotten me," I think, feeling sure that some environmental poison has attacked us both. My fear is almost entirely private. I reveal just the edges of it to my doctor, whom I am now seeing in follow-up visits every four or five weeks at his insistence. But I am intensely aware that I am already asking for and receiving more from all the people in my life than any one person could expect. And Andrew and I are just barely holding on to our lives as it is; I know I can't burden him with a whole new set of fears and worries. I can see in his own worry lines, his own preoccupation, that he is as close to falling apart as I am.

By June, my doctor wonders whether it might not be time for me to consider getting a little pharmaceutical help. At the very least, I need to try to break the cycle of night waking that I'm in: I go to bed and fall immediately asleep, only to wake at 2 or 3 a.m. to hours of sleeplessness. At first this happens only sporadically, but by the time Claire is eight months old, I am sleeping the whole night through perhaps only one night out of ten. Desperate, I agree, and he prescribes a very low dose of a tricyclic antidepressant, a drug that should help specifically with the night waking. Having never taken any kind of antidepressant before, I am wary of the effects the drug will have on me. And my wariness seems justified: not only are these drugs completely ineffective in keeping me asleep, they actually make me feel as though I'm on speed—my body is just sort of buzzing all the time. I want to stop taking them immediately, but my doctor tells me over the phone that such a sudden cessation would likely bring on seizures. Seizures—the coincidences just keep on coming. So there is a careful weaning after which he prescribes a drug in the Valium family which only makes me slow and stupid. And then, finally, Klonopin—a "homeopathic dose," he says. But it doesn't matter how little I'm taking; it matters only that I am now taking the same medication that Claire is on for her seizures. I can't ignore the coincidences anymore. And, though I'm finally sleeping a little better, the twitching is not going away.

A few weeks later I am sitting in an examination room recounting yet again my symptoms when this man who has been so tremendously patient with me suddenly seems to lose that patience. "Lisa," he says sharply, surprising me, "is there something really bad happening to you?" I look at him in confusion. "That's why I'm here," I say, "*You're* the one who's supposed to tell me that." "Lisa," he repeats, and he pronounces my name a little too forcefully, as some people do when they're speaking to someone whose native language is not their own, "is there something really bad happening to you?" "Do you want me to tell you?" I ask, grappling for some footing in this odd exchange, thinking that maybe he's come to the end of his diagnostic powers and is asking me to intuit what it is I'm suffering from. Again, he repeats his question, each word fenced off from the others. Confused and a little scared, I can only stutter, "I don't know, I just don't know anymore." Then the sharpness is gone and he says to me, as though he's resigned to the futility of this exchange and maybe even a little sad about it, "Lisa, something really bad *is* happening to you . . . but it isn't this." And I sit there in paralyzed silence as he gets out a pen and writes me a referral to a neurologist. Handing me the referral, he tells me to schedule my regular follow-up for four weeks out, and he walks out of the room, shutting the door quietly behind him.

※

In the days and weeks after this exchange the obvious began to dawn on me: the fact that my symptoms were imitating Claire's had nothing to do with an external event or any sort of mystery illness that was attacking me. The body has an amazing way of "thinking" for itself. And my body was doing the only thing it could do to connect me with my child—it was imitating her. Freud (1914) says that "parental love, which is so moving and at bottom so childish, is nothing but the parents' narcissism born again, which, transformed into object-love, unmistakably reveals its former nature" (91). The fact that I could not answer what was, in fact, a very simple question made it clear that I was stuck in this first-order parental narcissism that Freud describes: I had not been able to put any distance at all between Claire and myself. Trapped by a diagnosis, I had not managed the parental transition to object-love, even this counterfeit object-love that Freud refers to, and my body was acting out the narcissistic predicament I found myself in. I thought about the time before Claire was diagnosed, when I would spend hour after hour just trying to get her attention and feeling terrified about the yawning space between us, a space of unknowability. When she was diagnosed, I felt desperate about my realization that I would never be able to know what my own child was feeling, that each door to her lived, everyday reality was completely locked to me. My incapacity to accept that situation, to leave the narcissistic impulse behind and find another way to love my child, was now made manifest in what my body was doing. I will know her, my viscera seemed to be insisting, even if it means leaving the conscious mind behind.

Freud wrote "On Narcissism" in 1914, but he had been thinking about the concept of narcissism for a long time before that, and he thought about it for a long time afterward. Certainly the concept lies at the absolute center of object relations theory; the Introduction to "On Narcissism" calls it the "necessary intermediate stage between auto-eroticism and object-love" (69). If, in 1914, Freud was struggling to articulate the concept—he was said to have been deeply dissatisfied with "On Narcissism" (Strachey 1957, 70)—by 1920 he had lived with the concept long enough to transform it into the kind of richly narrative theory that characterizes his most memorable writing. It was one of these stories that I was especially drawn to as I began to work through what had happened in that examination room.

In *Beyond the Pleasure Principle* (1920), Freud tells the story of an eighteen-month-old boy, greatly attached to his mother, yet who, as Freud tells us with some admiration, "never cried when his mother left him for a few hours" (14). "This good little boy, however," writes Freud,

> had an occasional disturbing habit of taking any small objects he could get hold of and throwing them away from him into a corner, under the bed, and so on, so that hunting for his toys and picking them up was often quite a business. As he did this he gave vent to a loud, long-drawn-out "o-o-o-o," accompanied by an expression of interest and satisfaction. His mother and the writer of the present account were agreed in thinking that this was not a mere interjection but represented the German word *"fort"* ["gone"]. I eventually realized that it was a game and that the only use he made of any of his toys was to play "gone" with them. (14–15)

Watching the boy one day, Freud sees him take a wooden reel by the string and throw it over the edge of his curtained cot, uttering, as it disappears, the expressive "o-o-o-o." For the first time, however, Freud witnesses the child complete the "gone" game: the little boy pulls the reel back into the cot, declaring joyfully as it reappears, *"da"* ("there"). "The interpretation of the game then became obvious," says Freud. "It was related to the child's great cultural achievement—the instinctual renunciation (that is, the renunciation of instinctual satisfaction) which he had made in allowing his mother to go away without protesting. He compensated himself for this, as it were, by himself staging the disappearance and return of the objects within his reach" (15). The young boy had mastered the traumatic disappearance of his mother with a narrative: something is lost, something is found. It is the shortest story ever, but it is, even in its brevity, a kind of creative compensation both in act and in language—*fort* and *da* being among the very first words the child speaks—for something that clearly caused him a great deal of emotional pain, the most pain, perhaps, that a healthy toddler can feel.

The child's game is, of course, deeply narcissistic. It may be a kind of dress rehearsal of mature object love, but the child's own ego is still entirely at the center of the game: *he* throws the toy away, *he* reels it back. Furthermore, the game is played entirely for his own benefit; no one can play this game *with* him. But Freud's realization that a version of this game is played by adults under the name of artistic play indicates that the compensatory nature of the act of return—which is what most interests Freud in the *fort-da* game— is also a crucial part of the mature life of the ego. The fact that mature works of art, which, as Freud says, "are aimed at an audience" (1920, 17), can somehow, in the case of tragedy for instance, transform the most painful experiences into a highly enjoyable experience for the spectators is "convincing proof that, even under the dominance of the pleasure principle, there are

ways and means enough of making what is in itself unpleasurable into a subject to be recollected and worked over in the mind" (17).

Freud's move in this direction suggests not only that the playing of the
game allows the little boy to compensate for the temporary loss of his mother,
but also that the particularly narrative aspect of the game makes it so effective. Freud becomes interested in the child's game when he can finally understand it as a *story*. It is not a story if the only thing that happens in the plot
is "gone"; it becomes a story when the child completes the plot with the
return of the toy. But neither is the toy simply lost and found, for Freud's rendition of the game also places a great deal of emphasis on the fact that the
child *narrates* the story and that the narration consists of some of the child's
very first words. Though Freud does not say so directly, it is clear that part of
the child's triumph is linguistic and narrative. His words and the very brief
story they tell are a kind of compensation; they contribute to the child's
process of grieving. In fact, I need only look to the bottom of the page in
Freud's text for proof of the linguistic significance of the game and how that
relates to grief.

In a footnote that appears toward the end of his discussion of the *fort-da*
game, Freud writes, "When this child was five and three-quarters, his mother
died. Now that she was really 'gone' ('o-o-o'), the little boy showed no signs
of grief" (1920, 16n1). Freud does not say that the child is his grandson, that
the boy's mother was Freud's daughter Sophie. And yet here, buried in a footnote, is a startling and deeply moving expression of Freud's own grief at
Sophie's death. "O-o-o," he says, in parentheses, even though at almost six
years old the child would certainly be able to say "*fort*." The *fort-da* game of
the footnote is Freud's. His use of the child's prearticulate stammer in his
attempt to repeat the game testifies movingly to the profundity of Freud's
grief at the loss of his beloved daughter. In a sense, he needs to learn how to
talk again. He also needs to learn how to tell, for Freud's appropriation of the
game's narrative is notably incomplete: he cannot get past "gone."

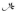

In their book, *The Brain and the Inner World* (2002), Mark Solms and Oliver
Turnbull, both neuro-psychoanalysts, provide us with an enormously sugges-
tive way of thinking about what the *fort-da* game teaches us about grief and
language. Through their work with patients with right-brain lesions, Solms
and Turnbull try to understand the relationship between the patients' disorders in spatial cognition, disorders that characterize right-hemisphere syndrome, and their fragile emotional lives. All of these patients exhibit a
marked inability to discern or comprehend actual physical space. They cannot, for instance, "draw a bicycle without misaligning the component parts;
they cannot copy a simple construction made with children's blocks; and they

cannot learn the route from their bed to the toilet" (260). Solms and Turn-bull also notice, however, that many of the patients discussed also present with anosognosia, the primary symptom of which is a complete unawareness of illness. These patients, many of whom are completely paralyzed on the left side of their bodies, insist that they are entirely well. As the authors say, "The lack of awareness of their incapacities, and the rationalizations con-cerning their problems, extend to the point of delusion. . . . These patients seem prepared to believe anything, so long as it excludes admitting that they are ill" (262).

The tendency has been to understand anosognosia as a manifestation of the problems in spatial cognition that are more obviously on display in peo-ple with damage to the right part of their brains: the patients insist that they are well because they have no perception of the left side of their bodies. Yet in their psychotherapeutic sessions with some of these patients, Solms and Turnbull observed something that forced them to think differently about how anosognosia is related to spatial cognition. Two of the patients discussed, for instance, while displaying what Solms and Turnbull refer to as "classical emo-tional indifference to their disabilities," are nonetheless surprisingly fragile emotionally. "In their psychotherapy sessions," explain the authors, "both patients burst into tears for brief moments during which they seemed to be overwhelmed by emotions of the very kind that are normally conspicuous by their absence. This gave the impression of *suppressed* sadness, grief, depen-dency fears, and so on, rather than a true *absence* of such feelings" (266; ital-ics in original). Solms and Turnbull conclude that, rather than an inability to *experience* negative emotion (which would suggest that the anosognosia can be explained physiologically, as a direct effect of the damage to the brain), these patients cannot *tolerate* negative emotion, particularly feelings of loss (which would suggest that the anosognosia is psychological in origin, that it is *indirectly* associated with the brain damage). Solms and Turnbull thus refer to the patients' anosognosia as a "failure in the process of mourning" (270).

In "Mourning and Melancholia" (1915), written shortly after "On Nar-cissism," Freud says that the normal process of mourning, the description of which Solms and Turnbull use as their benchmark as well, eventually "impels the ego to give up the object by declaring the object to be dead and offering the ego the inducement of continuing to live" (257). In other words, the ego needs to give up the dead love object and seek out a new one, for it is pre-cisely the ego's attachment to a new object that will testify to the desire for continued life. Given the particular issues associated with their patients' medical circumstances, the question for Solms and Turnbull thus becomes: how could the ego's inability to search out another love object—its inability to mourn properly—be related to the rather obviously displayed disorders in spatial cognition that are particular to right-hemisphere syndrome?[1] Here is their answer to that question:

> The right perisylvian convexity is specialized for spatial cognition. Damage
> to this area therefore undermines the patients' ability to represent the rela-
> tionship between self and objects accurately. This in turn undermines object
> relationships in the psychoanalytic sense: object love (based on a realistic
> conception of the separateness between self and object) collapses, and the
> patients' object relationships regress to the level of narcissism. This results
> in narcissistic defenses against object loss, rendering these patients inca-
> pable of normal mourning. They deny their loss and all the feelings (and
> even *external* perceptions) associated with it, using a variety of defenses to
> shore up their denial whenever the intolerable reality threatens to break
> through. (270; italics in original)

Simply put, proper mourning requires the perception, or more accurately, the
renewed perception, of *space*. Patients who have lost their ability to conceive
of space, even in the most literal way, are thus denied the ability to mourn
that very loss. Put slightly differently, a problem with *spatial cognition* is also a
problem with *cognitive space*, which, as I am introducing it here, means an
internal space of perception, a psychological prospect that produces a space
outside of the self and the desire to go there.

Solms and Turnbull's remarkable, and remarkably moving, investigation
of the inner life of neurological patients led me to consider anew the implications of the game Freud watches his grandson play. I started with the most
obvious way in which the *fort-da* game acts out the child's growing awareness
of the concept of space, the separateness between him and his mother: he
throws the toy. He doesn't just put his blanket over it, or cover his eyes to
make it disappear, he makes it literally *go away*. When he reels it back in he
conquers the very space that he has created. The physical game is still a
deeply narcissistic kind of activity: the little boy controls every aspect of it;
he plays it entirely for his own benefit. Yet notably, Freud is interested not
only in the events of the game but also in the way in which the child narrates
those events. And indeed, it is that narration which, to my mind, gets most
suggestively at the ideas of space and mourning that Solms and Turnbull have
introduced.

Language is inherently representational; its very nature, in other
words, is to *stand for* something else—an object, a concept, a feeling. To
use language deliberately, therefore, is an acknowledgment of space, of
the cognitive distance between the thing itself and that with which we
represent the thing. For the little boy, who uses some of his very first
words to narrate his game, the most significant—because it is the most
unconscious—acknowledgment of the space he sees opening up between
his mother and him comes in the use of language. That the words also tell
a story—a very short story, but a story nonetheless—suggests that the
child has in fact proceeded quite far in his unconscious acknowledgment

of distance, for the story functions as a form of consolation to the child—something is lost, something is found. The literary theorist Terry Eagleton (1996) puts it this way:

> Something must be lost or absent in any narrative for it to unfold: if everything stayed in place there would be no story to tell. This loss is distressing, but exciting as well: desire is stimulated by what we cannot quite possess, and this is one source of narrative satisfaction. If we could *never* possess it, however, our excitation might become intolerable and turn into unpleasure; so we must know that the object will be finally restored to us. . . . Our excitation is gratifyingly released: our energies have been cunningly "bound" by the suspenses and repetitions of the narrative only as a preparation for their pleasurable expenditure. (161; italics in original)

In *Beyond the Pleasure Principle* (1920), we remember, Freud talked about mature art as possessing "ways and means enough of making what is in itself unpleasurable into a subject to be recollected and worked over in the mind" (17). Even if mature art does that best, any complete narrative—as Eagleton defines it—accomplishes something of that by creating distance in its imitation of life. The child does not actually throw his mother away—a story that could never console because it is exactly what he fears—he throws a toy. The action of his story and the words he uses to narrate it are *imitative* of his fear, but they are not, significantly, the fear itself. Aristotle, the first and probably the greatest theorist of narrative, called this imitation or representation *mimesis*. And it is the "very contrivance and artifice of *mimesis*," says the philosopher Richard Kearney (2002), that "detaches us from the action unfolding before us, affording us sufficient *distance* to grasp the meaning of it all" (138; italics added). *Fort-da*, seen in this context, is perhaps best understood, then, as a game of mourning.

In this way, we might think of Freud's recollection of the *fort-da* game in the footnote he added after the death of his daughter as a way of rewitnessing the narrative act of consolation that, in his role as spectator, affords him some of the cognitive distance that he requires to do his own mourning. He cannot yet re-create the act of narrative consolation—his *fort* is not yet completed by a *da*—that will offer him "the inducement of continuing to live," but in his parenthetical "o-o-o," truly a first word as he has represented it, his ego takes a tentative step outside of the protective cocoon of narcissism toward the monumental work of mourning. It is a prearticulate expression of grief that Freud had almost certainly heard before, on the stage perhaps. For Freud's parenthetical howl is so like the similarly primitive "Howl, howl, howl" of Shakespeare's Lear over the dead body of his youngest daughter, Cordelia, as to be no mere coincidence. The echo is almost certainly unconscious, but there is no doubt as to the presence of Shakespeare in Freud's thinking and writing.[2]

⚜

Freud's narrative impasse, I came to realize, bears some resemblance to my own. In *Doctors' Stories* (1991, 123–47), Kathryn Montgomery Hunter discusses what she calls "narrative incommensurability," the fact that often doctors' stories about our illnesses and our own stories of our illnesses don't match. Hunter's book understands the difference between these two narratives as a detriment to the patient, yet in seeking out my doctor's advice and help I was in quest of exactly this difference. Almost certainly I knew that my physical response to being Claire's mom was ineluctable, but the narrative that made it so was too painful to articulate, too painful, even, to acknowledge. In seeking a "diagnosis"—terrified as I may have been about that—I was looking for another story, one that I could own even if I couldn't control it. Most doctors would, I think, have gladly cooperated with my quest: it is their job, after all, and a great deal of what makes their job interesting, to name and treat illness. Yet it was my doctor's very refusal to tell his own story about my illness that allowed me to regain my health. "Patients need more than the medical facts of their case," Hunter says, "they need to be able to translate that knowledge into the terms of their lives" (146). In my case, it was always and only about "the terms of my life"— that was the whole diagnosis. Amazingly, despite his considerable skill as a conventional practitioner of modern medicine, my doctor recognized that.

"I think I was mean to you last time." It is the first thing he says to me at our next appointment. I tell him that his cruelty, if that's what he thought it was, seems to have been necessary for I feel as if his question has quite literally saved my life. In the weeks and months since that appointment, as I slowly but certainly returned to health, I came to realize that my inability to recognize my own story was the result of my inability to pronounce *da*—to tell, to imagine, the whole of my and Claire's story. "Gone," I kept saying, "she is gone." And I had said it, or its equivalent, over and over and over again. There was no room for *da* at all. Unable to sustain the relentlessly fractional nature of this narrative event, my psyche, through my body, had begun to assert its own version of *da*: Claire would not be gone if I could become her, if I could imitate her. It was, in the long run, the wrong kind of imitation, not a healthy way of telling the story. I needed to find, as Kearney (2002) says, "sufficient distance to grasp the meaning of it all" (138), a better way to pull the reel back in.

The British psychoanalytic theorist D. W. Winnicott (1956), whose work on maternal-child relations owes much to Freud's theories of ego development, would no doubt have identified what I was going through as a (probably dysfunctional) version of "primary maternal preoccupation."[3] Winnicott describes a psychological, sometimes also somatic, condition in the weeks just before and after her child is born when the mother is in a "state of heightened sensitivity" (302) to the infant, a state that looks very much like the sort of parental narcissism Freud talked about. Winnicott sees this stage as absolutely necessary to the properly functioning parent-child relationship: the tiny infant, thoroughly helpless, needs a parent to be able to understand its needs and do the right thing. Primary maternal preoccupation gives the mother the special ability to do that. There is a fine line, though, between properly functioning primary maternal preoccupation and illness, as Winnicott makes explicitly clear when he calls it "almost an illness" and then goes on to say, in a parenthetical explanation, "(I bring in the word 'illness' because a woman must be healthy in order to develop this state and to recover from it as the infant releases her. If the infant should die, the mother's state suddenly shows up as illness. The mother takes this risk)" (302). The parenthesis speaks almost directly to my situation: my child did not immediately die, but my fears before the diagnosis and then the diagnosis itself functioned in much the same way as Winnicott imagines infant death would function. Claire could not release me; or perhaps more accurately, I could not release Claire, and what may have originally been a healthy and necessary identification with my child became, for a while, an illness that affected both of us.

I found the distance I needed first in other peoples' stories. Having given up fiction following Claire's diagnosis for the worst kinds of nonfiction—articles from medical journals mainly—I became, for a while, an absolutely fanatical reader of novels. They did not need to be novels about people in my own situation, for I found that, in fact, the plot of every novel—like the plot of the *fort-da* game—is in some significant way a story of loss. But the truth of it was, my compulsion to read had somewhat less to do with subject matter than it had to do with the simple fact of beautiful words on the page and the way they could draw me into the space that is the gap between the real and the expressed or imagined life. It was from that space—a cognitive space—that I could observe and reflect on the contours of loss without getting caught up in details that would take me back into the profound claustrophobia of my present life. I appreciated that the writers I was leaning on—Anne Michaels, Arundhati Roy, Allegra Goodman, Michael Ondaatje, Rohinton Mistry among others—knew not just what to tell, but *how* to tell. Richard Kearney (2002) describes this experience as the "curious conflation of empathy and detachment which produces in us—viewers of Greek tragedy or readers of contemporary fiction—the double vision necessary for a journey beyond the closed ego towards other possibilities of being" (13).

It was not a magic bullet; literature didn't make everything all better all of a sudden. Indeed, there were many times when I harbored all of the cynicism expressed by a character in a story by Lorrie Moore (1998): "I mean, the whole conception of 'the story,' of cause and effect, the whole idea that people have a clue as to how the world works is just a piece of laughable metaphysical colonialism perpetrated upon the wild country of time" (222). But the fact that that emotional outburst occurs in a *story* is an ironic testament to the ineluctable human need to participate in exactly that colonizing gesture. The "wild country of time" is a place where things only ever go missing; planting our narrative flags in its inhospitable soil and claiming a piece of its ground as our own, though perhaps ultimately a futile gesture, is nonetheless what we need to do to survive the pain of this life, to get to the "there" that must follow the "gone."[4]

I did, gradually but certainly, get better after my narrative revelation. I credit my return to literature with the restoration of the cognitive distance I needed to survive the trauma of Claire's diagnosis, to see my situation for what it was, to see Claire for who she was, and to understand my role as her mother for what it was: to admit to all the sadness but also to admit to my need and desire to survive that sadness. I carried (and still carry) a great deal of that sadness with me, but I nonetheless began to sleep better and eat better. I weaned myself off the Klonopin, and the twitches and light-headedness departed. There was no trip to the neurologist, there were no CAT scans, no MRIs, no muscle biopsies. Just a slow climb back to health. And an enduring sense of gratitude for, and the irony of, a medical doctor who was wise enough to give me a dose of my own medicine.

※

Claire Margaret Schnell Barnaby died at home, in the bed in which she was conceived, on June 1, 1998. She was eighteen months old and loved and treasured by more people than would seem possible for one so young and so compromised.

NOTES

1. Solms and Turnbull (2002, 270–71) note that, despite similarly devastating physical losses, patients who suffer from left-hemisphere syndrome do not present with anosognosia.

2. I am grateful to my colleague (and husband) Andrew Barnaby for pointing out to me this moving parallel.

3. I am grateful to one of the reviewers who read this paper for *Literature and Medicine* for drawing my attention to the Winnicott material.

4. Moore's wonderfully evocative phrase—"the wild country of time"—of course points to the issue of *temporal* distance in which theorists of narrative are at least as interested—if not more interested—as they are with the idea of cognitive distance that has been the focus of this chapter. And indeed, my own experience of grief and its association with narrative includes a profound sense of temporal as well as cognitive space. But that is the subject of another paper entirely.

REFERENCES

Eagleton, Terry. 1996. *Literary theory: An introduction.* Second ed. Minneapolis: University of Minnesota Press.

Freud, Sigmund. 1914. On narcissism: An introduction. In *The Standard Edition of the Complete Psychological Works* (hereafter S.E.), ed. and trans. James Strachey et al., 14:69–102. London: Hogarth Press, 1953–1974.

——. 1915. Mourning and melancholia. S.E., 14:239–60.

——. 1920. *Beyond the pleasure principle.* S.E., 18:3–64.

Hartman, Geoffrey H. 1995. On traumatic knowledge and literary studies. *New Literary History* 26:537–63.

Hunter, Kathleen Montgomery. 1991. *Doctors' stories: The narrative structure of medical knowledge.* Princeton: Princeton University Press.

Kearney, Richard. 2002. *On stories.* London: Routledge.

Moore, Lorrie. 1998. People like that are the only people here: Canonical babbling in peed onk. In *Birds of America*, 212–50. New York: Picador.

Solms, Mark, and Oliver Turnbull. 2002. *The brain and the inner world: An introduction to the neuroscience of subjective experience.* New York: Other Press.

Strachey, James. 1957. Introduction to Freud 1914. S.E., 14:69–71.

Winnicott, D. W. 1956. Primary maternal preoccupation. In *Collected papers: Through paediatrics to psychoanalysis*, 300–305. New York: Basic Books, 1958.

TEN

Imagining Immunity

ED COHEN

Imagination atrophies.
—Horkheimer and Adorno,
The Dialectic of Enlightenment

I HEAL THEREFORE I AM:
AN AUTOBIOGRAPHICAL OPENING

PROBABLY MORE than many people, I grew up in thrall to a metaphor—not that I knew this at the time. During the summer after eighth grade I began to experience uncontrollable diarrhea and wasting. Within the course of a few months, I went from being a husky, energetic, pubescent boy to a withered, incontinent, critically ill teen. Rather than starting high school with the rest of my cohort, I spent the fall adjusting to a different kind of institution: the hospital. After what felt like an eternity of probing, prodding, palpating, and x-raying, it was determined that I was suffering from an acute inflammatory bowel syndrome called Crohn's disease. When the doctors who were treating me tried to explain what Crohn's was, I heard the word "autoimmunity" for the first time. Now, for a thirteen-year-old I had a pretty big vocabulary, but this wasn't part of it, so they tried to break the word down for me. First one doctor told me: "Your immune system is attacking the lining of your small intestine. It's as if your body is rejecting part of itself." My face must have shown that I didn't get the concept, so another added: "Well, autoimmunity is like being allergic to yourself." Despite this clarification I was still adrift, so they tossed one more metaphoric life preserver my way: "It's as if you're eating yourself alive," they said. With this analogy they finally hauled me up onto the dry terrain of knowledge. Unfortunately, I lived on that cannibal island for almost twenty years. No doubt, the doctors who gave me these memorable images offered them as gifts of understanding. They really did seem to want to help. It is just that their metaphors weren't particularly safe for a thirteen-year-old's imagination. Or anyone's imagination, as far as I am concerned.

From my current perspective, I can see that one of my main medical problems was that the professionals who undertook my treatment didn't believe that metaphor had much to do with their practices. For them, the problems with my immune system were of the order of biochemical fact, as was my immune system itself. How they talked about it, how they thought about it, how they explained it, did not for them change the "it" to which they referred. The immune system was real: it did important things in the world and it was something medicine needed to know more about so that sick people like me could be helped. Not until a decade or so of medicalization later, after I had passed through another life-and-death encounter with my immune system, did I begin to glimpse that there might be problems of meaning as well as biology involved in my experience of living with an autoimmune disorder.

In my second year of graduate school, I was an acutely ill, twenty-three-year-old gay man living in the San Francisco Bay area. My doctors seemed unable to comprehend the complexity of my symptoms (which turned out to have been the result of an undetected bowel perforation that wreaked havoc within my abdominal cavity); consequently, they subjected me to a barrage of inconclusive tests that left no orifice unprobed. One day, after I had already submitted to exhaustive examinations by gastroenterologists, hematologists, radiologists, nuclear medicine experts, and infectious disease specialists, a new round of doctors came to my room to tell me about a deadly syndrome that had recently appeared among gay men in San Francisco. It seemed to be sexually transmitted and to destroy the immune system so that people died of horrible opportunistic infections. Then they asked me if I thought I might have it. Now given how sick I had been for the preceding ten years, it is probably no big surprise that sex had not been a major part of my life. Indeed, my response, "Not unless you believe in immaculate infection," provided the best laugh I have ever gotten from a medical audience.[1] Yet the force of their questions lingered. For years I had imagined that I suffered from an overzealous immune system that was attacking me from within, and now I was told that I might be suffering from a deficient immune system that could let otherwise harmless microbes overwhelm me from without. I just didn't get it. If the immune system was so real, then why could its effects be so contradictory?

During the ensuing months that I spent in the hospital, I had the leisure to consider the many things medical experts had been telling me about my illness. Slowly, it began to occur to me that there remained a bit of confusion both about what immunity was and about what biomedicine knew about it. Though I didn't perceive it then, retrospectively I believe that I encountered a contradiction deeply embedded in this metaphor, which limits the ways we imagine experiences inscribed under its name. At the time, however, I was much more focused on denying the gravity of what was happening to me, and so I tried to continue reading for my courses. Ironically—or prophetically, depending on how you like to interpret such coincidences—I was engaged in an independent study on the texts of Michel Foucault. Reading *Birth of the Clinic, Discipline and Punish,* and *The History of Sexuality* in my hospital bed affected me like a revelation. They gave me tools to reframe the ways my docile body was, and had been, enmeshed in the institutional plays of power/knowledge. They helped me to entertain the possibility that the "truth" of my illness might not be exhausted by the accounts that medical experts were giving me, much as I might desire that to be the case. For the first time in my extensive history of submitting to medical authority, I began to wonder if there might be something that the organism-that-I-am "knew" about my experience that might be important for my recovery, something that my doctors not only *did not* know, but that they *could not* know within their version of "the true." For the first time, I began to wonder how to make such a "knowledge" known to myself.

As a counterpoint to this intellectual awakening, my body was undergoing its own radical transformations. Descending into acute illness is an awesome process, materializing the organism's struggle to maintain its vitality even in the face of overwhelming challenges. Yet perhaps even more awesome than such physiological disintegration is the organismic capacity to return to health following such a metamorphic episode. After an artery in my small bowel ruptured, causing blood to start gushing out of my rectum and precipitating what I remember as a somewhat clichéd but nonetheless incredibly powerful out-of-body, near-death experience, I was rushed into emergency surgery where several feet of festering intestine were removed and abscesses in my liver were drained. While recovering from this surgery and receiving massive doses of IV antibiotics to help control the major infection that was ravaging my organs, I spontaneously began to put myself into trances—no doubt facilitated by all the drugs I was receiving. I would lie on my hospital bed, listening to tapes on my Walkman, and visualize wrapping a band of warm light around the surgical incisions. This was strictly pain management as far as I was concerned. No metaphysics was involved, since everything in my personal history mitigated against such a possibility. As I liked to say: my father was a physical chemist and my mother a communist, so materiality was all that mattered.

A few months later, when I was being discharged from the hospital, my surgeon told me that I had been one of the sickest people he had operated on in five years who was still alive, and that he had no idea how I had gotten well so quickly. His words stunned me—and not just because they broke through the denial that had sustained me during my hospitalization and made me consider how sick I had actually been. They also disoriented me because this was the first time I had ever heard one of my physicians admit that there were elements to healing that exceeded his understanding. For more than a decade I had trusted my physicians' knowledge implicitly, if perhaps unwisely (especially since I now realize that several of them were not terribly competent). Certainly, they seemed to know much more than I did about this strange and frightening phenomenon that had erupted in my bowels and disrupted my being. So what could the incredibly dashing and successful surgeon (who drove a blood red Porsche—to my mind the perfect metonym for his métier) mean when he said that he didn't understand how I had made the passage from the brink of death to the land of the living well with such alacrity? Reflecting on his comment years later in therapy, what struck me about his offhand remark was that what bioscience did not know about my experience might have been precisely what had enabled me to heal so rapidly.

Today I believe that what science does not and cannot know probably has as much to do with healing as what it does know. Now, don't get me wrong: I am incredibly grateful for the capabilities of Western medical practice and especially its most high-tech manifestations without which I would have died on several occasions. Moreover, I think that these practices excel the closer and closer we come to death (which is probably not unrelated to how the opening up of corpses functions both in biomedical history and in biomedical training). However, I am not so sure that they are as adept at addressing the ongoing experiences of illness that many of us diagnosed with chronic diseases endure, let alone at helping us imagine what healing from them might entail. And this assumes of course that we have access to such medical resources in the first place—which is not something that many people in the world today can presume.

Over the last twenty years, I have focused considerable attention on healing. Indeed, given how sick I had been throughout adolescence and early adulthood, my radical recovery and ongoing remission from the symptoms of Crohn's (with a few lapses here and there during periods of high anxiety and stress) has been quite miraculous—albeit a miracle that requires lots and lots of upkeep. By and large, these healing efforts have taken place outside the ambit of medical rationality. Among numerous nonmedical modalities, I have tried and deeply benefited from psychotherapy, guided imagery, massage, bodywork, somatics, meditation, acupuncture, herbs, homeopathy, rolfing, tai chi, yoga, movement workshops, auric cleansing, and psychic counseling, to name a few. Beyond their specific benefits, which were quite significant, these practices have collectively taught me to appreciate and *to value* the organismic capacity for healing. Moreover, they have helped me to recognize what I would now call "corporeal intelligence," an intelligence that obtains both beneath and beyond the order of the individual, and which went unrecognized and unappreciated throughout my extensive and intensive encounters with biomedicine.[2] In fact, so long as my attention was exclusively focused on the insistent problems with my immune system, healing seemed to be a non sequitur.

Of course, there is nothing inevitable about this exclusionary attention; however, I do believe there is something systematic about it. Having had my imagination not only shaped by, but thoroughly invested in, the bioscientific understanding of Crohn's disease, it never occurred to me to consider that healing had been rendered anachronistic within the increasingly high-tech discourse of immunology. Only years later, when I had the good fortune to visit one of the twentieth-century's experts on Crohn's, a very eminent and very elderly gastroenterologist, who also happened to be the father of a good friend of mine, did I entertain this possibility. Chatting with Dr. J. about the changing protocols for Crohn's during his long career and the continuing uncertainties about what causes the condition or how to treat it—other than symptomatically—I was brought up short by his question: "You've done better than ninety-nine percent of the patients I've seen over the years, so what do you think has enabled you to do so well?" Like my surgeon's comment a decade earlier, Dr. J.'s question catalyzed my thinking about how my experiences of illness had been limited by the medical frame through which I had learned to make sense of them. Indeed, though I wasn't able to respond adequately to his question at the time, it sparked me to consider why healing had remained occluded so long as I remained attached to my immune system as the source—if not the cause—of all my physical problems. If Dr. J. were to ask me this question today, I think I might reply: "I not only learned to value healing, but I learned that healing is itself a value."

IMMUNITY TO THE RESCUE;
OR, THE DEMISE OF HEALING

Throughout most of recorded history, healing was understood to be a "natural" quality of the organism, albeit one that also needed human support and encouragement. From antiquity until the middle of the nineteenth century, almost all cultures recognized that nature exercised a curative power on the organism, a power that medicine sought at best to emulate or to enhance. Within the Hippocratic tradition (the prevailing philosophy of healing in the West), this force was known as *vis medicatrix naturae*, the healing power of nature. According to this worldview, healing was imagined as a natural manifestation of the organism's inherent elasticity: it incorporated the organism's most expansive relations to the world, embracing the forces that animated the cosmos as a whole. Those seeking to facilitate the healing process attempted (at best) to encourage nature's course by addressing the imbalances between microcosm and macrocosm that kept symptomatic crises from resolving favorably. Thus, natural healing traditionally expressed the immersion of living beings in the universe and affirmed their fundamental connection to the matrix from which they arose and to which they would one day return (Neuburger 1926).

By the end of the nineteenth century, however, the *vis medicatrix naturae* had fallen out of favor among Western bioscientists. Deemed unduly vitalistic by the emerging reductionist paradigms of scientific medicine (which increasingly sought biochemical explanations for biological processes), healing became a more and more anachronistic notion. Instead, Western medical rationality embraced a new image, adopted from a very old legal doctrine, to describe how organisms survive illness: "immunity." Taken from Roman Law, this metaphoric innovation fundamentally reconceived the prevention and amelioration of illness. Bracketing healing as an improperly fuzzy premise, scientific medicine used the heretofore primarily juridical and political rubric "immunity" to incorporate what it now saw as the more properly "natural" function of the organism: "self-defense." This metaphoric substitution proved highly productive for the science of medicine since it restricted the complex, contradictory, and yet entirely necessary intimacy of organism-environment to a single salient type of engagement: aggression/response. Furthermore, it imagined the individual organism as the site within which a cellular struggle for survival (a.k.a. disease) took place, while simultaneously defining a hostile microbial agent as the dreadful "cause" against which the organism must wage its relentless war with death. Instead of manifesting the organism's essential connection to the world in which it lived, immunity refigured medicine as a powerful weapon in the body's necessary struggle to defend itself from the world.

Certainly, many of us now take this reinterpretation to be definitive. Most of us who rely on biomedical treatments accept the idea that our "immune systems" ought to "defend" us against disease (even as we are also increasingly aware that they do not always live up to this promise). While few of us have any deep understanding of its complexities, we generally presume that the immune system represents the front line in our incessant battle with the hostile forces of disease. Despite our ready acceptance, however, "immunity" is not an inevitable choice of images for our capacity to live as organisms among other organisms of various sizes and scales—nor, for that matter, is "self-defense." Instead, both terms derive from theories created by Western legal and political thinking to account for the complex, difficult, and at times violent ways that humans live among other humans. Only later, much later, do they get applied to the animate world more generally. Both concepts are saturated with modern presumptions about personhood and collectivity, and each represents a different strategy for accommodating the frictions and tensions (if not outright contradictions) between "the one" and "the many" that characterize modern political formations. Indeed, both immunity and self-defense have played central roles in framing what we would now understand as "liberal" or "democratic" governance, and thus have critically shaped the economic and political horizon within which we live. So how did they end up in biomedicine anyway?

Here is some background information: in the pre-Christian era, "immunity" finessed a problem of citizenship that arose as "Rome" expanded militarily beyond the Latin plain to encompass much of the Mediterranean basin. Inhabitants of some conquered cities could receive the rights of citizens, and yet because their territories were deemed "immune," they could neglect the obligations—primarily taxation and military service—incumbent on all ordinary Roman citizens. In this context, immunity conferred a flexible form of legal belonging that responded to political challenges the Romans faced when attempting to assimilate their new conquests within the purview of Roman laws. Over the next two millennia, immunity served almost exclusively as a political and legal concept (and a crucial one at that), adapting itself to new historical contexts in which it continued to rectify contradictions engendered when European states used "the law" to enforce social pacification and coherence. In particular, immunity has historically enabled the law to negotiate among competing powers and interests: first between church authorities and political rulers, then between monarchs and their nations, and subsequently between citizens and governments, between local and national jurisdictions, and among nations themselves.

Compared to immunity, "self-defense" was a relative latecomer to the pantheon of Western political thinking, emerging only during the early modern period. Yet over the last 350 years it has profoundly informed our reflection on the freedom and liberty of citizens. Canonized by Thomas Hobbes in *Leviathan* (1651) as the first "natural right," "self-defense" negatively affirmed one's primary relationship with one's body as a kind of "self-ownership." For Hobbes (and for Locke after him) human bodies, or what he calls "life & limbs," are "held in propriety" as "dearest to a man" (382–83); moreover, they must continue to be "held," if they are to continue to confer "propriety." The possible interruption of such "holding" then comes to be imagined violently as a taking away, a theft, or a plundering. In order to remain alive amid the "natural" condition that Hobbes famously characterized as the "perpetuall warre of every man against his neighbor" (296), one needed continually to protect the "property" that is one's "life" and thereby prevent others from taking hold of it. In this world where human bodies must be "held in propriety," or owned, to be or remain human, "self-defense" named the "rational" obligation of self-preservation in a "natural" world where (social) behavior made humans into physical, political, and economic threats to each other.

Though gesturing toward very different, if not actually mutually exclusive, forms of human coexistence, both "immunity" and "self-defense" weave the domains of law and politics together. In so doing, their trajectories seem to swerve decidedly away from the natural world toward the social. While growing within the shadow of "natural law," both immunity and self-defense reveal internal contradictions that political uses of law must finesse in order to maintain their coherence and authority. Almost nothing about either of these concepts suggests that they correspond to any naturally occurring biological phenomena whatever. So how then could the awkward confluence, the hybrid formulation, that defines "immunity" *as* biological "self-defense" have been so rapidly assimilated into modern medical thinking as one of its central metaphors? Moreover, given the seeming impropriety of using explicitly juridico-political terms to elucidate biological phenomena, how did this metaphoric translation come to make sense? And what consequences did this translation have both for the practice of medicine and for the experience of healing?

The word *immunity* was transplanted into bioscience a little more than a hundred years ago in order to describe the ways in which multicellular organisms systematically mediate relations with the environments replete with other living beings in which they exist. Within this paradigm, "self-defense" constitutes the most significant form of such mediation, and "immunity" describes the organism's activities toward this end. Needless to say, there is no physical connection that grounds the analogy between the political and biological concepts at play here. Moreover, as with all transformative metaphors, rhetorical success depends upon the way the metaphoric terms both retain and resolve the tensions that exist between the categories they bring into relation. When immunity first began to appear sporadically in medical texts during the middle of the nineteenth century, it knew nothing of self-defense. Rather, it was used figurally to indicate a nonspecific tendency that spared or "exempted" an organism from infections or contagions afflicting other organisms sharing the same milieu. In this context, the metaphorical efficacy of immunity for medicine was constrained by the unresolved incongruity of the terms it mobilized. At that time, immunity did not significantly increase medical understanding because the force of the legal concept, which underscores exemption and distinction, overtly clashed with prevailing humoral and environmental explanations, which stressed continuity and connection among organisms and their environments. Hence, immunity appeared in these early biological deployments as at best a paradoxical, and not particularly helpful, metaphor. By the end of the century, however, political, philosophical, and scientific developments had significantly changed the context for biological understanding. So much so that when the concept was reinvoked in the early 1880s and used to explain the miraculous results of Pasteur's vaccination experiments, it rapidly transformed the basic understanding of how organisms—and especially human organisms—endure.

Only during the last one hundred years, then, has a term that first appeared in Roman law come to serve as the metaphoric crux for some of the

most powerful techno-scientific endeavors in human biology. Its naturaliza-
tion provided, and continues to provide, a conceptual frame that informs how
scientific medicine addresses and transforms human bodies. By facilitating
the application of biochemical theory to organismic function, immunology
has successfully shaped the "objects" of twentieth and now twenty-first-cen-
tury biomedicine (in the double sense of its epistemological domains and its
therapeutic aims).[3] Today immunity literally underwrites the project of scientific medicine as it has been incorporated in our culture since the end of
the nineteenth century. It is a trope that seems to make biochemical reductionism self-evidently the best—if not the only—way of understanding the
complex, and at times contradictory, engagements of organism and environment. Yet "immunity" as a metaphor disturbs the "truth" of immunity as bioscientific concept precisely insofar as we forget the metaphoricity that makes
this truth seem true.[4]

Both the conceptual limitations and the geopolitical limits of Western
biomedical practice may stem in part from the ways a defensive sense of
immunity has superseded healing as the privileged metaphor for the vital
interplay of organism and environment. During most of Western—and non-
Western—history, healing defined a quality that was manifested in a multi-
plicity of practices, only some of which were recognizable as "medical" in the
sense that we now understand it. Indeed, it seems that scientific medicine was
institutionalized in the West as a simultaneously technological and economic
enterprise precisely by abjuring healing as an explicit value. Instead, in the
wake of the turn toward interventionist biotechnologies and their theoriza-
tion through the tropes of attack and response (e.g., "the war on cancer," "the
war on AIDS"), Western medical practice appears to have taken as its *raison
d'être* the fortification of the isolated and vulnerable body—not surprisingly,
the very locus that metonymically defines the individual as the atom of Western politics. With the advent of the modern biomedical era, healing became
largely reduced to events that were believed to represent the body's self-
defense, events that then were themselves analyzed primarily in terms of the
biochemical reactions that crystallized within them. Concomitantly, health
care became the (commercial) activity of supporting the individual's battle
against disease precisely insofar as it enabled the victor to return to the more
"productive" engagements of normal social life.

Unfortunately, while this model led to the development of numerous
effective treatment protocols, treatments that became the major selling
points for scientific medicine specifically and bioscience generally, it also
took infectious disease as the paradigmatic example of the pathogenic
encounter itself. Not surprisingly, then, bioscience has had more limited success in either understanding or treating numerous serious and chronic illnesses that are not readily encompassed within this model (e.g., cancers and
autoimmune illnesses), while it has had its most heroic achievements in both

preventing and circumventing the deleterious effects of pathogenic contagions. Yet as the recent appearance of antibiotic-resistant strains of formerly
treatable illnesses (such as TB) or the pandemics of infectious illnesses for
which no vaccines are available (such as AIDS) portend, even this "triumph"
may not be as clear-cut as once was hoped. Moreover, numerous medical apo-
ria—such as the failure to develop effective treatments for numerous debili-
tating and deadly "tropical" illnesses (e.g., malaria) that affect parts of the
world not amenable to huge profit making by the biotech industries, or the
transformation of one of modern medicine's most trumpeted successes (i.e.,
the elimination of smallpox) into the condition of possibility for one of the
deadliest bioweapons—also threaten to undermine the credibility of Western
medicine's triumphal claims (Silverstein 1999). However, I am not really
interested in disputing the "successes" of Western medical practice, without
which (I reiterate) I and many, many others around the world would not be
alive. Instead, what I would like to foreground are some consequences of taking the metaphors that underwrite immune discourse as immutable truths
rather than as metaphors, albeit generative ones.

When bioscientists at the end of the nineteenth century banished healing both as a natural capacity of the organism and as a productive metaphor
for medicine, they substituted the idea of immunity as an organismic activity
responsible for protecting the individual body against the threatening world
in which it necessarily lives. As a result, the embodied subject comes to be
figured more in terms of the strategic vulnerabilities that expose it to illness
and death, and less in terms of its capacity for vitality and aliveness. Instead,
physicians themselves—and by extension bioscientists and the health care
corporations for which they increasingly work—come to serve as agents of
the healing principle, which is reconstituted as an epistemological effect
rather than a biological possibility. The theoretical premise that drives the
transformative labors of a Pasteur, or a Watson and Crick, or a Salk, or the
ongoing efforts of the normal laboratory bioscientist, or even the daily struggles of the practicing physician, presupposes that these biomedical practices
incorporate the power of healing as manifest through knowledge. "Better
cures through better knowledge" could be the logo of the biotech enterprise
that underwrites our contemporary "health care industry" (which the pharmaceutical giant Pfizer made quite clear with its ad campaign: "Making life
better through technology"). As a result, healing becomes understood as a
process actively instigated by biomedical understanding and treatment, but
only passively aroused in the person being "treated."

THE VALUE OF HEALING

Yet what if we were to reclaim the metaphor "healing" for ourselves? Or what
if we were to consider the imaginary effects that metaphor evokes as part of

the healing process? Or even more powerfully, what if we were to affirm healing *as* metaphor?[5] In the history of Western medicine, the imagination has proved a powerful counterpoint to the desire for biological determinism. As the historian and philosopher of science Isabelle Stengers (Nathan and Stengers 1995) has demonstrated, at the end of the eighteenth century bioscience propelled itself across the threshold of scientificity by devising an epistemological technology that allows it to distinguish between its own "real cures" and the "false" practices of charlatans. The legacy of this technique is widely evident today in what is called "double-blind testing," which provides the industry standard for determining acceptable therapeutics. Unfortunately, what goes largely unappreciated by this paradigm is that which it explicitly excludes: the dismissively named "placebo effect." The irony here resides in the fact that the reason biomedicine excludes the placebo is not because it is *not* therapeutically effective but precisely because *it is*. However, since the effects a placebo produces are not determinant, they are hard to reproduce reliably and hence to appropriate profitably. Thus, instead of providing the basis for properly medical technologies, these imaginary effects are metaphorically bracketed as "placebos" and thereby declared to be less interesting—*and less real*—since they are deemed merely "imaginary" (Cohen 2003). Yet if, as Donna Haraway (1997) reminds us, "a research program is virtually always also a very mobile metaphor," then we can also welcome the significance of her insight that "metaphors are tools and tropes. The point is to learn to remember that we might have been otherwise, and might yet be, as a matter of embodied fact" (39).

In order to entertain one such "otherwise," we might consider both what metaphor itself offers as a mode of healing and what the metaphor "healing" has to offer as a particular trope. By reanimating healing as an explicitly metaphorical technology, I want to suggest that there may be a material payoff to the imaginary effects that biomedicine has excluded under the name of the placebo. That is, healing may provide a metaphor that connects human corporeality and imagination by traversing the unknown—and perhaps unknowable—dimensions that lie in between. Of course, metaphor is hardly unknown to bioscience; however, its role is understood to be primarily instrumental, not transformational. Before a metaphor becomes epistemologically "robust"—to invoke the quality that science attributes to its most successful poetic borrowings—its purchase on the imagination is patent. The meanings held in tension by the trope are largely available because they are provisional and hence still vibrant. At this early stage of the circulation of a metaphor, people must actively engage with the troubling uncertainties evoked by the disparate terms that it brings into relation in order to realize its potential to augment their understanding. This imaginary engagement actually gives rise to material effects by transforming the resources available for literally "making sense" of the world. Evoking the most concrete form of *poesis*, we might say that metaphor operates as a transformational technology by producing and reproducing similarities among differences. Hence, its success depends upon the density and elasticity of the connections established among terms that simultaneously must be defined and maintained as distinct. In other words, metaphor thrives on tension. If there is no distance, no separation, no incommensurability among the elements that are rhetorically linked, there is no metaphor, just tautology.

Metaphor emerges, then, within the spaces of not-knowing opened up between related differences. Erupting from the abyss of the unknown, metaphor surges toward knowledge. The unknown is essential here since it is the precondition for the emergence of the known. Yet, in metaphor, the known does not replace the unknown but grows from it and is nourished by it. If the animating unknown is exhausted or denied, metaphor dies and its corpse petrifies, turning either into cliché or truth. None of this is especially problematic either for bioscience or for rationality more generally. Metaphor's transitivity feeds upon its transience: new metaphors yield new ways of knowing. The problem arises only when the generative unknown—or indeed unknowable—aspect of metaphor is "forgotten," thereby effacing its troubling powers and reducing it to a transparent instrument for knowledge.

In advocating healing as metaphor, I want to call attention to the generative potential that the unknown and the unknowable may harbor for our experiences of illness and disease. When I was lying in my hospital bed imagining bands of warm light wrapped around my surgical incisions, I was entering into an experience that was entirely unknown to me. Yet the power of that imagining remains palpable decades later. This metaphorical practice articulated possibilities that exceeded what I "knew" of my illness, especially as that knowledge had been inscribed within me by the skillful hands of the doctors who saved my life. The knowledge dripping into my veins in the form of the antibiotics that biochemically addressed the bacteria making themselves at home in my abdomen did not convey much to me about the process that I inhabited and that inhabited me. Rather, only as I began to consider healing as a creative possibility that exceeded the domain of medical intervention, as a metaphor that might suture the gaping wound between the unknown dynamics of the human organism and the reflexive activities of human understanding, could I begin to appreciate and value it.

In the hospital, you learn that your "job" is to get well. How you do that, however, is not entirely clear. Certainly, being a "good" patient—taking all your meds, eating your meals, voiding on demand, offering up your veins, minding the doctors' instructions, being polite to the nurses—is deemed a necessary condition. But is it a sufficient one? And what if your illness remains intractable? What resources are available to us if we cede to our physicians all knowledge about our experience? In recent years we have become increasingly aware of the limits of biomedicine to address the organismic suffering we encounter as living beings. The explosion of what are called "alternative," or "complementary," or "nontraditional," or "adjunctive" therapies bears witness to needs that remain unaddressed or underaddressed by biomedical protocols.[6] While the efficacy of any of these nonscientific possibilities is certainly open to question—as are the effects of biomedicine themselves—what seems less questionable is that collectively these supplemental practices recall the healing capacities that biomedicine has increasingly bracketed over the last two centuries. By engaging the nondeterminable (or not yet determined) aspects of our organismic capacities, these healing modalities invite us to recognize and reanimate our relation to metaphor, to embrace it as what I like to call an *imaginary technology*, precisely insofar as they confound the conceptual transparency that makes biomedicine seem so true. When we go to the acupuncturist, herbalist, masseuse, bioenergy specialist, or shaman, for example, we not only avail ourselves of the particular skills that these practitioners possess, we also engage the possibility that biomedical knowledge does not exhaust the promise of healing transformation. In addition to any specific therapeutic results, then, the resurgence of nonmedical healing traditions may help us begin to appreciate the unknown, if not unknowable, dimensions of our biological existence as having valuable potential for our well-being.

As a properly "enlightened" practice, medical knowledge seeks to circumscribe the frightening unknowns that diseases embody. In this sense, biomedicine manifests one of the powerful contradictions that cut across what Horkheimer and Adorno labeled "the dialectic of enlightenment." They describe this paradox precisely: "Man imagines himself free from fear when there is no longer anything unknown. . . . Nothing at all may remain outside, because the mere idea of outsideness is the very source of fear" (1944, 16). While I am most certainly in support of the knowledge-effects that biomedicine offers us, and I am most happy to be a poster child for its successes, what I would like to reclaim is the affirmative potential that the unknown, the outside, has for helping us to reimagine what we believe we already know. In affirming "healing as metaphor," I hope to suggest both that *healing* provides a powerful metaphoric potential—that is, it augments our capacity to reconnect our imaginations and our organisms—and also that *metaphor* provides a powerful healing potential—that is, it supports our capacity to transform our relations to ourselves and to the worlds in which we live. But what do I really mean by this? I must confess that I really don't know. However, it seems to me that it is a potentially productive kind of not-knowing, a kind of not-knowing that asks us to engage imaginatively with the organisms-that-we-are in the service of our vitality and aliveness. By valuing our capacity for both material and imaginative engagements with ourselves and our worlds, we body forth the transformational possibilities that we metaphorize as healing.

By appreciating the healing capabilities of metaphor, we affirm our productive relations to the very unknown that enables metaphor to mean. "Healing as metaphor" is only a metaphor, then, but perhaps it can become a metaphor that heals.

NOTES

1. A real irony of this question resides in the fact that my greatest risk of HIV infection at this point in my life was from the multiple blood transfusions I had received in the very Bay Area hospital where I was being treated.

2. Don Johnson (1983) uses the phrase "somatic genius." I prefer "intelligence" with its etymological resonance of "gathering in-between." That is, intelligence as that which we reap from the places between certainties, as the harvesting from the fecundity of the un- or not-yet-known. I thank Emily Conrad for her explication of this idea.

3. Alfred Tauber and Leon Chernyak (1991; see also Tauber 1995) describe the transition from healing to immunity:

> It is apparent that the idea of healing power is quite different from . . . immunity. The former does not imply, as does the latter, that the healing power is exercised by a special subsystem in order to restore the integrity of the organism. On the contrary, it implies that the integrity, as an essence underlying particular physiological processes, acts on behalf of the processes. After Metchnikoff, the immune idea argues for a special activity (a subsystem) of the whole that performs the functions of a personal physician in respect to the whole. The normal activity of this special part takes place when the normal (the integrity) is violated. Quite opposite to that, the healing power of Nature is nothing else but the expression of the whole on behalf of its parts (in order to prevent their extreme deviation under the influence of cosmic tendency). (119)

4. For the classic analysis of metaphor and/as "truth," see Nietzsche's "On Truth and Lie in a Non-Moral Sense" (1873).

5. In her famous polemic *Illness as Metaphor* (1978), Susan Sontag takes exactly the opposite tack. Her approach is to abjure metaphor entirely and to exhort us to leave illness to the capable hands of our literal-minded physicians. Presumably she is thinking here of her own experience with cancer that occasioned the book in the first place, though we only find this out ten years later in a sequel, *AIDS and Its Metaphors*. Ironically, Sontag's highly literary text cautions us against invoking our imaginations in the service of our own well-being. For her, the social stigmatization that has historically followed in the wake of tuberculosis and cancer provides proof that metaphors are used against those who suffer from these diseases, and hence it is not "morally permissible" to use such metaphors. Therefore, she concludes that disease must be "de-mythicized" so that science may reign. Of course, it is hardly fair to take Sontag to task for her partial sense of history, especially when it comes to the history of bioscience; however, it does seem a bit odd that a professional writer and critic would so quickly cede metaphor as a possible resource.

6. Given the large amounts of money that Americans currently spend out of their own pockets for various forms of "alternative" healing practices—conservatively estimated at twenty-seven billion dollars in 1997, the same amount spent out of pocket on all U.S. physician services—it appears that there is already a marked and market recognition on the part of consumers of some insufficiencies in the biomedical paradigm. See Eisenberg et al. (1993; 1998).

REFERENCES

Cohen, Ed. 2003. The placebo disavowed; or unveiling the biomedical imagination. *Yale Journal for the Humanities in Medicine* (www.info.med.yale.edu/intmed/hummed/yjhm/).

Eisenberg D. M., R. C. Kessler, C. Foster, F. E. Norlock, D. R. Calkins, and T. L. Delbanco. 1993. Unconventional medicine in the United States. Prevalence, costs, and patterns of use. *New England Journal of Medicine* 328:246–52.

Eisenberg, D. M., R. B. Davis, S. L. Ettner, S. Appel, S. Wilkey, M. Van Rompay, and R. C. Kessler. 1998. Trends in alternative medicine use in the United States, 1990–1997: Results of follow-up national survey. *Journal of the American Medical Association* 280:1569–75.

Haraway, Donna. 1997. *FemaleMan© meets OncoMouse™: Feminism and technoscience.* New York: Routledge.

Hobbes, Thomas. 1651. *Leviathan.* Ed. C. B. Macpherson. London: Penguin, 1968.

Horkheimer, Max, and Theodor Adorno. 1944. *The dialectic of enlightenment.* Trans. John Cummings. New York: Continuum, 1972.

Johnson, Don. 1983. *Body.* Boston: Beacon Press.

Nathan, Tobie, and Isabelle Stengers, eds. 1995. *Médecins et sorciers.* Paris: Éditions des Laboritires Synthélabo.

Neuburger, Max. 1926. *The doctrine of the healing power of nature throughout the course of time.* Trans. L. J. Boyd. New York, 1932.

Nietzsche, Friedrich. 1873. On truth and lie in a non-moral sense. In *Philosophy and truth: Selections from Nietzsche's notebooks of the early 1870s.* Trans. Daniel Breazeale. Amherst, NY: Humanities Books, 1979.

Silverstein, Ken. 1999. Millions for Viagra, pennies for diseases of the poor: Research money goes to profitable lifestyle drugs. *The Nation,* July 19, 13–19.

Sontag, Susan. 1978. *Illness as metaphor.* New York: Farrar, Straus and Giroux.

Tauber, Albert. 1995. *The immune self: Theory or metaphor?* New York: Cambridge University Press.

Tauber, Albert, and Leon Chernyak. 1991. *Metchnikoff and the origins of immunity: From metaphor to theory.* New York: Oxford University Press.

ELEVEN

A Perspective on the Role of Stories as a Mechanism of Meta-Healing

KIMBERLY R. MYERS

> And I'm standing on the edge of some crazy cliff. What I have to
> do, I have to catch everybody if they start to go over the cliff. . . .
> That's all I'd do all day. I'd just be the catcher in the rye. . . .
> —J. D. Salinger, *The Catcher in the Rye*

THE CORE OF NARRATIVE medicine is story—the story a patient tells about his illness and how that story gets told and heard. As a physician reads or listens to this illness narrative, she scrutinizes her patient's text for nuances that might inform a diagnosis made on physical examination. Accurately interpreting symptoms inscribed on the body and described on the page enables a physician to mitigate or even eliminate the physical pain caused by disease. However, especially with chronic or catastrophic disease, a patient's psychological suffering is at least as urgent as his physical pain; and a physician must attend to this dimension of healing as well. Psychoanalysis, known from the start as "the talking cure," has revealed that the very act of telling one's story contributes to his psychological healing, so it stands to reason that providing the patient a place to tell his story of illness—apart from any physical cure it might effect—is simply good medicine. For both their diagnostic and therapeutic potential, then, words function as a mechanism of healing.

This chapter explores a unique perspective on "meta-healing" with words, not through traditional academic analysis but based on my dual position as a person with chronic illness and as editor of a volume of illness narratives entitled

Illness in the Academy: A Collection of Pathographies by Academics (Myers 2007), a project that grew out of my experience as a Fellow in the 2002 National Endowment for the Humanities Summer Institute, "Medicine, Literature, and Culture." I should clarify from the outset that I am trained in neither psychoanalysis nor medicine, and I will offer no new theoretical constructs for either psychoanalysis or narrative medicine. What I offer instead of conclusions, however, are observations that I believe shed light on some fundamentals of how we use words in talking ourselves through trauma into healing. Moreover, I am aware that just as I attempt to analyze the stories and experiences of others, my own words and perspectives can be profitably analyzed for whatever human truths they reveal.

As is perhaps true with all academic passions, my interest in narrative medicine was born out of personal experience. In October 1993, I began a journey of disease, illness, and healing that would influence my personal life and my career as an academic far more than I could ever have suspected at the time. As I was preparing for doctoral comprehensive exams in English at the University of North Carolina, I was diagnosed with Inflammatory Bowel Disease and thus took on the challenge of learning to live a whole new way— or rather, *many* new ways, as this disease continually modulates in presentation, intensity, and duration of activity. In the pages that follow, I describe how my experience with illness and my belief in the healing power of words have led me to the pathographies project, an enterprise designed to provide an opportunity for healing for myself and others.

The therapeutic power of words was critical to me during the days, weeks, and months between the first presentation of symptoms and the diagnosis, a period filled with both high-pitched anxiety and simmering dread. While my personal life was organized according to various doctors' appointments, medical tests, and lab results, my life as a teacher and scholar of literature was comforting and familiar; it was life as I had known it, life before "the fall" (from health). Reading and discussing literature with my students was soothing to me, not so much because it was a temporary escape from the demands of living the life of a patient—though it was that, too—but because the very words held sway over me in a different way. Passages about living life intensely and with intention, passages about death, those about illness and impotence and incapacity now had a new significance in my life. Literature had long since shown me intellectually and philosophically that I was not alone in facing life-altering bodily change, but now I understood these truths more profoundly, "in the deep heart's core," to borrow a phrase from W. B. Yeats's 1893 poem "The Lake Isle of Innisfree." As John Keats aptly observed in a letter to his friend J. H. Reynolds dated May 3, 1818, "axioms in philosophy are not axioms until they are proved upon our pulses" (Bush 1959, 273). The Romantic poet wrote these words while he was caring for his brother Tom, who was suffering from the tuberculosis that would ultimately take his life. Having studied medicine, Keats could now appreciate the difference between illness in the abstract and that which had become all too personal and concrete. No doubt this understanding would deepen when he himself began manifesting symptoms of tuberculosis; it would end his life, too.

But perhaps it was William Wordsworth's "Ode: Intimations of Immortality" (1807) that meant most to me at the time—not just because Wordsworth captures so eloquently the sense of loss that had come with illness, but also because his words had become my mantra for how to live this new kind of life. Toward the end of the poem, Wordsworth writes:

> What though the radiance which was once so bright
> Be now for ever taken from my sight,
> Though nothing can bring back the hour
> Of splendor in the grass, of glory in the flower:
> We will grieve not, rather find
> Strength in what remains behind. . . .

I was of two minds one Friday morning as I stood before three dozen college students discussing with them the implications of Wordsworth's meaning in this poem. There was the professional me, contextualizing the loss of one's youthful and radiant "celestial light" in terms of William Blake's categories of Innocence and Experience; and there was the private me, telling myself at the very moment I spoke Wordsworth's words aloud that I, too, chose not to dwell on the irrevocable loss—that I, too, would find strength somewhere in this part of me that remained. In that space where I was neither entirely objective academic nor subjective mourner of loss, I was aware that just as words were healing a part of what was broken in me, for others struggling with illness words would in some way transform what was lost into something found. I wondered what I might do, given my training with words, to facilitate such healing.

Years passed as I completed the PhD, accepted a tenure-track position, and consequently moved across the country to Montana. My disease was relatively well managed for the first few years of this new life, which was especially fortunate in that it afforded me a respite from many of the emotional and logistical burdens of sickness and left me the time and energy to establish myself professionally. Searching for a meaningful way to combine my training in language and literature and my identity as a person with chronic illness, I began to explore medical issues in literature: medical ethics in Stephen Crane's novella *The Monster*, and the joint influence of Hinduism and medical science in Yeats's decision to undergo the controversial Steinach operation (genital surgery for sexual rejuvenation). I was eager to deepen my understanding of this cross-disciplinary field, and consequently proposed and chaired two special sessions on Literature and Medicine at a regional Modern

Language Association meeting. During this time, I was struck by the fact that an unusually large number of students who dropped by my office were sharing stories of illness—either their own or that of a close relative or friend. It seemed the perfect time to provide a forum in which to explore issues of health and illness, and I designed a course in Literature and Medicine as a means of empowering myself and my students. This was the beginning of what I would later come to call "meta-healing."

The term *meta-healing* is currently used primarily in the realm of alternative medicine.[1] Neal Mahr (2003), founder of an organization called Freedom Unlimited, defines meta-healing as "a process in which many modalities or methods are brought in to facilitate the multi-dimensional restoration of an individual." He explains, "The body knows best how to heal itself. We simply restore the condition in which the body can access that self-healing ability that is more optimum, more encompassing and longer lasting." While my definition does not necessarily exclude any of these particulars, it is a much narrower concept. In much the same way that "meta-analysis" is an analysis of the analyses that have gone before, so is "meta-healing" a means of healing that occurs in observing or facilitating the healing of others. Specifically, in providing my students with an opportunity to share their stories of illness, I would be transforming the seeming senselessness and futility of my own compromised health into something productive. In turn, I would discover, if not a meaning for my illness, then at least a purpose to it; creating something of value would restore a sense of agency in the face of my loss of control—in Yeats's words from "Lapis Lazuli" (1938), "gaiety transfiguring all that dread." As it turned out, I would need such meta-healing more than I knew.

Ironically, after living a fairly normal life for several years, my disease flared just before I began teaching the first of two Literature and Medicine seminars, and I spent most of that semester discussing medical issues in the abstract in class while living them all too concretely outside class. Toward the end of the term, I decided to write my own pathography, which I had wanted (and needed) to do for years. As part of our study of narrative medicine, I gave my students this pathography and asked them to respond to it in any way they thought meaningful. At that time, they did not know that I had written it, nor did they know of my illness. I wanted to keep it that way in order to preserve what I believed to be an important professional boundary; I did not want my students to be apprehensive that I might collapse in class or subject them to some similar (though highly unlikely) embarrassment. After reading the pathography, some students wrote analyses of its literary/rhetorical strategies; some connected it to the materials we had been reading by Rita Charon (2001), Arthur Frank (1997), Anne Hunsaker Hawkins (1999), Arthur Kleinman (1998), and others. But the writings that really captivated me were the "in kind" responses in which students told their own stories of illness. This had been an impromptu exercise, so I was amazed at the eagerness and facility with which these students wrote. It was almost as if they had needed to tell their stories as much as I had.

What these students wrote was as powerful as anything we had been reading, and I asked four of them to share their pathographies. Their reading had a marked effect on the class; things seemed risky (in the way that meaningful things nearly always are), and we all recognized that a new kind of learning was transpiring. That evening as I was reflecting on the surprisingly powerful combination of intellectualism and catharsis that pervaded the class, it occurred to me that I had asked my students to demonstrate a kind of courage that I had not possessed. I decided to claim my story the next class. It was probably the most vulnerable moment of my life when I admitted to students that this was my story, especially since it contained such intimate details of my physical and emotional struggle. But a remarkable thing happened: a bond formed among the members of our class (I had unmistakably become one with my students in this enterprise) that surprised all of us and dramatically influenced the nature of their final projects, creative reflections on the service/experiential learning they had completed during the preceding weeks.

Following her scholarly and clinical research on grief and the grieving process, one student wrote a twenty page short story illustrating the grief she experienced after her sister died in a car accident the previous summer. Having worked with AIDS patients, another student wrote a series of journal entries from the perspective of a young adult dying of AIDS. Another produced a professional-quality documentary videotape on "The Healing Powers of Faith," complete with original script and background music to complement his interviews with survivors of purportedly fatal diseases and accidents. Sometimes the emotional import of the projects overwhelmed the students as they were presenting to the class. When this happened, that person's neighbor simply took over and continued to the end whatever she could read aloud. Something significant had happened in this class, something I had not expected nor could have anticipated. In their exit interviews for the course, all nineteen students commented on the community we had forged—one of intellectual probing that had also fostered significant personal growth. Their comments affirmed Virginia Woolf's assertion in her 1939 essay, "A Sketch of the Past": "It is only by putting it into words that I make it whole; this wholeness means that it has lost its power to hurt me; it gives me, perhaps because by doing so I take away the pain, a great delight to put the severed parts together" (72).

I continue to marvel that just at this point in my journey deeper into the therapeutic potential of words, a colleague forwarded to me an announcement of the National Endowment for the Humanities 2002 Summer Institutes. Never in my life has there been a more powerful example of what Carl Jung calls "synchronicity" than the opportunity to join twenty-four other

scholars and teachers interested in precisely the concerns that had been my
overt focus for the past year and a guiding force in my life for a decade. I have
said repeatedly that the month I spent at the Milton S. Hershey Medical
Center of Pennsylvania State University as a Fellow in the Institute "Medicine, Literature, and Culture" was the most intellectually invigorating and
personally gratifying experience of my life; and I have discussed some of the
transformative events of that time in an article called "Coming Out: Considering the Closet of Illness" (Myers 2004).[2] But for the purposes of the chapter at hand, I would like to focus on only one significant outgrowth of that
Institute: the pathographies project.

In late fall of 2002, I issued a call for submissions from academics in any
discipline. The organizing principle for this collection is how one's discipline
influences the way he or she understands and processes the experience of illness, and I suggested that pathographies be around fifteen pages in length. I had
no idea what to expect in terms of the interest in such a project, so I was pleased
when I started receiving inquiries. At first, there were a dozen or so; then, the
correspondence increased dramatically. Because I was—and still am—so committed to the value of this kind of work, I vowed to treat each person and his
or her story not only with professional courtesy, but also with the appropriate
human attention. From my own experience I was, of course, keenly aware of
how vulnerable one is when divulging illness of any kind, and I knew that there
was some therapeutic value just in sharing one's story with another person,
whether or not it was ultimately published to a large readership.

Several times, e-mail conversations progressed into telephone conversations, some lasting for more than an hour. The kind of instant connection
afforded by illness encouraged and pleased me, but it also intimidated me
somewhat. I had expected to handle these illness narratives much as I have
handled other professional texts: as documents to be refined in terms of
argument and illustration. But suddenly, here were colleagues I had never
met who were sharing with me details of their most intimate life experiences. It was easy, yet strange, to sympathize—sometimes even empathize—
with a total stranger in this way, and for the first time I had a glimpse of what
physicians and therapists must experience on a regular basis. The obvious
difference was that I had had no professional training in such matters, and I
wondered about my ability to be of any help. But because for years I had
been committed to following this path of language and medicine wherever
and as far as it would take me, I was humbled by such eager response to this
work and excited that people would risk vulnerability for the possibility of
healing themselves through telling their own stories. Aside from my tasks as
editor, my responsibility was to witness the stories—merely to be present for
the people who were telling them. I was glad for this charge because it meant
that something powerful was emerging for other people . . . and also, recip-
rocally, for me.

Several people I spoke with over the course of four months evinced a keen desire to tell their stories of illness and also an equally keen apprehension about the ramifications of doing so. Again, from my own experiences in the classroom, at the NEH Institute, and within my own academic institution, I understood how strong these misgivings were—and often for good reason.[3] I listened with dismay to one young scholar who told me about watching his friend, a fellow graduate teaching assistant, die of AIDS. His department did nothing to commemorate this person's death; so as a gesture of protest, he came out as a gay man, HIV positive, and subsequently lost his teaching position and financial support. His mission since then had been to tell his story as widely as possible, and he was glad for a new forum to discuss the politics of illness. I spoke several times with an associate professor who was trying to decide whether she should make public her struggle with anorexia nervosa. She wanted to write her story, but she thought it best to remain anonymous in case she might be compromised professionally by such candor. In the end, she decided that the risk of exposure was too great, and she did not send a pathography. Another scholar similarly requested anonymity and sent a remarkable essay about vaginismus, a relatively common but not widely discussed malady. She was very clear that a primary reason she wanted this story to be known was so that others who shared her condition would not feel isolated and silenced, as she had. For the first and last of these three scholars, their healing went beyond merely giving voice to their illness; they, too, were practicing meta-healing in offering something of value to others and, in doing so, transforming their loss.

In the end, I received more than ninety pathographies. I had expected, if I were fortunate, to receive twelve, at most. While the volume of material was daunting, it also affirmed the value of the project, and I began to read with an eagerness uncommon even for me. I was completely unprepared for what happened next, however: the sheer magnitude of fear and grief recounted within these pages overwhelmed me. Even though most of the stories contained ample hope and even humor, I was riddled with a sense of impotence at not being able to mitigate any of the suffering. I felt like Holden Caulfield trying to catch everybody who was about to go over the cliff and knowing all I could do was stand there, arms open wide. Though of course no one had asked me to be a counselor, much less savior, hearing these stories made me restless, aware of how much of our inner tragedy goes unacknowledged even while our bodies receive the best medical attention. Inundated with images of such profound illness, I lost sight of the conviction I had had all along: to provide a place for healing for author, reader, and, yes, editor too. How ironic that one who had been so excited about this idea of meta-healing was suddenly afflicted with discomfort that bordered on depression. Again, I was mindful of what physicians and therapists surely must feel even despite having undergone a training that attempts to preclude such visceral identification with their patients and clients. For the first time in my illness experience, I understood "upon [my] pulse" why compassionate detachment is beneficial and utterly necessary for both doctor and patient.

I am confident that much of my response stemmed from the fact that I am not fully healed nor will my body ever be completely cured. As a person with chronic illness, I still wrestle with physical discomfort and all the misgivings surrounding disease; so immersing myself in the illness of others is challenging. It is very much like an observation made in one of the pathographies. This person, suffering from panic disorder, humorously questions the wisdom of choosing university life where one is continually scrutinized and evaluated by students and colleagues alike. Why would someone who has to undergo so many medical tests, wait not so patiently for the results, and confront her limitations on a daily basis voluntarily commit herself to a project that entails countless hours enmeshed in stories fraught with the same tensions? The answer is this: that the gift in simply being there is valuable not because it is *easy*, but precisely because it is so difficult. Venturing into the shadowlands full force is the gift one gives not only to another, but also to oneself.

Fortunately for me, the passage of several weeks' time and talking about my unexpected reaction with a colleague in the field of medical humanities enabled me to overcome my hesitancy in working with the pathographies I had received. I was able to regain a confidence that even if I could not do everything, I could do *something* to promote healing. Since then, having corresponded with those whose essays are included in the collection both about the details of their stories and the technical aspects of style, I have grown to understand the paradox of intimacy and detachment surrounding the illnesses of others. With the completion of this project, I trust that we now all share a sense of having furthered our own healing through words.

The implications of what I write here are certainly not novel, but I think they may be worth remembering. First, there are ways for those not trained in medicine or psychotherapy to facilitate healing. Whether it be in the classroom or with our friends and colleagues, providing a safe place for discussing the realities of living with illness is hugely beneficial; one need not have all the answers or an ability to "cure," for it is now a commonplace that active listening is therapeutic, just as is merely speaking (or writing) one's story. Furthermore, even for those who understand that proactively processing illness entails spending time in the presence of one's deepest fears, it is wise not to underestimate the many unexpected ways anxiety and reticence can manifest themselves. Acknowledging the surprise and frustration surrounding such setbacks, and giving oneself the time and space necessary to stabilize, are good strategies to overcome what might seem insurmountable resistance to the very processes that ultimately promote healing. And finally, for those of us who are neither physicians nor therapists, I believe it is important to recognize that while trained professionals are paid to contend with our greatest physical and psychological problems, they are nevertheless human beings with their own stories, their own misgivings. The compassion that we expect in a medical setting should likely go both ways, even if we patients merely refrain from expecting our doctors or therapists to be entirely selfless at all times. Perhaps what we could contribute to *their* well-being is an understanding that they might be exhausted after a long call, for instance, or grappling with their own frustrations in caring for an aging parent or sick spouse. Perhaps we might enhance our own healing in facilitating the healing of others.

NOTES

1. The concept of *meta-healing* appears in a wide range of thought and practice—from the more common domains of holistic health and psychotherapy, to the more esoteric practices of "*conjuring* healing" with its emphasis on cosmic forces.

2. This essay appears as part of a two-volume edition of *Journal of Medical Humanities* (Winter 2004 and Spring 2005) devoted to the work of the NEH Fellows and guest-edited by co-director of the Institute, Anne Hunsaker Hawkins.

3. I offer an extended examination of the processes and politics of "coming out" as a person with illness in the essay mentioned in note 2.

REFERENCES

Bush, Douglas, ed. 1959. *Selected poems and letters of John Keats*. Boston: Houghton Mifflin.

Charon, Rita. 2001. Narrative medicine: A model of empathy, reflection, profession, and trust. *Journal of the American Medical Association* 286:1897–1902.

Finneran, Richard, ed. 1996. *The collected works of W. B. Yeats Volume I: The poems: Revised*. Second ed. New York: Scribner's.

Frank, Arthur. 1997. *The wounded storyteller: Body, illness, and ethics*. Chicago: University of Chicago Press.

Hawkins, Anne Hunsaker. 1999. *Reconstructing illness: Studies in pathography*. Second ed. West Lafayette: Purdue University Press.

Kleinman, Arthur. 1998. *The illness narratives: Suffering, healing, and the human condition*. New York: Basic Books.

Mahr, Neal. 2003. Meta-healing. http://www.freedomunlimited.net/Meta_Healing.htm accessed 20 August 2003.

Myers, Kimberly. 2004. Coming out: Considering the closet of illness. *Journal of Medical Humanities* 25:255–70.

———. 2007. *Illness in the academy: A collection of pathographies by academics*. West Lafayette: Purdue University Press.

Van Doren, Mark, ed. 2002. *Selected poetry of William Wordsworth*. New York: Modern Library.

Woolf, Virginia. 1939. A sketch of the past. In *Moments of being: Unpublished autobiographical writings*, ed. Jeanne Schulkind, 61–137. New York: Harcourt, Brace, Jovanovich.

TWELVE

The Discourse of Disease

Patient Writing at the
"University of Tuberculosis"

JEAN S. MASON

ON MAY 26, 1937, the Adirondack mountain weather seemed so "fine" that seventeen-year-old Bill Hastings wrote to his Aunt Peggy and Grandpa, "Summer is here!" Barely graduated from high school, Bill had contracted tuberculosis and been sent to "cure"[1] at the famed Trudeau Sanatorium in Saranac Lake, New York. Bill's parents felt confident this northern New York sanatorium would, in fact, cure their son's TB in time for him to enter Annapolis in September. Like many TB patients "taking the cure," Bill instinctively turned to writing to relieve long hours of loneliness and anxiety. Bill's letters paint a detailed picture of sanatorium life from a patient's perspective. "Now that summer is here my entire day is spent out on the porch. I have my radio outside too. The other day I went to the dentist to have a couple of cavities filled. It was a nice day and I enjoyed getting out for that half hour." Typical of sanatorium patients, Bill obsessed about his temperature and weight, and reported these vital statistics in a letter to his Dad on June 6: "My temps this week have been 99.1, 99, 98.6, 98.7, 99, 99. Lost a pound this time—probably the heat." Bill continued to enthuse about the fine spring as he wrote, "We are still having grand weather here—makes you glad to be alive." Sadly, Bill Hastings died a few days after writing these words. But Bill's letters live on as part of a substantial collection of writing by TB patients who cured in Saranac Lake before "wonder drugs" eliminated the sanatoria movement in the mid-twentieth century. Both implicitly and explicitly, these TB "pathographies" suggest how patient narratives can contribute to a more inclusive, informative, and insightful discourse of disease.

By the time Bill Hastings cured in Saranac Lake in the 1930s, the village had become known as the "university of tuberculosis" for its leading role in the treatment and research of TB. The Saranac Lake collection contains a significant database of patient writing, centered on a single disease, framed within a specific time, and located in a relatively controlled setting. Largely unexplored, this archive includes correspondence, diaries, poems, manuscripts, memoirs, newsletters, reunion memorabilia, and ephemera including postcards and photographs. Archival material suggests the important role that writing played in the daily curing regimen of many sanatoria patients, and it allows us to incorporate more patient narratives into a historiography traditionally dominated by medical practitioners.

A sense of sanatoria culture in general and Saranac Lake in particular is essential to understanding the setting that prompted these patients to write. Picture, for a moment, the world where TB victims such as Bill Hastings lived. Until 1944 and the discovery of streptomycin, the "white plague" killed more people than any other disease on earth (Reichman 2002, xii). Imagine HIV as an airborne contagion, or SARS as a widespread affliction. Primarily a disease of the lungs, the tubercle bacillus flew from one person to another on the airwave of a laugh or a sneeze. Known variously as TB, consumption, or phthisis, the result was the same. If the bacillus found a receptive resting place in your lungs, that nagging cough you thought was a cold progressed to symptoms similar to bronchitis or influenza. As the disease took its course, you experienced variously fever, cough, congestion, breathlessness, weight loss, weakness, and even haemorrhaging as indications of your probable fate. Your demise might be as brief as months or as lengthy as years. And, of course, you infected any number of unlucky breathers who happened to share your airspace. Your best chance for recovery was to join the thousands of other afflicted souls in a pilgrimage of hope. Destination: the tuberculosis sanatorium.

The sanatoria movement started in Germany and Switzerland in the mid-1800s, spread rapidly to North America where it began as an ad hoc initiative, developed a character of its own, and grew to immense proportions. From the late 1800s to the mid-1900s, millions of North American TB sufferers spent time in sanatoria practicing curative regimes based principally on climate, rest, diet, and, sometimes, surgical intervention. TB patients might find themselves taking the cure close to home and loved ones, or far from friends and family in a world devoid of modern telecommunication. Depending on their finances, health seekers could be incarcerated in an inner city fortress with gulag-like conditions, introduced to the wonders of nature in little more than a tent, ensconced behind gilded gates noshing gourmet fare, cloistered among well-meaning religious philanthropists, or nestled cozily among forest pines in a mountain hideaway—like Bill Hastings in Saranac Lake.[2]

Saranac Lake led North America in establishing and institutionalizing tuberculosis treatment and research. In 1873, young Dr. Edward Livingston Trudeau, recently diagnosed with tuberculosis, discovered the region's health-giving properties. Anticipating death, Trudeau went to Saranac Lake to die surrounded by memories of youthful vacations spent fishing, hunting, and exploring in the Adirondack Mountains. Instead of dying, Trudeau revived and regained a remarkable degree of health in a surprisingly short time. This pattern repeated itself several times over a period of six years. Each time Trudeau left Saranac Lake, his tuberculosis recurred. Each time Trudeau returned to Saranac Lake, he regained strength and spirit. In 1876, against all advice, the urbane Doctor Trudeau of New York City moved himself, his wife, Charlotte, their two infants, and his medical practice to this remote mountain wilderness that was home to only a few hundred loggers and wilderness guides.

A naturally curious intellectual, Trudeau's interest in tuberculosis went beyond his own experience. He gathered information on developments in Europe—the emergent sanatoria movement, and Koch's claims of isolating the tubercle bacillus in 1882. In 1884, with approximately four hundred dollars donated by sympathetic friends, Trudeau founded North America's first successful TB sanatorium—the Adirondack Cottage Sanitarium—to provide "suitable accommodations in the Adirondacks for patients of moderate means."[3] The first cottage, called "Little Red," consisted of "one room, fourteen by eighteen, and a porch so small that only one patient could sit out at a time. Little Red was furnished with a wood stove, two cot-beds, a washstand, two chairs and a kerosene lamp" (Trudeau 1914, 169–70). The first two patients were Alice and Mary Hunt, sisters who worked in the factories of New York City. Local workers hauled water up the hill from the Saranac River. Little Blue and Little Green soon followed Little Red. Relying on philanthropy and good will, Trudeau acquired land, built cottages, recruited and trained caregivers, instituted research, and contributed his own medical services for free.

In addition to founding a sanatorium, Edward Trudeau became the first person in North America to isolate the tubercle bacillus. Trudeau and his colleagues opened the first research facility in the world devoted solely to TB, founded a school of nursing dedicated to educating nurses in the care of TB patients, established the first institutionalized occupational therapy facility in the world, and supported the development of other local curing initiatives. The "university of tuberculosis" incorporated patient care, scientific research, medical training, and patient rehabilitation—in many ways an exemplary model of community-based health care. Patients and practitioners moved freely and naturally between their traditionally separate worlds since many patients contracted TB as practitioners, came to Saranac to cure, and stayed on afterward to practice health care again. Lay patients sometimes took up health care–related careers as a result of their Saranac experience, and remained in the community after regaining health. The vision and methods of Edward Livingston Trudeau and his colleagues attended to psychological as well as to physical needs and they reflect, in many ways, today's turn toward holistic medicine. E. L. Trudeau ultimately succumbed to TB in 1915. He lived long enough, however, firmly to establish "America's magic mountain," a remarkable community of healing founded on tuberculosis.[4]

By 1920, the population of Saranac Lake had grown from several hundred to more than six thousand—a population comprised mainly of tuberculosis patients and caregivers, many filling both roles at different times during their stay. By 1930, the Trudeau Sanatorium occupied sixty buildings on ninety-three acres. Other local sanatoria soon followed Trudeau's example. At its peak in the 1920s, 1930s, and 1940s, Saranac Lake was home not only to Trudeau, but also to Ray Brook State Sanatorium, Will Rogers Sanatorium for patients in the theater industry, Stony Wold Sanatorium for women, Gabriel's Charitable Sanatorium operated by the Sisters of Mercy, and an entire village consisting largely of private cure cottages.

Tuberculosis wove a socioeconomic tapestry unimaginable under ordinary circumstances, and created a culture that would challenge the most intrepid anthropologist. Saranac Lake health seekers ranged from the rich and famous, including Robert Louis Stevenson, Albert Einstein, Walker Percy, Christy Mathewson, Norman Bethune, Rollo May, Stephen Crane, Bela Bartok, and Manuel Luis Quezon Antonia y Molina (former President of the Philippines), to countless indigent and unknown sufferers. (Bartok's and Einstein's health problems eventually proved to be unrelated to TB.) Unlike many other sanatoria destinations, TB victims were welcomed in Saranac Lake, not stigmatized or confined outside village limits. TB was the heart of the community. A 1951 letter from village Mayor Alton B. (Tony) Anderson typifies the welcome new patients received. Anderson's message reassured and comforted new arrivals, "We know from the experience of others, including myself, who have come to Saranac Lake and regained health, due to the environment and competent medical and other attention which you receive here that at some future time you will be able to resume your normal mode of life." Perhaps even more important, Anderson's letter gave patients a sense of hope and belonging within the community: "When you are able to participate in our local activities we have many social and fraternal organizations which will be happy to be of service to you and aid in making your stay in our midst beneficial and enjoyable." The tone set by Edward Livingston Trudeau's personality and the geophysical isolation of Saranac Lake combined to create a unique opportunity for community building and health care. Together, diverse refugees from the "white plague" built an unusual and thriving society of doctors, nurses, patients, merchants, professionals, schools, libraries, newspapers, a radio station, churches, undertakers, entertainers, athletes, artists, and sundry support workers that stands in marked contrast to the culture of illness both historically and at present.[5]

Within this generally supportive environment, however, TB patients shared a common challenge—long hours of enforced idleness. Patients spent a large portion of their days, and even nights, lying on outdoor porches in specially designed "cure chairs" breathing the mountain air. Even today, most Saranac Lake homes reflect this architectural heritage. The "village of a thousand porches" still bears witness to an economy built literally on air. One of the features of many "cure chair" designs was a flat, extra-large, wooden armrest constructed to accommodate writing.

One of the first patients to leave evidence of daily writing is sixteen-year-old Evelyn Bellak. Imagine opening the stiff dusty covers of a 1918 diary that preserves the story of a young girl stricken with TB and sent far from home to cure. Evelyn Bellak cured at Ray Brook State Sanatorium. Evelyn begins her diary on Tuesday, January 1, 1918, with the words, "Well, Diary, I'll introduce myself. My name is Evelyn. I'm 16 years old. I have tuberculosis and at present time am in the Ray Brook Sanatorium trying to get cured." Evelyn wrote faithfully every day for nearly an entire year. Evelyn's diary describes activities common to many teenagers. Evelyn attended religious services, concerts, movies, and parties at the sanatorium and occasionally in the village. Evelyn kept a detailed record of the time she spent "curing" each day, which to her signified literally the precise time she spent outside lying in her cure chair. Like Bill Hastings, Evelyn Bellak obsessed about her weight and temperature, noting fluctuations almost daily. Although nothing in the content of Evelyn's diary suggests a particular effect of writing in relation to tuberculosis, her diary is representative of a collection of patient narratives that simply record the ordinary existence of sanatorium life with little reflection on its impact or the recording process. The very plenitude of these works, however, suggests that they played a significant role in patients' lives if no more than as a way to pass time. Taken together, these narratives help to flesh out the patients' perspective and the minutiae of sanatorium life at a basic level.

While many patients kept private diaries like Evelyn Bellak or wrote letters like Bill Hastings, others were drawn to more typically expressive media, such as poetry. Some even chose to publicize their writing, particularly in small local presses that sprang up in response to demand. One such patient is Herbert Scholfield. In 1892, Scholfield had recently begun his career as a young teacher in New Jersey when he contracted tuberculosis and left for Saranac Lake. Scholfield lived as a semi-invalid for thirty years. The 1919 publication *Sonnets of Herbert Scholfield*—containing 133 sonnets in all—merits attention for three reasons.

First, each sonnet displays a remarkable level of technical accomplishment. Scholfield's sonnets conform to the Elizabethan tradition of meter and rhyme, form a complete sequence on a single theme, employ typical literary conventions such as the quest, the guide, the dream, and the idealized female, and exemplify the narrative development of a sonnet sequence. Second, the narrative development in Scholfield's *Sonnets* traces the speaker's process of coming to terms with tuberculosis in a deeply reflective way. And third, the speaker describes explicitly the role that writing played in this process. Stating his purpose to offer cheer and comfort in the "Prologue," the speaker of Part 1 begins his exploration of the tubercular process when he imagines his life had he not contracted TB. Fantasies of courting, marriage, family, and old age are rendered in heartbreaking detail. Part 2 explores the reality of a life half-lived. Part 3 examines the speaker's diminished options and declares a commitment to writing. The final Part 4 embraces resolution through the immortality of verse. In particular, sonnet 91 in Part 3 depicts clearly the place of writing in the speaker's world:

> O poesy, thou art a path for me
> Through the dark forest tangle of my days;
> Thou art a stream and I am borne by thee,
> Thy life my pain of loneliness allays;
> Thou art a hidden cleft deep in the earth,
> Through which the waters of my love are led
> In yearning hope that they may yet find birth
> And some far vale may yet by them be fed.
> Why must my path the lonely forest keep?
> Why winds my stream through endless solitude?
> Why must my love be ever buried deep
> And my own heart its tenderness seclude?
> Nature hath willed it thus; yet kind was she
> Giving thy way for an escape to me.

Scholfield leaves no doubt as to his understanding of the importance of writing in his curing regimen. Scholfield died in Saranac Lake two years after publishing his sonnets and thirty years after contracting TB.

Like Herbert Scholfield, thirty-five-year-old Adelaide Crapsey wrote poetry to counteract the long hours of unwelcome passivity. Because Adelaide was severely ill, she was confined to bed in a private cure cottage with infrequent outside contact other than her doctor and nurse. Adelaide could do little other than write. In contrast to her letters, which disguised distress beneath a veneer of sophisticated "bons mots," Crapsey's poetry provided a private outlet where this atypically liberated woman could confide her fears and frustrations. Adelaide graduated from Vassar in 1901 and taught poetics at Smith College when tuberculosis forced her to seek the cure in Saranac Lake in 1913. Writing poetry was not new to Adelaide. She had earlier invented a highly compressed verse form she called the "cinquain" and written a number of poems, but published only a single poem before contracting TB. As a technically minded English professor, Crapsey approached poetry more from a critical than an expressive perspective. Considered her more serious life work, Crapsey left two-thirds of *Analysis of English Metrics* complete at the time of her death in 1914. When faced with tuberculosis, however, Adelaide turned to the expressiveness of poetry. Although she considered many of her poems works in progress, Adelaide arranged them in careful order as she sensed the end approaching. Crapsey's seventy poems were published posthumously as a collection eight years after her death. Near the end of her collection, Adelaide placed "The Lonely Death":

> In the cold I will rise, I will bathe
> In waters of ice; myself
> Will shiver, and shrive myself,
> Alone in the dawn, and anoint
> Forehead and feet and hands;
> I will shutter the windows from light,
> I will place in their sockets the four
> Tall candles and set them a-flame
> In the grey of the dawn; and myself
> Will lay myself straight in my bed,
> And draw the sheet under my chin.

As sad as we may find this poem, it gives voice to the patient's experience, and we may speculate that the writing gave Adelaide emotional release and, perhaps, a sense of being heard. The collection's final poem, "The Immortal Residue," suggests the palliative value Adelaide Crapsey placed on her writing: "Wouldst thou find my ashes? Look / In the pages of my book; / And, as these thy hand doth turn, / Know here is my funeral urn." This single collection (1922) of Crapsey's poems brought the deceased poet some attention. Crapsey's evident promise and her tragic end prompted three biographies (Osborn 1933; Butscher 1979; Alkalay-Gut 1988). Unfortunately, none of these studies examines critically how writing figured in Crapsey's (albeit unsuccessful) curing process.

John Theodore Dalton arrived in Saranac Lake seven years after Adelaide Crapsey had come and gone. Dalton read and admired Crapsey's poems while curing at Trudeau. Dalton's health problems had begun when he could not seem to recover fully from the influenza epidemic of 1918. Friends said it was his training in the Students' Army Corps during the Great War that sapped John's health. But John graduated from Dartmouth and went abroad to study classics at Cambridge. By 1923 he tested positive for tuberculosis and left Cambridge for Saranac Lake. Perhaps it was John's admiration of Adelaide's poetry or his love of classics that prompted him to write poems, plays, and songs to pass the time and amuse fellow patients. But Dalton did not seem to place much literary value on his own poetry. Friends often rescued poems written on scraps of paper that John tossed into the wastebasket. It was apparently the writing process that John valued. When he died in 1927 at the age of twenty-nine, John's friends prepared and published a small volume of forty-nine poems he had scribbled while at Saranac Lake. They called it *Land of Dreams*.

John Dalton's verses display a gentle bantering of the personnel and paraphernalia attached to curing, and a delicate mockery of his own suffering. The poem, "Write Verse"—beginning with its ironic title—shows an understanding of the therapeutic value of both laughter and writing in its whimsical tone:

> In summer things are all my way;
> It's flower growing time.
> For, when I want a big bouquet,
> I've always got a dime.
> But when the snow begins to fly
> I haven't got a chance;
> The other fellow's flower-talk
> Still breathes the same romance.
>
> Oh, daffodils and crocus buds
> And orchids pink and blue!
> Oh, roses red and violets
> And white carnations too!
>
> The other fellow sends her these:
> I've but an empty purse.
> Aw gee! What can a fellow do
> But write her flowery verse? (1930, 43)

John Dalton's ironic sense of life didn't fail him even when he chose to invoke his muse. Dalton acknowledged his bond with Crapsey's experience in "You've Shown the Way," subtitled "To Adelaide Crapsey—Once of Saranac": "Thanks, Adelaide, you showed the way; / I'm sorry you're not here to-day. / Perhaps I'd make your verse less sad, / And you could make mine far less bad" (5). John Dalton's fellow-patient, Bob Davis, sums up his friend's reliance on writing while curing: "Valiantly he fought the white plague with song and story" (Rinehart 2002, 99).

Humor and writing likewise helped patient Edward E. Locke to confront tuberculosis. Locke spent eight years in Saranac Lake during the 1930s and

1940s. Locke left behind a manuscript entitled *Smiles: A Novelty-Souvenir-Book Picturing Life in the Adirondacks*. Locke's manuscript contains poetry, prose, sketches, and cartoons. In the Introduction, Locke declares:

> These tales were mostly written when "sitting out" on the porch taking the cure. Numbed fingers frequently held a pen in which the ink was frozen. It was always at such times that brilliant thots [*sic*] came to me—but alas before the ink would flow, the thots [*sic*] had flown.

Locke's avowed purpose in writing *Smiles* was to "cause a few smiles." Although his intention was comic relief, Locke seems uncannily perceptive when, in "The Saranac Mind," he describes how the "writing mindset" descends upon sanatorium patients:

> Saranac Lake where the air is so pure,
>> That's where you go to take the cure,
> You hire a porch that is two by four,
>> And on it you dwell six months or more,
> For a week you think of things galore,
>> Of business, or troubles by the score;
> Of pleasures and each boyhood prank,
>> But after that your mind's a blank:
> For it only takes one week I find,
>> To develop the genuine "Saranac mind."

Locke's description of the "Saranac mind" alludes to an environment of natural beauty and freedom from ordinary stress that allowed patients the relative luxury of release through healthy self-expression despite the extraordinary circumstances in which they found themselves. Speaking for himself and others who turn to laughter and writing for relief, Locke comments in his Introduction that "the freedom with which we write and speak of our troubles is not born of a hardheartedness or a callousness to the situation. . . . [F]or we all know, that no physical improvement is possible, where the body is governed by a depressed mind." Locke expresses a straightforward understanding of the mind-body connection in healing and the role that writing may play in it.

For some Saranac Lake patients, the chance to write and publish locally was literally a lifeline. One of the most innovative schemes for turning writing into dollars was hatched by Beanie Barnet and his Trudeau Sanatorium roommate Seymour Eaton Jr. When Beanie and Seymour complained of feeling down, Seymour's father suggested they write inspirational messages to cheer each other up. Beanie and Seymour soon realized they could never pursue demanding careers, so the two decided to publish small chapbooks of these inspirational messages to cheer others and make money. Together they launched their *Trotty Veck Messages* series in 1916.

A character in Charles Dickens's short story "The Chimes," Trotty Veck delivered messages of cheer to townsfolk, despite the frailties of his health. Barnet and Eaton fashioned themselves after Dickens's character and became "Trotty Vecks." Their *Trotty Veck Messages* contained short selections of prose and verse steeped in wisdom and humor. Quotations came from the widest imaginable range of sources from antiquity to current events to local lore. Shakespeare shares the spotlight with an old Adirondack guide in an issue devoted to the theme of "Friends." Shakespeare counsels, through Polonius, "Those friends thou hast, and their adoption tried, / Grapple them to thy soul with hoops of steel, / But do not dull thy palm with entertainment / Of each new hatched unfledged comrade." Equally confident of his counsel, "The old Adirondack guide says he does not mind long sermons as long as they do not wake him up."

Trotty Veck Messages became an instant success—an antidote for both TB and the Great War. Barnet and Eaton sold four thousand copies the first year of 1916. Sadly, Seymour Eaton died in 1918. But Beanie Barnet carried on. By 1966 the *Adirondack Daily Enterprise* reported that *Trotty Veck Messages* had sold four million copies worldwide. Beanie had arrived in Saranac Lake in 1907 expecting—like Edward Livingston Trudeau—to die. Instead, Beanie cured, wrote, stayed, employed others, and lived in Saranac Lake as both patient and ex-patient until he died there in 1977, aged ninety (Hotaling 1980–1981, 4–7). Surely writing played a key role in Barnet's ability to cope with the challenges of TB. Certainly his widely distributed *Trotty Veck Messages* integrated the patient's voice into the discourse of this particularly widespread disease.

Martha Rebentisch cured in Saranac Lake on her own terms. Martha's father checked her into the Trudeau Sanatorium in 1927 when she was in her late twenties. In 1931, unimproved and frustrated after the usual curing regimen and several attempts at surgical intervention, Martha spotted an ad in the "local paper." It read "Wanted: To get in touch with some invalid who is not improving, and who would like to go into the woods for the summer" (Reben 1952, 1). Martha contacted the advertiser, Fred Rice, a local guideboat builder in his sixties known in Saranac Lake for his opposition to the sanatoria movement. She checked out of Trudeau Sanatorium and embarked on Fred's alternative naturalistic cure. Fred packed his guideboat with supplies, brought Martha aboard, and headed for Weller Pond, a two-hour paddle through two of the Saranac lakes and up the Saranac River.[6] Fred installed Martha onshore in one tent, himself in another. Martha spent the next six summers camping on Weller Pond, and wintering with Fred and his family in their humble cottage. Martha whiled away her long uninterrupted hours by writing. She filled her journals with the minutest details of a life surrounded by water, trees, flowers, fish, animals, insects, birds, sunshine, wind, rain, rainbows, and, most of all, fresh mountain air. As Martha camped and wrote, her health slowly improved. As a result of her Weller Pond regimen, Martha recovered from TB and joined the community of Saranac Lake where she continued to write until her death in 1964.

Martha's journal writing was so copious that she eventually published three books based on her journals under the name Martha Reben. *The Healing Woods*, *The Way of the Wilderness*, and *A Sharing of Joy* record the process that Martha believes cured her tuberculosis. Exactly when she became tuberculosis-free is uncertain. In *The Healing Woods* (1952), Martha writes: "I wish I could say that I was cured of tuberculosis during my second summer in the woods, but the truth is that I never knew when this came about. It was more than ten years after I first went into the woods before I had an X-ray taken or had a medical examination of any kind. These tests confirmed what I had already guessed—that I no longer had tuberculosis" (249). It is impossible to say exactly what cured Martha's TB, but her experience certainly suggests both the woods and her writing played significant roles. Reben (1955) comments specifically on the need she felt to write in *The Way of The Wilderness*: "I would not exchange a single hour of my freedom for something I did not need. I would cut living to the bone and buy time for writing and studying with the things I did without" (272–76).[7]

Perhaps the most fascinating patient narrative I've encountered belongs to Isabel Smith. Smith contracted TB in 1928 as a young nurse trainee in New York City. She was speedily packed off to Saranac Lake where she remained bedridden for twenty-one years. Finally, in 1950, new "wonder drugs" left Isabel Smith cured but frail. During her curing years, Smith wrote copious journals and letters and, ultimately, published her memoir, *Wish I Might*, in 1954. Smith's memoir provides two compelling insights into the role of patient narratives.

In the first place, Smith speaks directly to the power of writing in healing, and gives an eloquent explanation of this process. During her twenty-one years as a patient, Smith led a painful and precarious existence. Yet, as is also evident in her memoir and according to all who knew her, Smith's optimism and engagement with life were inspirational (Streeter 1963, 5–6). How did Smith maintain such optimism in the face of despair? Smith writes in her memoir of a pivotal event early in her curing process:

> One day I picked up a notebook from the shelf over my bed. Its pages were blank and I wondered why it had come there in the first place. Then I had a wonderful idea. It would be my Trouble Book. In it I would set down all my tumultuous, chaotic thoughts just as they came. . . . Once my problems and worries had become tangible words on a page, I discovered that I could deal with them almost as impersonally as if they belonged to someone else. . . . Writing in my Trouble Book provided me with a means for taking action of a sort, even when it did not amount to more than pushing a pen. And when I closed its pages I always felt relieved and released, as if whatever I had confided to it was now no longer *here*, but *there*. (1955, 62)

In her "Trouble Book," the first letters of which inevitably evoke her illness, Smith articulates explicitly and clearly what many TB patients apparently sensed and practiced—writing supports healing. Formal research has begun to theorize what patients such as Isabel Smith have known intuitively and practiced informally. Notably, groundbreaking articles in the *Journal of the American Medical Association* report positive results using writing in clinical settings (Smyth, Stone, Hurewitz, Kaell 1999; Spiegel 1999). Gabriele Rico (1991) and Louise De Salvo (1999) combine rigorous research with personal experience to reveal the therapeutic power of writing. Psychologist James Pennebaker's (1990) experiments with expressive writing suggest the healing potential of writing as a means for "opening up." Charles Anderson and Marian MacCurdy's (2000) collected essays from a variety of researchers and disciplines explore the interpenetration among writing, health, creativity, and learning. Joseph Gold (2002) and Mark Turner (1996) draw on the latest scientific findings to establish a biological basis for narrative. Increasingly, studies attest to the therapeutic value of writing.[8]

Secondly, in her detailed descriptions of the many curing practices she underwent, Isabel Smith provides us with an opportunity to examine some of the multiple dimensions that constitute the discourse of disease. As part of her TB treatment, Smith submitted to a surgical procedure known as pneumothorax. The purpose of pneumothorax was to collapse a diseased lung by means of air forced through a needle between the ribs into the pleural cavity surrounding the lung. Medical experts thought that collapsing the lung allowed it to rest and recover. As the body absorbed the air, regular refills were required to keep the lung at rest. The following examples portray this procedure from each of three perspectives—the scientific report, the clinical record, and the patient narrative.

In 1940, about the time Isabel Smith underwent pneumothorax, physicians at the Trudeau Foundation published a *scientific report* on *Artificial Pneumothorax: Its Practical Application in the Treatment of Pulmonary Tuberculosis.* Chapter II, "The Physiology of Artificial Pneumothorax," describes how the procedure affects the normal respiratory cycle:

> When, as in artificial pneumothorax therapy, quantities of 300 to 500 cc. of air are introduced into the pleural space at intervals of a week or thereabouts, striking alterations in the dynamics of respiration occur. The nature and the extent of these changes depend upon the quantity of air introduced and the state of the mediastinum, pleurae and lungs. . . . Artificial pneumothorax therapy frequently relieves dyspnea by reducing toxemia. "Selective" artificial pneumothorax may relieve dyspnea in subjects with a low vital capacity, by reducing the residual air in the healthy portion of the collapsed lung and improving the ventilation of the contra lateral lung. (Packard, Hayes, and Blanchet 1940, ch. 2)

A *clinical record* in the form of a Pneumothorax Chart was kept for each patient undergoing treatment. A typical chart recorded the patient's name, number, side and site of needle insertion, and method of anesthesia on the front of the chart. The reverse side was divided into five columns that recorded the date, the amount of air administered, the pressures before and after, and the administering doctor. The charts I have seen include only these bare facts with no space for additional comments. Details of each treatment were recorded meticulously on each patient's "pneumo" chart.

Isabel's own narrative tells this patient's experience of pneumothorax. Smith describes waiting for x-ray results as her condition worsened and then experiencing her first treatment. She writes:

> I held my breath, waiting for my report and I prayed that it might be all right. Perhaps I had just caught cold. Within twenty-four hours I saw Dr. Trudeau's car pull up in front of the house.[9] And when I saw Miss Taft, his office nurse, getting out followed by that meaningful mahogany case containing the pneumothorax apparatus, my heart sank. I knew the answer. When the two of them walked into my room, Dr. Trudeau's face was so grim and his manner so gruff that I had no word to say. I simply turned over on my stomach ready for what I knew was to come. And the hollow needle was already inserted in my anesthetized back before I ventured a cautious question. "I guess my X ray didn't look so good?" I murmured, feeling like a bug being pinned to a board. "No, Izzy. It was punk," he replied. Even as he spoke, air was beginning to pour through the needle into the space beyond the pleural lining of my chest wall, thus gradually inducing my lung to collapse. Not that I felt it as far as the lung was concerned. I felt only the tugs and pulls of pain where adhesions were trying to hold the lung fast to the pleura. But Dr. Trudeau's skill and gentleness— he is a great hand with the needle—made this initial treatment much easier than it might have been. It was not really more than six or eight minutes— although it seemed much longer to me—before only a tuft of cotton on my back marked the puncture where my pneumothorax treatments had begun, and the general area in which I would receive from time to time, like an inner tube, further refills of air. The needle had not made a sound as it entered my back and the minute break in the skin healed in a day. But as I lay bolstered high on my pillows that night, with every breath making me wince (the adhesions are sometimes stubborn the first few days), I knew that all my hopes for the future had collapsed along with my faithless lung. (Smith 1955, 51)

Both the scientific report and the clinical record contain literal, decontextualized facts. They are devoid of the expressive dimension related by Smith's narrative. Rita Charon presents a model of narrative medicine that argues for "respect for the narrative dimensions of illness and care-giving" (2001, 1901). Although Charon's counsel is directed primarily to medical practitioners, the notion that narrative brings an essential way of knowing to the experience of illness can also be understood within the context of patient narratives. On a more global scale, Anne Hunsaker Hawkins (1999) directs us to consider the cultural value when patients' voices assume their logical place in medical discourse: "Not only, then, does pathography restore the phenomenological and the experiential to the medical encounter, but it also restores the mythic dimension that our scientific, technological culture ignores or disallows" (23).

The use of metaphor by Smith and others—though perhaps at odds with Susan Sontag's (2001) argument that metaphor can distort our understanding of disease—does restore a certain phenomenological and even mythic dimension implicit in the complexity of the medical encounter. Smith's movement from the literal to the figurative in describing her pneumothorax treatment reflects Gold's and Turner's contention that the human capacity for language and knowing is inherently metaphoric. As Gold argues, "When people search for metaphors to explain themselves they are working hard to communicate; they are overcoming the *limitations of literal language*" (2002, 202).

I do not mean to imply that practitioners intentionally and routinely ignore or are insensitive to patients' experiences. The Saranac Lake community health initiative, in fact, suggests quite the opposite in this instance. What I want to argue is that the scientific, the clinical, and the patient discourses, when taken together, as I have tried to exemplify here, can provide a historiography that incorporates multiple perspectives of experience, and recognizes the particular types of valid knowledge each one contains. I would also suggest that the inclusion of patient narratives in the discourse of disease and the therapeutic value of writing are not mutually exclusive. For some patients, perhaps the act of expression through writing is enough. For others, the knowledge of being heard, and even remembered, seems to be an integral part of the therapeutic experience. Ultimately, a multidimensional discourse of disease benefits patient, practitioner, and all those who seek to understand illness. Patient narratives form an integral part of narrative medicine.

Narratives such as those of Bill Hastings, Evelyn Bellak, Herbert Scholfield, Adelaide Crapsey, John Dalton, Edward Locke, Beanie Barnet, Martha Reben, and Isabel Smith speak in particular and powerful ways about both unique and collective experiences at the "university of tuberculosis." Their writing represents only a small part of the Saranac Lake collection, and a tiny fraction of what must exist worldwide in relation to tuberculosis and other diseases. Like a stone tossed into a mountain pond, "patient writes" create multiple ripples of engagement within the discourse of disease.

NOTES

1. Both "curing" and "taking the cure" were common expressions used in conjunction with time spent at TB sanatoria whether or not the patient actually recov-

ered. I adopt that usage in this article, which is based on research supported by a three-year grant from the Social Sciences and Humanities Research Council of Canada.

2. See Dubos (1987); Caldwell (1988); Bates (1992); Rosenkrantz (1994); Rothman (1994); Ott (1996); Daniel (1997); Dormandy (1999).

3. Victoria E. Rinehart explains the difference between "sanitarium" and "sanatorium" with reference to tuberculosis: "'Sanitarium' is derived from the Latin word *sanitas*, which means health. In Dr. Trudeau's time, 'sanitarium' was used in relation to all chronic care institutions. However, because of its close link with the word 'sanity' it was often linked to institutions that treated mental disorders. 'Sanatorium' comes from the Latin word *sanare*, which means to heal. Therefore, at the turn of the century it became the preferred word for the treatment of consumptives" (2002, 155). The Adirondack Cottage Sanitarium was renamed the Trudeau Sanatorium after Trudeau's death.

4. It is interesting to note that Edward Livingston Trudeau's son, Dr. Francis B. Trudeau, assumed his father's role of leadership at the Trudeau Sanatorium and in the community. Dr. Francis B. Trudeau's son, Dr. Frank Trudeau Jr., became the third generation to assume the role occupied by his grandfather. The original cure cottage, "Little Red," today stands as a monument on the grounds of what has become the Trudeau Institute. The Institute is successor to the Trudeau Sanatorium's research facility, the Saranac Laboratory. In a new location several miles from the old Lab, the Institute is a modern biomedical facility devoted to immunology and identified by the Institute for Scientific Information as one of the ten most influential independent research institutes in the United States. The original Lab premises was donated to Historic Saranac Lake, and is being developed as a museum devoted to Trudeau, tuberculosis, and Saranac Lake.

5. See De Sormo (1974); Mooney (1979); Taylor (1986); Caldwell (1988; 1993); Morris (1998).

6. There are three lakes in the Saranac chain of lakes that incorporate the name "Saranac": Lower Saranac, Middle Saranac, and Upper Saranac. Lower Saranac is closest to Saranac Lake village. Fred paddled Martha through Lower Saranac and Middle Saranac. Weller Pond is accessed by guideboat (Adirondack type of canoe) directly from Middle Saranac.

7. See Reben (1952; 1955; 1963) and Tisdale (2000).

8. See also Kleinman (1989); Herman (1992); McNiff (1992); Progoff (1992); Fox (1997); Frank (1997); Foehr and Schiller (1997); Rainer (1998; 1999); Hawkins (1999); Elbow (2000); Mattingly (2000); Charon (2001); Charon and Montello (2002) Nelson (2001); Brody (2002); Lepore (2002); Zimmerman (2002).

9. Smith refers here to Dr. Francis B. Trudeau, the son of Dr. Edward Livingston Trudeau.

REFERENCES

Alkalay-Gut, Karen. 1988. *Alone in the dawn: The life of Adelaide Crapsey*. Athens: University of Georgia Press.

Anderson, Alton. 1951. Welcome letter to patients. Saranac Lake, NY: Historic Saranac Lake.

Anderson, Charles, and Marion MacCurdy. 2000. *Writing and healing: Toward an informed practice*. Urbana, IL: National Council of Teachers of English.

Barnet, Beanie. 1916–1966. *Trotty Veck messages*. Saranac Lake, NY: Currier Press.

Bates, Barbara. 1992. *Bargaining for life: A social history of tuberculosis, 1876–1938*. Philadelphia: University of Pennsylvania Press.

Bellak, Evelyn. 1918. *Fond memories of Ray Brook: A diary*. Saranac Lake, NY: Saranac Lake Free Library.

Brody, Howard. 2002. *Stories of sickness.* New York: Oxford University Press.

Butscher, Edward. 1979. *Adelaide Crapsey*. Boston: Twayne.

Caldwell, Mark. 1988. *The last crusade: The war on consumption, 1862–1954*. New York: Atheneum.

———. 1993. *Saranac Lake: Pioneer health resort*. Saranac Lake, NY: Historic Saranac Lake.

Charon, Rita. 2001. Narrative medicine: A model for empathy, reflection, profession, and trust. *Journal of the American Medical Association* 286, no. 15:1897–1902.

Charon, Rita, and Martha Montello, eds. 2002. *Stories matter: The role of narrative in medical ethics*. New York: Routledge.

Crapsey, Adelaide. 1922. *Verse*. New York: Knopf.

Dalton, John T. 1930. *Land of dreams and other poems*. New York: Knickerbocker Press.

Daniel, Thomas. 1997. *Captain of death: The story of tuberculosis*. Rochester: University of Rochester Press.

De Salvo, Louise. 1999. *Writing as a way of healing: How telling our stories transforms our lives*. San Francisco: Harper Collins.

De Sormo, Maitland. 1974. *The heydays of the Adirondacks*. Saranac Lake, NY: Adirondack Yesteryears.

Dormandy, Thomas. 1999. *The white death: A history of tuberculosis*. Rio Grande, OH: Hambledon Press.

Dubos, Rene, and Jean Dubos. 1987. *The white plague: Tuberculosis, man, and society*. New Brunswick: Rutgers University Press.

Elbow, Peter. 2000. *Everyone can write: Essays toward a hopeful theory of writing and teaching writing*. New York: Oxford University Press.

Foehr, Regina Paxton, and Susan A. Schiller. 1997. *The spiritual side of writing: Releasing the learner's whole potential*. Portsmouth, NH: Boynton/Cook.

Fox, John. 1997. *Poetic medicine: The healing art of poem-making*. New York: Tarcher/Putnam.

Frank, Arthur. 1997. *The wounded storyteller: Body, illness, and ethics*. Chicago: University of Chicago Press.

Gallos, Philip L. 1985. *Cure cottages of Saranac Lake: Architecture and history of a pioneer health resort.* Saranac Lake, NY: Historic Saranac Lake.

Gold, Joseph. 2002. *The story species: Our life-literature connection.* Markham, ON: Whiteside.

Hawkins, Anne. 1999. *Reconstructing illness: Studies in pathography.* West Lafayette, IN: Purdue University Press.

Herman, Judith. 1992. *Trauma and recovery.* New York: Basic Books.

Hotaling, Mary B. 1980–1981. Beanie Barnet and the Trotty Veck messages. *Center for Adirondack Studies Newsletter* (Winter-Spring):4–7.

Kleinman, Arthur. 1989. *The illness narratives: Suffering, healing, and the human condition.* New York: Basic Books.

Lepore, Stephen, and Joshua Smyth, eds. 2002. *The writing cure: How expressive writing promotes health and emotional well-being.* Washington, DC: American Psychological Association.

Locke, Edward E. n.d. *Smiles: A novelty-souvenir-book picturing life in the Adirondacks.* Saranac Lake, NY: Historic Saranac Lake.

Mattingly, Cheryl, and Linda Garro, eds. 2000. *Narrative and the cultural construction of illness and healing.* Berkeley: University of California Press.

McNiff, Shaun. 1992. *Art as medicine: Creating a therapy of the imagination.* Boston: Shambala Press.

Mooney, Elizabeth. 1979. *In the shadow of the white plague: A memoir by Elizabeth Mooney.* New York: Thomas Y. Crowell.

Morris, David. 1998. *Illness and culture in the postmodern age.* Berkeley: University of California Press.

Nelson, Hilde Lindemann. 2001. *Damaged identities: Narrative repair.* Ithaca: Cornell University Press.

Osborn, Mary Elizabeth. 1933. *Adelaide Crapsey.* Boston: Humphries.

Ott, Katherine. 1996. *Fevered lives: Tuberculosis in American culture since 1870.* Cambridge: Harvard University Press.

Packard, Edward Newman, J. N. Hayes, and S. F. Blanchet, eds. 1940. *Artificial pneumothorax: Its practical application in the treatment of pulmonary tuberculosis.* Philadelphia: Lea and Febiger.

Pennebaker, James. 1990. *Opening up: The healing power of expressing emotions.* New York: Guilford Press.

Progoff, Ira. 1992. *At a journal workshop: Writing to access the power of the unconscious and evoke creative ability.* Los Angeles: Jeremy Tarcher/Putnam.

Rainer, Tristine. 1998. *Your life as story: Discovering "new autobiography" and writing memoir as literature.* New York: Jeremy Tarcher/Putnam.

Reben, Martha. 1952. *The healing woods.* New York: Thomas Y. Crowell.

———. 1955. *The way of the wilderness*. New York: Thomas Y. Crowell.

———. 1963. *A sharing of joy*. New York: Harcourt Brace.

Reichman, Lee, with Janice Hopkins Tanne. 2002. *Timebomb: The global epidemic of multi-drug-resistant tuberculosis*. New York: McGraw-Hill.

Rico, Gabriele Lusser. 1991. *Writing your way through personal crisis, pain, and possibility*. New York: Jeremy Tarcher/Putnam.

Rinehart, Victoria E. 2002. *Portrait of healing: Curing in the woods*. Utica: North Country Books.

Rosenkrantz, Barbara Gutmann. 1994. *From consumption to tuberculosis: A documentary history*. New York: Garland Publishing.

Rothman, Sheila. 1994. *Living in the shadow of death: Tuberculosis and the social experience of illness in American history*. New York: Basic Books.

Scholfield, Herbert. 1919. *Sonnets of Herbert Scholfield*. New York: Alfred A. Knopf.

Smith, Isabel. 1955. *Wish I might*. New York: Harper Press.

Smyth, Joshua S., Arthur A. Stone, Adam Hurewitz, and Alan Kaell. 1999. Effects of writing about stressful experiences on symptom reduction in patients with asthma or rheumatoid arthritis. *Journal of the American Medical Association* 14:1304–09.

Sontag, Susan. 2001. *Illness as metaphor and AIDS and its metaphors*. New York: Picador.

Spiegel, David. 1999. Healing words: Emotional expression and disease outcome. *Journal of the American Medical Association* 14:1328–29.

Streeter, Edward. 1963. Frail conqueror. *Family Weekly*, March 10, 5–6.

Taylor, Robert. 1986. *Saranac: America's magic mountain*. Boston: Houghton Mifflin.

Tisdale, Betty. 2000. *Martha Reben, Adirondack writer*. Saranac Lake, NY: Historic Saranac Lake.

Trudeau, Edward Livingston. 1914. *An autobiography of Edward Livingston Trudeau, M.D.* Garden City, NY: Doubleday.

Turner, Mark. 1996. *The literary mind: The origins of thought and language*. New York: Oxford University Press.

Zimmerman, Susan. 2002. *Writing to heal the soul: Transforming grief and loss through writing*. New York: Three Rivers Press.

PART IV

Acts of Reading

THIRTEEN

The Teaching Cure

JEFFREY BERMAN

IT WAS "FRÄULEIN ANNA O.," Bertha Pappenheim, who coined the expression "the talking cure" to describe verbal therapy. The first patient in what
became psychoanalysis, she jokingly referred to her treatment with Josef
Breuer as "chimney-sweeping" (Breuer and Freud 1895, 30), which left her
free of distressing feelings for several days. The talking cure is now more than
a century old, and although its demise has long been predicted and, in some
cases, devoutly wished for, psychoanalysis remains alive and well. It has taken
that century for the talking cure to spawn "the writing cure," and in recent
years two books have been published with that title, one written by Mark
Bracher (1999), a noted Lacanian literary critic, the other edited by two psychology professors, Stephen Lepore and Joshua Smyth (2002). Both books
affirm the growing recognition of the therapeutic value of writing. In 2002,
Professor Sophie Freud, Sigmund Freud's granddaughter, gave a stimulating
lecture to students in my "Literature and Healing Arts" class on "the reading
cure"—since published (2003) in *American Imago*—in which she discussed the
importance of bibliotherapy to her personal and professional development.

In light of the talking cure, the writing cure, and the reading cure, can
we now speak about "the teaching cure"? Surely my title raises more questions
than answers. Can any pedagogy, psychoanalytic or otherwise, have a curative effect, and, if so, for what "malady" can the teaching cure be used? To
what extent can education—which Sigmund Freud (1937) called an "impossible" profession in that "one can be sure beforehand of achieving unsatisfy-
ing results" (248)—truly heal? What precautions must be used to prevent the
teaching cure from becoming countertherapeutic? These are some of the
questions I would like to explore in the present chapter.

THE SMALL ROOM: "GIVE HER PSYCHIATRIC
ATTENTION . . . AND SHE'LL JUST WALLOW IN SELF"

Before discussing my own teaching experiences, I want to look at a literary representation of college teaching, one of the most moving academic novels about how a teacher's empathy makes a difference in her students' lives. May Sarton's 1961 story *The Small Room* describes a young assistant professor's first teaching experience at an elite women's college in New England. The novel is fascinating in several ways. First, it explores the student-teacher relationship, including the complex and often unruly transference-countertransference dynamics that are rarely acknowledged by educators. Second, *The Small Room* focuses on the personal aspects of teaching, especially the elusive qualities that contribute to the art of teaching. Third, the novel analyzes the different roles teachers play in the classroom, particularly the role of therapist, for which they are seldom trained or prepared. Fourth, the novel is a cautionary tale about the benefits and risks of teacher interventions in students' lives. And finally, *The Small Room* dramatizes many of the similarities between teaching and psychotherapy, both of which have far more in common with each other than teachers or therapists are wont to admit.

Published shortly before the birth of the women's movement, *The Small Room* contains several minor details—and one major detail—that reveal how different higher education is today. Appleton, which resembles Wellesley College, is an institution that prides itself on teaching, and for Lucy Winter, who has just received her PhD in English from Harvard University, Appleton represents her initiation into the profession. Lucy entered a doctoral program so that she could be near her fiancé, a student at Harvard Medical School; but when she abruptly breaks off the engagement, she decides, albeit reluctantly, to look for a teaching position. Neither Lucy nor Sarton could realize that the early 1960s was one of the few sellers' markets for professors. To anyone in the humanities who has been unlucky enough to be on the job market in the last thirty years, the ease with which Lucy lands a job at Appleton, considered the "pristine well, the essence of female institutions of learning" (1961, 12), must seem a fantasy—especially since the twenty-seven-year-old assistant professor, with no publications or burning desire to write, is promised tenure and promotion "in a year or so." Another detail that strikes contemporary academics as strange is the question that she is asked during her on-campus interview: "You are not planning to marry in the immediate future?" (12)—a query that violates current antidiscrimination laws. Unlike today's students, who wear jeans and sweatshirts to classes, for Appleton students the "unrequired but almost universal uniform [is] . . . short pleated skirts and blazers" (30). Neither students nor teachers think twice before lighting up cigarettes during conferences. Teachers drink more alcohol than do their students, a detail that contemporary students would find archaic.

But what most separates us from the world of Appleton is that the college does not yet have a resident psychiatrist to counsel its students. This is the emotionally charged question that drives the novel's plot, for when Lucy discovers that one of the college's most brilliant students, Jane Seaman, has plagiarized an essay, the campus is polarized around the issue of whether to expel her, as college regulations demand, or recommend that she see an off-campus psychiatrist who will help her uncover the unconscious motives behind the self-destructive act—an act that the novel's proponents of psychiatry assert confirms the urgent need for a resident therapist to help Appleton's troubled undergraduates. Adamantly opposing the hire of a psychiatrist are Jane's mentor, Professor Carryl Cope, an internationally famous medieval scholar, and Carryl's closest friend and lover, Olive Hunt, an eccentric member of Appleton's Board of Trustees who has threatened to change her will leaving a multimillion dollar donation to the college, which desperately needs the money to ensure its survival.

It is hard for us to imagine a college or university without a counseling center, yet this is the situation at Appleton slightly more than forty years ago. Why the fierce opposition to psychiatry? Both Carryl Cope and Olive Hunt offer what they regard as irrefutable reasons why Appleton's students would be harmed by a mental health professional. To begin with, the opposition is a generational issue: as the college president explains, Olive Hunt "comes of the old-fashioned school which thinks you pull yourself up by your own bootstraps"; a moment later he elaborates that this is precisely what she did years ago when she was in a psychological crisis: "I suspect that she may have had some sort of breakdown herself, after her father's death, and that she pulled herself out of it on sheer guts" (57). Olive has no use either for therapists or students who need their services: "What the girls need," she states imperiously, "is not more 'help'—ugh, how I loathe that word!—but greater demands on their intellects and souls" (78–79). When Lucy tells her about a freshman, Pippa Brentwood, who is grieving her father's recent death, neglecting her personal appearance, and spending a great deal of time crying, Olive Hunt replies unempathically:

> So did I when I was her age. . . . I suspect that I rather enjoyed it. I got out
> of it, not because I had a professor who took a personal interest in me, but
> because I did have (thank God!) a professor who made me take an interest
> in a subject. It happened to be Greek. Give her psychiatric attention—for I
> presume what you are saying is that you would be glad to turn this weeper
> over to someone else and take her back when she combs her hair and stops
> crying—give her *that*, and she'll just wallow in *self*. (79–80)

Whereas Olive Hunt believes that the appointment of a resident psychiatrist will discourage professors from making challenging demands on their students' intellects and souls, Carryl Cope asserts that there are people such as Pippa who shouldn't be in college because of psychological problems. Carryl is less opinionated than Olive Hunt but no less psychologically obtuse, at least until the end of the novel, when she undergoes a change of heart. Unlike Lucy, who tries to teach all her students, Carryl is devoted only to the most extraordinary. "I teach for the singular, for the exceptional," she maintains; "I teach for the one in a hundred, one in a thousand maybe" (75). Believing that the price of excellence is "eccentricity, maladjustment if you will, isolation of one sort or another, strangeness, narrowness" (69), Carryl is devastated by the seemingly inexplicable behavior of her star student, Jane Seaman, whom she has been grooming as a disciple. Carryl's solution is to hush up the plagiarism so that her protégée's career will not be destroyed; she cannot imagine that Jane committed plagiarism as an unconscious rebellion against the authority figure who has been trying to control her life. Carryl is so invested emotionally in Jane that she threatens to resign if the college recommends psychiatric help for her student—thus ironically demonstrating that the faculty might also need psychological counseling.

Lucy Winter, the novel's sympathetic heroine, intuits the reasons behind Jane Seaman's plagiarism, Olive Hunt's and Carryl Cope's implacable opposition to psychiatry, Pippa Brentwood's mourning, and the complex dynamics of the student-teacher relationship. Lucy's psychological and pedagogical insights identify her with the authorial point of view, but what makes her a compelling, believable character are her self-doubts and vulnerability, along with her self-effacing personality and empathic understanding. Recognizing that Jane's paper on *The Iliad* is plagiarized from an essay by Simone Weil appearing in an obscure English publication, Lucy asks her to explain why she resorted to intellectual theft. "I just got tired of being pushed so hard, tired of the whole racket, tired of having a brain, tired of coming up to the jump and taking it again and again. Lost my nerve" (102). Lucy listens nonjudgmentally to her student's explanation and, without using the word *transference*, helps her see that her anger toward the increasing demands placed upon her by Carryl Cope is a repetition of her disappointment with her divorced parents, who have apparently neglected her. In Lucy's view, Jane has sought love and approval through intellectual achievement, but when that fails to fulfill her deeper longings, she sabotages herself by committing a crime that she knows will lead to eventual discovery and expulsion. Lucy thus interprets Jane's plagiarism as a psychological cry for help, and she urges her to seek professional treatment to expand her self-awareness. At first Jane angrily rejects her teacher's words, concluding that "[y]ou're just like everyone else who has read a little Freud and thinks he can paste a label on things and solve them with a label" (161), but she gradually overcomes the fear of exploring her unconscious motivation and agrees to go with Lucy to New York City to visit a psychoanalyst with whom she begins treatment.

Lucy also helps Carryl Cope explore countertransference issues, namely, how and why the intense demands that she has placed on her young protégée have been damaging to both of them. Lucy again functions as a psychoanalyst, tactfully suggesting to her senior colleague that what Jane needs most from her professor is not more intellectual knowledge, as Carryl believes, but understanding of a different kind. Carryl initially rejects this interpretation, denying that she has unduly pressured her student. Nor does she realize that her effort to cover up the plagiarism will make the situation worse. Only gradually does she recognize that she has "refused to recognize the whole person in Jane Seaman" (232). As the novel closes, Carryl realizes that she has been too involved with her student's success and failure, and she discovers that teachers must preserve a delicate balance between involvement and detachment. "Part of the art of teaching," a colleague observes, "lies in how this pseudo-intimacy is handled" (40–41)—a pseudo-intimacy that is as problematic in the student-teacher relationship as it is in the patient-analyst relationship.

Contemporary readers may believe, as I do, that Lucy's psychoanalytic interpretation of Jane Seaman's plagiarism is too neat. Plagiarism is now so common that few teachers seek to discover the underlying psychological motivations behind it; moreover, the problem of how to respond to plagiarism would still remain even if that motivation could be determined. Another problem with *The Small Room* is that few assistant professors would have the courage—or foolishness—to confront a senior professor's lifelong pattern of relating to students. Nor is it credible that Olive Hunt, so contemptuous of psychology, should agree with Lucy that Carryl Cope sees Jane as a younger version of herself. Both Carryl and Olive accept many of Lucy's psychoanalytic interpretations at the end of the novel, further straining credibility.

"THERE MUST BE A SUBJECT BETWEEN US"

Lucy's attitude toward her "weeper," Pippa Brentwood, is also puzzling. Lucy recoils in horror when Pippa tells her, after their first class, that her father has died recently; Lucy is unnerved by what she regards as her student's inappropriate "plea for sympathy" (Sarton 1961, 38). She dreads to see Pippa in conference "because she is clearly incapacitated by some private woe" (79). Lucy's explanation to an older colleague hints at her discomfort with the personal aspect of teaching: "What depressed me, I think, was that I tried to say something about learning and teaching, and the only result was that a girl wanted to tell me about her father's death" (39). The colleague's response indicates that she too is critical of the student's tears: "Pippa Brentwood . . . does tend to dramatize . . . and I'm afraid her father's death, sudden and tragic as it was, has given her rather a chance to indulge herself" (39). This judgment of grief as a form of self-indulgence seems to reflect the authorial point of view.

Pippa's tears strike at the heart of the novel, for they signify what Lucy calls the "old universal wound" (49). Lucy knows all about this wound because of her disappointment with her own father, a successful surgeon who seems to derive more pleasure from his career and hobbies than from his family. Pippa's tears penetrate Lucy's defenses, awakening her deepest psychological conflicts. Throughout the novel Lucy struggles to empathize with her students without being overwhelmed by their problems; at times she prefers to relate to Pippa only as a student, while at other times she speaks more personally, acknowledging her own vulnerability. "She found herself speaking quite gently now about the load of guilt children always do carry around about their parents, and how self-blame can, after a point, become self-indulgence. 'It's the human condition, Pippa'" (49). Lucy's words have a therapeutic effect on Pippa, as the narrator observes: "It was touching to see the immense relief in the face of innocence before her, relief like some clear dawn taking the place of disintegration and darkness." Pippa thanks her teacher with the words, "I knew you'd understand. I knew you'd help" (49–50). But Lucy still fears personal involvement with her student, and Pippa seems just as needy as ever: "You won't refuse to see me?"—a question that sets up the following dialogue:

> "On professional matters, Pippa, I'll always be here. This has been an excursion outside them."
>
> "I'm a terrible nuisance, I guess," Pippa said hopefully.
>
> "No," Lucy summoned dispassion to her side as if it were a guardian angel. "But you are, perhaps, confusing me with someone else, an imaginary someone, let us say, 'a father confessor and friend.' I don't see myself in that role, I'm afraid." Lucy got up and stood with her back to the window. It was meant to be a dismissal.
>
> "You sound so hard," Pippa said in an accusing voice.
>
> "I'm not hard," she shot back, fatally on the defensive. "I'm too vulnerable. I have never been a teacher before. And I don't believe in college teachers being amateur psychoanalysts." She recovered herself firmly. "There must be a subject between us, Pippa, an impersonal subject," she said, facing the girl squarely.
>
> "Well," Pippa, accepting defeat, gathered her books together as slowly as possible, "but if I could just see you when I get desperate? I'll try not to, I really will," she added eagerly.
>
> "I'm not a monster, after all," Lucy said, and left it at that. (50–51)

Lucy is not a monster, though she does strike me as surprisingly fearful of empathizing with her student's distress. Perhaps Lucy's youth and professional inexperience heighten her vulnerability, making empathy dangerous, but what most surprises me is May Sarton's portrayal of Pippa's grief as a form of self-indulgence. There's something comical about the number of times Pippa "wails" in her teacher's presence. Pippa has every right to cry over her father's recent death, yet the novel depicts her tears as excessive. Later, Pippa again begins to cry in Lucy's office, this time because of the accurate perception that Carryl Cope is playing favorites by trying to conceal Jane's plagiarism, but now the narrator tells us that "Pippa's tears, this time, could not be pushed aside as self-indulgent" (133). "It takes some courage to face out the self-righteous indignation of your peers," Lucy observes, adding, "My sympathy is with Jane." Once Lucy acknowledges her own confusion and self-doubt, she senses that the "intimacy which this painful interview was establishing between her and Pippa, far from feeding a 'crush' as she had feared it would, was rooted now in mutual respect" (135–36). Both feel better after their discussion, and the chapter closes with Lucy wondering "whether crisis may be one of the climates where education flourishes—a climate that forces honesty out, breaks down the walls of what ough[t] to be, and reveals what *is*, instead" (138).

"TEACHING IS MORE THAN JUST A SUBJECT"

May Sarton provides readers of *The Small Room* with a degree of closure at the end without fully resolving the pedagogical questions raised by the novel. Lucy receives an appreciative note from Jane indicating her progress at the sanitarium where she is being treated: "They say I shall get well, and I am try-ing" (Sarton 1961, 210). Pippa is also doing well: she turns in a thoughtful essay on Emerson and Thoreau, and she seems to be in control of her grief. "You've taught me a lot," she gratefully tells Lucy, who is pleased with her academic progress. Yet Lucy is still troubled by the degree to which her stu-dent's academic growth depends upon her personal feelings toward the teacher. "Oh Pippa. . . . Do it for the thing itself, not for me," to which Pippa responds firmly, "For you as well. . . . Teaching is more than just a subject, you know. It's a person, too. You can't get away from that, even if you want to" (212). Lucy clearly *wants* to escape from the personal element in teaching, fearful that it will result in a loss of boundaries in the student-teacher rela-tionship. Her final realization is that teaching is always personal but must never be the main focus of education. "There was no avoiding the issue: the most detached teacher in the world infused her detachment, and if one stu-dent or another received this as a personal message, well, maybe one had to accept that that was one way of learning. No wonder teaching was called an art, the most difficult kind of art in which the final expression depends upon a delicate and dangerous balance between two people and a subject. Elimi-nate the subject and the whole center collapses" (212–13).

The Small Room raises intriguing pedagogical questions that are as impor-tant today as they were when the novel was published. It remains one of the most authentic fictional studies of the student-teacher relationship. Carryl Cope speaks for all of her colleagues when she observes that the "relation between student and teacher must be about the most complex and ill-defined there is" (83). Sometimes this complexity is gently satirized, as when Lucy tells her students on the first day of the semester that "[y]ou will discover . . . that you appreciate teachers rather a long time after you have suffered from them" (34). The narrator is well aware that "teaching is first of all teaching a person" (104), an insight that affirms teaching the whole person. Teachers can never predict when a story will speak to its readers, but sometimes it is only when a student is experiencing a crisis. Thus, it occurs to Lucy that "it was perhaps only at points of conflict that some door in the lazy attention was finally forced open, and people became educable—at least if the conflict were not too intense or deeply buried" (131).

Lucy learns a great deal about teaching, and as the novel closes, she has made the kind of difference in her students' lives that her own teachers made in hers. Indeed, during her first day of class she tells her students about the "great teachers" who have had a transformative effect upon her. Despite differences in teaching styles and subjects, they were all humble and respectful. One teacher was "devastatingly honest, with a kind of honesty that forced him to ask questions rather than to make statements, and to question himself as seriously as he did us" (35). Another teacher failed Lucy on a midterm but told her that her paper contained an original idea that many of the A exams did not have. And a third teacher "wore his learning so lightly that he forced you to wear yours with at least an attempt at a sense of proportion" (37). Lucy embodies these same qualities, along with the recognition that "there are as many kinds of good teachers as there are of artists" (110).

May Sarton has indicated that *The Small Room* was based on her own college teaching experiences. Although she never attended college, she taught composition at Harvard from 1950–1953 and creative writing at Wellesley College from 1959–1964. She wrote to a friend in 1961 that *The Small Room* "was a kind of love letter to the profession of teaching . . . but I was anxious both not to be snide (as so many novelists have been when dealing with college life) nor sentimental" (2002, 92). Mark Fulk notes that her "advocacy here—revolutionary at the time—for the use of professional counselors on campus ties in with her own commitment to become more candid, honest, and open with herself, and to model that openness for others" (2002, 84). She stated in an interview that she loved teaching but decided to leave the profession when she was fifty-five because "it takes exactly out of you what writing does" (Ingersoll 1991, 47).

Curiously, Sarton's attitude toward psychoanalysis in *The Small Room* is more positive than her statements elsewhere suggest. In a letter written in 1947, she complained that "Freudianism . . . excuses everything one may do or be" (1997, 274)—a statement that echoes Pippa's sentiments in the novel. Sarton also objected to the psychoanalytic bias against homosexuality. "I would be an anti-Freudian in that I never believed that a homosexual was a cripple" (Ingersoll 1991, 71).

The world has changed profoundly in the last forty years, and nowhere is this change better seen than in the fact that today's students visit college counseling centers in record numbers. The question today is not whether a college should appoint a resident psychiatrist but whether it has the resources to hire enough mental health professionals to treat all the students who seek counseling. Few novelists could have predicted in the early 1960s how many future college students would suffer from clinical depression, suicidal ideation, anxiety and panic attacks, eating disorders, and drug and alcohol addiction. Pippa's grief over her father's death anticipates the anguish of countless students whose families have been shattered by divorce and who may have lost contact with one or both of their biological parents. If, as the novel suggests, psychological counseling is essential to a student such as Jane Seaman, what about the students sitting in our classrooms who are in more desperate situations?

MY OWN SMALL ROOM

May Sarton's novel affirms the value of the talking cure, but I want to suggest how college teachers can avail themselves of the writing, reading, and teaching cures. To do so, I need to give a brief history of the evolution of my approach to teaching and what academic life is like in my own small room. Like Lucy, I believe that teaching depends upon a "delicate and dangerous balance between two people and a subject." I also believe, as she does, that professors should not have to "take on the students' personal problems" (Sarton 1961, 79). But unlike Lucy, I believe that the subject students may write about is their own lives. Since the middle 1970s, when I began teaching a course on literature and psychoanalysis, I have encouraged students to make connections between fictional characters and their own lives. This "life writing" has taken many forms, including introspective diaries in my psychoanalytic courses, reader-response diaries in my literature courses, and self-disclosing essays in my expository writing courses. *Diaries to an English Professor* (1994) explores the ways in which undergraduates use psychoanalytic diaries to probe conflicted issues in their lives. *Surviving Literary Suicide* (1999) investigates how graduate students respond to suicidal literature, including the dangers of romanticizing a subject in literature that we would never wish to glorify in life. *Risky Writing* (2001) describes how teachers can encourage students to write safely on a wide range of subjects often deemed too personal for the classroom, including the breakup of the family, eating disorders, sexual abuse, and depression. My most recent book, *Empathic Teaching* (2005), focuses on the ways in which a pedagogy of self-disclosure can enable teachers to make a difference in their students' lives.

The teaching cure depends upon the creation of a safe and empathic classroom in which students know that they will not be attacked by their classmates or teacher. The only prerequisite I list for my writing courses is empathy: the desire to understand another person's point of view. One cannot completely know another person, but one can attempt to know as much as possible. I ask my students to be empathic and nonjudgmental when responding to a classmate's essay, and I model this behavior myself. Students soon discover that they can write on the most personal subjects without fearing that their feelings will be invalidated.

Teachers who encourage students to write about their lives must be sensitive to the potential dangers of such writing, and in *Risky Writing* I describe in detail the many protocols I put into place to minimize the possibility that students will become at risk. For example, students decide on the degree of self-disclosure, and they can avoid writing on any topic they deem too dangerous or personal. I usually do not grade their self-disclosing writings, and I never psychoanalyze my students' diaries or essays. Instead, I praise my students' efforts toward self-analysis and raise clarifying questions that enable them to develop their diaries and essays. I also make grammatical and stylistic suggestions in my expository writing courses. One of the most distinctive aspects of my approach to writing is that students have more freedom to write on personal topics than they would with other instructors. They know that I will read carefully every essay and help them find the best words to express themselves.

As valuable as it is for my students to engage in personal writing, it is even more valuable when they share their writings with classmates. In my literature courses, I read about five psychoanalytic or reader-response diaries aloud before returning them to the students. I always read these writings anonymously, and there is no class discussion. Students reach their own conclusions about the writings read aloud. Those who do not want me to read aloud their writings simply write the word "no" on the bottom of their entries. In the beginning of the semester there are usually a handful of students who do not want me to read aloud their writings, but by the end of the semester there may be only one or two in a class of forty. The diaries that I read aloud are powerful, moving, and insightful; students tell me in their anonymous evaluations written at the end of the semester that the diary component is the most interesting part of the course. If students in my expository writing courses wish to share their essays anonymously with classmates, I read the papers aloud, and there is no class discussion. Whenever possible, I prescreen essays to make sure they are not too painful to read aloud or hear.

One can imagine what May Sarton's characters might write about in introspective diaries. A student such as Pippa Brentwood would almost certainly write about her anguish over her father's death. If she was incapacitated by grief, then writing would be one of the best ways to work through her feelings. Jane Seaman might write about anger toward her absent parents, and Lucy Winter might write about her uncertainty whether she made the right decision to become a college professor. Olive Hunt might write about the self-destructive pride that alienates her from the college to which she has devoted her life. Carryl Cope might write about her aversion to psychiatry. If she resented the necessity to write a psychoanalytic diary, all she would need to do is to write a one-sentence comment—Bartleby's "I would prefer not to."

What do my own students write about? During the years in which I was writing *Diaries to an English Professor*, I collected several thousand diaries from my literature and psychoanalysis students, who enthusiastically granted me permission to use them for my research. (I have also received approval from my university's Institutional Review Board, which must monitor all human research.) It was daunting to reread all these diaries in an effort to decide how to organize the book, but it did not take long for me to realize that I would devote a chapter to each of the major subjects about which my students wrote. The chapter "Sins of the Fathers" explores how students write about the ways in which divorce has affected their families. "Hunger Artists," whose title comes from the Kafka story we read in class, focuses on how college students, mainly women, describe eating disorders, including anorexia and bulimia. In "Sexual Disclosures" students write about sexual abuse and homophobia. And in "Suicide Survivors" students write about the ways in which depression and suicide have affected their lives, including not only relatives' and friends' experiences but their own as well.

I never anticipated when I first started writing *Diaries to an English Professor* that it would be the first of several books on the subject of the teaching cure. An overwhelming majority of students tell me that they enjoy the opportunity to write about their lives, and many of them reach important breakthroughs in their understanding. They achieve not simply intellectual understanding but emotional understanding as well—what Daniel Goleman (1995) calls "emotional intelligence." Personal writing enables them to write about conflicts that in many cases they have never acknowledged before, and to construct their own interpretations of and solutions to these problems. Writing helps them to memorialize loss and pay tribute to beloved relatives and friends who are no longer living. Students discover that they are not alone and that others can identify with their feelings. Hearing their classmates' writings enables them to understand other points of view and to respond empathically in subsequent diaries.

How do my students feel about personal writing? At the close of *Risky Writing* I describe the results of the anonymous questionnaires I asked each of the 105 students who were enrolled in the five different expository writing courses I taught between 1995 and 1999. The results demonstrate that a large majority of students believed not only that their writing skills improved significantly but also that the course was helpful in more personal ways:

> Sixty-four percent believed that the course helped them to cope with personal problems. Fifty-nine percent believed that the course heightened their

self-understanding, and seventy percent believed that the course heightened their understanding of classmates. Sixty-three percent indicated that the course heightened their empathy. . . . Fifty-three percent believed that the course heightened their connection with their classmates, and sixty-eight percent believed that the course heightened their connection with me.

The students also indicated that they experienced therapeutic relief as a result of writing. I defined "therapeutic relief" as "feeling better about yourself, more in control of your problems." Eighty-six percent indicated that they experienced therapeutic relief as a result of writing. Ten percent of these people felt the relief would be temporary, forty-nine percent permanent, and forty percent were not sure whether it would be temporary or permanent. Sixty-one percent experienced therapeutic relief as a result of reading their classmates' essays, and fifty-one percent experienced therapeutic relief as a result of reading about fellow students' lives in *Diaries to an English Professor*. (Berman 1994, 235–36)

These findings are consistent with a study conducted by Hans Strupp and Suzanne Hadley in 1979 and reported recently by Andrew Solomon in his book *The Noonday Demon: An Atlas of Depression*:

> In an important study done in 1979, researchers demonstrated that any form of therapy could be effective if certain criteria were met: that both the therapist and the patient were acting in good faith; that the client believed that the therapist understood the technique; and that the client liked and respected the therapist; and that the therapist had an ability to form understanding relationships. The experimenters chose English professors with this quality of human understanding and found that, on average, the English professors were able to help their patients as much as the professional therapists. (2001, 111)

Strupp and Hadley conclude that the results of their investigation were "consistent and straightforward. Patients undergoing psychotherapy with college professors showed, on average, quantitatively as much improvement as patients treated by experienced professional psychotherapists" (Solomon 2001, 451–52). An important qualification made by Strupp and Hadley, but not emphasized sufficiently by Solomon, was that the college professors (who came from a variety of disciplines, including English, history, mathematics, and philosophy) were selected "on the basis of their reputation for warmth, trustworthiness, and interest in students" (Strupp and Hadley 1979, 1126).

THE USES AND ABUSES OF PSYCHOANALYSIS

Where does psychoanalysis fit into my teaching? I find psychoanalysis indispensable for understanding fictional characters and their relationship to their authors and readers. For example, in *The Small Room* fathers have a stronger influence on their daughters' development than do their mothers, an observation that may be partly explained by the fact that psychoanalysts placed more emphasis on oedipal rather than preoedipal relationships in the late 1950s, when Sarton was writing the novel. Thus, one learns a good deal about Lucy's, Pippa's, and Carryl's fathers but almost nothing about their mothers. But that doesn't explain why father-daughter relationships seem strained in *The Small Room*: Margot Peters's (1997) biography reveals Sarton's conflicted relationship with her own father, an eminent historian of science who failed to give his daughter the support and approval she needed. Psychoanalysis offers us insight into the erotic attachments among Appleton's teachers and students. Olive tells Lucy, for instance, that Carryl "loved Jane" (Sarton 1961, 204), a disclosure that takes on greater significance when we realize that Olive herself loves Carryl. In her next novel, *Mrs. Stevens Hears the Mermaids Singing*, published in 1965, Sarton disclosed her own lesbianism. Even without this biographical knowledge, we can infer that Olive and Carryl are both lesbians, but we know little about Jane Seaman's sexual orientation. Does Carryl's love for Jane contain a homoerotic element, and, if so, does her student welcome or fear this desire? We can ask these questions without fear of harming a real character. Psychoanalytic critics who limit their "practice" to analyzing fictional characters or their long-dead authors pay low malpractice insurance, and there are few if any penalties to wild analysis.

Psychoanalysis is much more dangerous, however, when used to describe real people, especially students in a literature or writing class. My guiding principle is to do no harm, and the way I achieve this is by not telling students more about their lives than they know themselves. I would not presume to psychoanalyze students whom I caught plagiarizing, as Lucy Winter does with Jane. However accurate Lucy may be when she tells Jane that her essay was "full of hatred and self-hatred, hatred of the intellect, hatred of all those critics who can prove themselves superior to the artist they analyse because they can analyse him" (Sarton 1961, 164), I would be reluctant to make such a comment, fearful that my words would be psychologically intrusive.

If we do not psychoanalyze our students, what value does psychoanalysis have to the writer and teacher? Phillip Lopate addresses this question in his delightful essay "Couch Potato: My Life in Therapy." Both writing and psychotherapy involve "the cultivation of observation and detachment, the attention to language and its subtexts, the necessity for empathy" (2000, 80). Lopate adds that his personal psychoanalysis was important both to his writing and teaching:

> In my case, I knew I lacked the *Sitzfleisch* [stamina] to sit hour after hour listening to other people's problems. But I often wonder whether I would have made a good therapist. What I did become was a teacher. Even more than

helping me with my writing, psychotherapy gave me important tools as a pedagogue. I learned, for instance, that the best thing to do in conference with a student was simply to listen and keep my mouth shut, offering an empathetic grunt. I also learned to monitor my gut responses to a student, checking for the unearned fondness or disgust triggered by physical appearance, tone of voice, or resemblance to someone I knew. Finally, I learned to discount student crushes on me as an inevitable transference. (80–81)

Lopate's comments on teaching suggest an intersubjective model of education in which teachers listen without offering advice or judgment and remain empathically attuned to their students. The teacher's role in this process is not passive but active: teachers observe their reactions to students' writings and guard against the projection or incorporation of inappropriate feelings. Empathy is the key element here, and the teacher's greatest challenge is to allow students to disclose painful or shameful experiences without becoming traumatized. Students feel heightened empathy when they share difficult experiences with classmates and discover how much they have in common with each other.

Educators who practice the teaching cure must be aware of the countertransference issues that arise in the classroom. They must heed Freud's warning in *The Ego and the Id* to avoid the temptation to "play the part of prophet, savior and redeemer to the patient" (1923, 50n)—or student. They must be aware of their own rescue fantasies so that they do not try to "save" their students' lives or impose their own agendas onto them. Educators can guard against boundary violations by listening to their students without offering personal advice, by maintaining necessary distance, and by avoiding an "erotics of pedagogy" advocated by Jane Gallop (1997), in which teachers compromise their judgment by becoming romantically or sexually involved with their students.

Reader-response diaries are an excellent way for students to make connections between literature and life. Students might explore how Primo Levi's *Survival in Auschwitz* helps them to understand the Holocaust's impact on their own family, or how William Styron's *Darkness Visible* increases their knowledge of clinical depression, or how D. H. Lawrence's *Sons and Lovers* relates to their own family dynamics. It was only when I read my students' diaries on Vladimir Nabokov's *Lolita* that I realized how and why sexually abused readers find the novel so problematic. I have received many powerful diaries on all of these stories, and they have been a revelation to everyone who has heard them.

Whether we realize it or not, all teaching is personal. As Lucy's colleague notes, "after a month of watching you and listening to you in class, your students know you better and more intimately than you will ever know them. They feel related to you, you see" (Sarton 1961, 40). Relational knowledge is greatly expanded in the self-disclosing classroom; students know their teacher better, and they have a greater understanding of their classmates' lives. And teachers have a greater knowledge of their students.

Contrary to Lucy's fears, teachers would not have to take on their students' personal problems. Students do not want their teachers to give them personal advice but rather to take them seriously, which means to listen attentively. Personal writing allows students to combine feeling and thought in ways that are not often associated with "academic" writing. Students sometimes cry in my classes when reading or hearing emotionally charged diaries or essays, and sometimes I cry myself, but I don't have "weepers" like Pippa Brentwood. Tears are as natural and appropriate to the classroom as are smiles, and they indicate that students and teachers are responding to education not only with their minds but also with their hearts, psyches, and souls.

I realize that my approach to teaching is controversial and that there is the potential for harm. The title "Risky Writing" suggests that teachers must establish protocols or ground rules so that students can write safely about dangerous topics. Before concluding, I would like to to summarize and then respond to some of the objections that have been raised by educators.

By encouraging personal writing, aren't you telling your students that their academic work is less important?

No, because the psychoanalytic and reader-response diaries they write are in addition to the extensive class readings, papers, and exams that they write in my courses. The personal writing component in my literature courses is extra work for my students and myself—work that is rarely onerous. In my expository writing course, students are expected to turn in forty pages of writing, typed and double-spaced. By underlining every grammatical and stylistic error, and by spending at least a third of every class on revisions, I emphasize the importance of good writing. Students discover that no matter how "personal" an essay is, it must be well written and therefore academically acceptable.

Isn't there the danger of pressuring students into self-disclosure?

Yes, but students determine the degree of self-disclosure in their writings. If these writings are not graded, and if students have the option not to write on any topic that is too personal, then this criticism can be avoided.

Isn't there the temptation for the teacher to play the role of therapist?

Yes, but teachers can avoid this danger by limiting comments to grammatical and stylistic revisions, clarifying questions, and supportive statements. My students neither want nor expect me to psychoanalyze their writings; they know that I am their English teacher, not a therapist. They don't ask me for personal advice nor do I offer it.

Don't you find yourself overwhelmed by your students' problems?

No, because although they write about problems, they also write about how they have dealt with these conflicts in the past or intend to deal with them in the future. Students who write about difficult personal problems usually reveal the determination to solve them. The vast number of diaries are not depressing but uplifting.

Aren't you afraid that being caring will make you into a caregiver?

No, because students don't expect me to intervene in their lives. They want me to read carefully their writings and to respond as an English teacher, not therapist. I know what it is to be a caregiver, and I have never felt the obligation to be a caregiver to my students.

For example, I always give my home telephone number to my students and tell them that they are free to call me about academic issues. Few call me at home, and the telephone calls are never about personal issues.

Aren't you afraid when you receive a diary or essay indicating that the student may be at risk?

I'm not afraid, but I'm concerned, and when this situation arises I recommend that the student visit the counseling center. This may happen once a semester. I believe that all teachers, no matter on what level they teach, should know the signs of depression and suicidal thinking and know how to respond appropriately. It does not take much effort to recommend a student go to the counseling center.

Don't you need to be unusually empathic to use this approach to teaching?

I don't regard myself as unusually empathic, and none of my colleagues is ready to canonize me. In fact, like nearly every professor living in such a fiercely contested and litigious age, I have found myself caught in the crossfire of destructive departmental wars. I suspect that many colleagues are distressed more by colleagues' than students' incivility.

Empathy can be learned, along with other befriending skills, such as listening carefully and remaining nonjudgmental. Just as empathy allows us to understand another person's point of view, so does empathic teaching allow us to understand our students. And we can help them to increase their empathic understanding of both others and themselves. This is, in my view, the goal of education.

THE TEACHING CURE

To return to the question I raised at the beginning of this essay, for what "malady" can the teaching cure be used? May Sarton raises a similar question in *The Small Room*. "And what was teaching all about anyway? If one did not believe one was teaching people how to live, how to experience, giving them the means to ripen, then what did one believe?" (1961, 51). How to live? This is the same question that Joseph Conrad raises in *Lord Jim*. If the question is unanswerable, or capable of limitless answers, then the more we raise it in our classes, the better able we are to cope with the vicissitudes of life. Literature and psychoanalysis are two of the best ways to learn more about ourselves and others and to preserve these provisional truths for those who come after us. When we study the question "how to live" in the small room of college classrooms, libraries, and analysts' offices, we realize, in Lucy's words, that "[w]e are all more vulnerable than we can afford to admit" (95). Freud's statement at the end of *Studies on Hysteria* comes to mind here:

> When I have promised my patients help or improvement by means of a cathartic treatment I have often been faced by this objection: "Why, you tell me yourself that my illness is probably connected with my circumstances and the events of my life. You cannot alter these in any way. How do you propose to help me, then?" And I have been able to make this reply: "No doubt fate would find it easier than I do to relieve you of your illness. But you will be able to convince yourself that much will be gained if we succeed in transforming your hysterical misery into common unhappiness. With a mental life that has been restored to health you will be better armed against that unhappiness. (Breuer and Freud 1895, 305)

Lest this statement seem unduly cynical, I would add that the talking cure, the writing cure, the reading cure, and the teaching cure can remind us not only of life's sorrows but also of life's joys. As the fictional "Sigmund Freud" observes in D. M. Thomas's novel *The White Hotel*, "Long may poetry and psychoanalysis continue to highlight, from their different perspectives, the human face in all its nobility and sorrow" (1981, 143n). Psychotherapists, writers, and teachers all have a role to play in exploring the tragedies and triumphs of life, and the small rooms in which they work all look out to a vast world that is limited only by the human imagination.

REFERENCES

Berman, Jeffrey. 1994. *Diaries to an English professor: Pain and growth in the classroom.* Amherst: University of Massachusetts Press.

———. 1999. *Surviving literary suicide.* Amherst: University of Massachusetts Press.

———. 2001. *Risky writing: Self-disclosure and self-transformation in the classroom.* Amherst: University of Massachusetts Press.

———. 2005. *Empathic teaching: Education for life.* Amherst: University of Massachusetts Press.

Bracher, Mark. 1999. *The writing cure: Psychoanalysis, composition, and the aims of education.* Carbondale: Southern Illinois University Press.

Breuer, Josef, and Sigmund Freud. 1895. *Studies on hysteria.* In *Standard edition of the complete psychological works of Sigmund Freud* (hereafter S.E.), ed. and trans. James Strachey et al., vol. 2. London: Hogarth Press, 1953–1974.

Freud, Sigmund. 1923. *The ego and the id.* S.E., 19:12–66.

———. 1937. Analysis terminable and interminable. S.E., 23, 216–53.

Freud, Sophie. 2003. The reading cure: Books as lifetime companions. *American Imago* 61:77–87.

Fulk, Mark. 2002. *Understanding May Sarton.* Columbia: University of South Carolina Press.

Gallop, Jane. 1997. *Feminist accused of sexual harassment.* Durham: Duke University Press.

Goleman, Daniel. 1995. *Emotional intelligence.* New York: Bantam Books.

Ingersoll, Earl, ed. 1991. *Conversations with May Sarton.* Jackson: University Press of Mississippi.

Lepore, Stephen, and Joshua Smyth. 2002. *The writing cure: How expressive writing promotes health and emotional well-being.* Washington, DC: American Psychological Association.

Lopate, Phillip. 2000. Couch potato: My life in therapy. In *Tales from the couch: Writers on therapy,* ed. Jason Shinder, 75–87. New York: William Morrow.

Peters, Margot. 1997. *May Sarton: A biography.* New York: Knopf.

Sarton, May. 1961. *The small room.* New York: Norton, 1976.

———. 1997. *May Sarton: Selected letters, 1916–1954.* Ed. and Intro. Susan Sherman. New York: Norton.

———. 2002. *May Sarton: Selected letters, 1955–1995.* Ed. and Intro. Susan Sherman. New York: Norton.

Solomon, Andrew. 2001. *The noonday demon: An atlas of depression.* New York: Simon and Schuster.

Strupp, Hans, and Suzanne Hadley. 1979. Specific vs. nonspecific factors in psychotherapy: A controlled study of outcome. *Archives of General Psychiatry* 36:1125–36.

Thomas, D. M. 1981. *The white hotel.* New York: Viking Press.

FOURTEEN

Reading, Listening, and Other Beleaguered Practices in General Psychiatry

NEIL SCHEURICH

MOST PEOPLE INVOLVED in teaching narrative medicine know the experience of working with medical students, residents, or even colleagues who simply cannot summon much interest in the subject. They may be polite about it, and if there is an assignment, they may well read the material and engage in perfunctory discussion. But no sense of passionate or vital interest develops. Generally, of course, such individuals are not serious readers on their own time, and clearly they are not impressed by the values that the instructor locates in reading. Often such persons are quite competent students or physicians as well as outwardly successful in their personal lives. Is it presumptuous, then, to think that they are missing out on something crucial?

For a while I felt a certain déjà vu when working with what I would call the unreflective student. At length I realized that the experience was parallel to a common clinical situation: the patient who seems likely to benefit from psychotherapy but who has no inclination for it. Not infrequently, patients reject psychotherapy not for financial or other logistical reasons, but rather because they simply prefer the idea of medication or see no value in considering their lives in a systematic way. Often such patients are not trying to be difficult; they genuinely fail to appreciate any outstanding virtues of psychotherapy. If they seek medication to treat their symptoms, is it an unwarranted imposition of opinion to feel that something may be amiss?

To be sure, students, residents, and colleagues are not patients, nor is reading literature congruent to undergoing or providing psychotherapy, even if it is widely recognized that there is a narrative aspect to both. But the question of why either process should be valued supersedes both literary criticism and purely clinical prudence. Why read? Why discuss intimate details of one's life with a stranger designated as a therapist? Within English departments and psychoanalytic institutes, respectively, an avid interest in such matters goes without saying, but advocates of both literature and psychotherapy often find themselves struggling to convey the worth of those experiences to unconvinced general audiences. In seeking to make this case, I shall propose that literature and psychotherapy, while obviously distinct in a number of ways, share a group of core values that are widely seen as endangered within psychiatry as well as within contemporary culture.

LITERATURE AND PSYCHOTHERAPY
IN THE NEW PSYCHIATRY

In contemporary general psychiatry, as in society at large, both literature and psychotherapy, because they are very much situated in a marketplace of ideas (the figure of speech is apt), require justification. This was not always so, of course. When psychoanalysis and other psychotherapies were central to psychiatry, both authors and fictional characters served as ideal clinical material. For this and other reasons, psychiatry and narrative modes long enjoyed a natural kinship. Indeed, insights from fiction and film continue to inform much psychoanalytic literature, but psychoanalysis is increasingly marginalized in mainstream psychiatry.

Proponents of narrative medicine have not often emphasized psychiatry, perhaps in the belief that the importance of narrative should be self-evident in that discipline. However, as evidence-based practice, managed care, and standardized diagnosis have brought psychiatry closer to general medicine, the relevance of literature and even psychotherapy to psychiatry have become far from obvious. Residents and medical students face crowded curricula and must master prodigious amounts of information. While I know of no data on the subject, many veteran therapists of my acquaintance remark that incoming psychiatry residents seem to have less interest or background in the humanities than those of past decades. Perhaps not coincidentally, one frequently encounters residents or even attending psychiatrists who wish to confine themselves to "medication management" and leave psychotherapy to social workers.

Is it worth the time and effort to incorporate literature or psychotherapy into psychiatric practice? One need not be a psychoanalyst or pine for the bygone days of a primarily psychoanalytic psychiatry to assent to this question. I aim to show that reading in general, utilizing literature for psychiatric training and understanding, and engaging in the peculiar process of psychotherapy all share common justifications that stem from the virtues of narrative form.

AESTHETICS AND NARRATIVE MEDICINE

Naturally enough in an increasingly evidence-based milieu, proponents of narrative medicine have tried to demonstrate the instrumental value of literature. There is a pressure to market literature, so to speak, by positing its value as information or as ethical admonition. These advocates assert that literature provides clinical case material that trainees may not have the time or opportunity to encounter in actual practice or that it can enhance a caring attitude by fostering empathy. To be sure, this approach has often been both nuanced and compelling, and the "literature" on literature and medicine is by now considerable.[1] However, those who care about literature often have misgivings about its use as a means to the end of task completion, even one as subtle and multifaceted as psychiatry. In their view, fiction and poetry should function as more than parable.

"Serious readers"—by which I mean those who read for more than diversion, although obviously most serious readers enjoy the activity as well—do not read merely to acquire information or to become virtuous. What kind of approach to a work of literature is simultaneously relevant to the practice of psychiatry and linked to more general notions of aesthetic experience? I would suggest that beyond any usefulness as clinical material, literature proves crucial to psychiatry for the same reason that it is important for life. In both cases, literature is not primarily about improved task completion but rather offers alternative modes of being in the world.

Narrative medicine recapitulates the venerable project of justifying literature and the other arts. As Arthur Danto explains in *The Philosophical Disenfranchisement of Art* (1986), ever since Plato advocated the political control of poetry, philosophers and critics have tended to explicate art and to reduce it to more fundamental terms. Richard Rorty (1989), for instance, has argued that a primary function of literature is the cautionary depiction of cruelty, that is, to open our eyes to the realities of evil and of human vulnerability. Martha Nussbaum (1990) posits that fiction serves as a branch of moral philosophy, one whose narrative form and emotional content appeal specifically to human understanding.

Invocations of the alleged usefulness of art have been countered by spirited defenses of its autonomy. Kant's aesthetic theory is famously based on the notion of disinterestedness. In her essay "Against Interpretation" (1964), Susan Sontag protests against reductive forms of interpretation that threaten to usurp the work of art itself, advocating an "erotics of art" in place of hermeneutics. Even more radically, Stanley Fish (1998) has maintained that the reading of poetry is a self-contained professional discipline, of no relevance whatever to one's political or moral beliefs. He implies that since no meaning transcends a given "interpretive community," every activity is imbued with significance. Philosophy is on a par with, say, plumbing, as both disciplines serve equally important functions in society. According to such thinking, art is a hermetic enterprise and quite literally amoral. Any interpretive community that places a high value on literature or other arts has no special prerogative to export its preferences to the wider culture.

Claims that art is autonomous are countered by charges of irrelevance and escapism. If art has no implications at all beyond itself, then what makes it different from hobbies, or any other pleasurable pastimes? If this is the case, then opera and epic poetry, like bowling or professional wrestling, are merely activities that some people choose to pursue for fun. Of course, devotees of the arts like to believe that their pursuits do possess a wider significance than this.

There have been attempts to balance the autonomy and the relevance of art. Clifford Geertz (1997) discusses how artists and critics, who tend to argue from a perspective in which the general merit of the arts goes without saying (perhaps not least because it is the source of their livelihood), often lose sight of the fact that any form of creativity only exists within a cultural network of meaning. This echoes John Dewey's pragmatic view (1934) that art cannot justifiably be abstracted from individual experience. Such thinkers point out that throughout most of world history art was assumed to be bound to cultural practices. The notion of "fine art" detached from all other interests has arisen only in the last two centuries, and primarily in the West. Barbara Herrnstein Smith (1991) maintains that aesthetic experience always entails a degree of evaluation and engagement. While we don't usually read fiction for information or any other concrete end, we do expect some kind of benefit inasmuch as there are various other endeavors that offer competing claims on our time and energy. When readers choose to read, they are to that extent most certainly engaged rather than detached.

Many philosophers have arrived at the belief that art teaches *something*, but not necessarily specific moral precepts. Dewey (1934) theorizes that the arts function to enlarge the sphere of human possibility, and he concludes *Art and Experience* by claiming that "imagination is the chief instrument of the good. . . . The moral prophets of humanity have always been poets even though they spoke in free verse or by parable" (348). George Santayana (1955) holds the position that aesthetics establishes the realm of positive values, those things that are the ends of life, whereas morality has a necessary but secondary and negative function, that of removing obstructions to those positive values. Heidegger (1950), whose aesthetic theory was similarly visionary, writes that art "unconceals" the truth of "Being" and that "towering up within itself, the work opens up a world and keeps it abidingly in force"

(672). Jean-Paul Sartre (1948) regards reading as a challenging, imaginative act that broadens the scope of human freedom. Such accounts echo those of writers such as Sidney, Shelley, and Emerson who have championed the transformative aspects of literature.

More recent commentators have touted reading at a time when visual media and passive consumption seem to monopolize our lives. According to Sven Birkerts (1999), "The finished work, the whole of it, then enables the reader to project a sensible and meaningful order or reality, one that might be initially at odds with the habitual relation to things" (108). Harold Bloom (2000) has asserted that we read "in order to strengthen the self, and to learn its authentic interests" (22), but he insists that the point of reading is not to improve others or society. In "Why Literature?" (2002), Mario Vargas Llosa, dumbfounded and alarmed by the decline of serious reading, mourns the increasingly prevalent notion that reading is a "luxury" for which even educated people cannot seem to find the time. These critics see literature as neither a solipsistic pursuit nor a shortcut to compassion or other attributes. Rather, reading is a mode of being in which time appears to slow down and one's attentiveness and flexibility of perspective expand. As Kafka famously but violently put it, "A book must be an axe for the frozen sea within us" (qtd. in Manguel 1996, 93). Like friendship or love, reading has a spiritual function, the ends of which are inseparable from the means. In referring to such experiences as spiritual, I mean that they help one to articulate the ultimate meanings by which one chooses to live. Friendship, love, and reading all may have favorable consequences, but if one merely focuses on results, the point of the activity is lost.

What is there to say, then, of those who read purely for relaxation or not at all? Even if one believes that virtue depends upon moral imagination, and not merely adherence to a series of admonitions, any simple correlation between reading and morality is questionable. It would be ludicrous to claim, for instance, that English professors are inherently more virtuous than, say, physics professors, and countless literary types in the history of the world have been scoundrels. Conceivably, it could be argued that reading consumes time and energy that might otherwise be devoted to actively improving the world. Other things being equal, we cannot conclude that the nonreader is any less virtuous than the devoted reader. Indeed, the mischievous nonreader could suggest that the avid reader is naturally more wicked and less imaginative than others since he needs such extensive moral instruction. Of any given reader who *is* a wise, virtuous person, it is impossible to say which came first, practice or personality. The reader can probably only suggest that the nonreader suffers from a kind of spiritual blind spot, that something worthwhile has been missed. I will propose that spirituality in the broadest sense is germane both to reading and to the experience of psychotherapy. It is to the latter's embattled status in contemporary psychiatry that I now turn.

JUSTIFYING PSYCHOTHERAPY

Just as many nonreaders sail through life without obvious detriment, increasingly many psychiatric patients who successfully obtain pharmacological relief come to view their appointments with psychiatrists as little more than a means to medication. Some biologically oriented psychiatrists would argue that any psychotherapy that fails to show objectively measurable clinical benefit (generally via standardized rating scales) is dispensable and quite possibly a waste of time and money. Remarkably paralleling the situation of literature and medicine, recent attempts to justify the role of psychotherapy within psychiatry begin with utilitarian arguments but have not ended there. By "psychotherapy" I intend neither psychoanalysis nor any other specific technique, but rather the very broad category of clinical interventions attending primarily to a patient's subjectivity, motivation, and capacity for internal change.

As alleged support for the legitimacy of psychotherapy, brain-imaging studies have demonstrated that the talking cure produces specific and discernible neurological changes. For instance, positron emission tomography has revealed that cognitive and behavioral therapies affect the metabolic rate in a specific area of the brain in patients with obsessive-compulsive disorder (Baxter et al. 1992). The point of this research has been to show that talking does not influence a disembodied "mind" or "spirit," but rather the same organ affected by somatic therapies.

Supporters of psychotherapy have also acceded to the demands of evidence-based medicine. Glen Gabbard (2002) defends the clinical effectiveness of psychoanalytic therapies, but acknowledges that a major evidence-based initiative is needed to show this clearly. Gabbard (2001) has also spearheaded the claim that psychiatrists, supposedly trained to contend with all three components of the "biopsychosocial model," are uniquely positioned to provide psychotherapy. He appeals solely to considerations of effectiveness and cost, however, and omits broader philosophical concerns.

Other voices, many of them outside of medical psychiatry, reject the very terms of the debate and have advocated a quite different rationale for psychotherapy. Eric Johnson and Steven Sandage (1999) argue that no psychotherapy worth its name can avoid engaging with general questions regarding the vital concerns of life. They understand psychotherapy less as a narrowly clinical intervention than as one of many human endeavors of meaning construction. As such, its borders with narrative, philosophy, and religion become fuzzier than ever. Psychotherapy can be viewed as an alternative expression of the human need for significance, and therefore valuable far beyond its effects on clinical symptoms. In opposition to claims that psychotherapy merely heightens attention to the self, Jeremy Holmes (1996) holds that, if properly conducted, it enhances awareness of all moral considerations, including those of other persons.

At the same time, interest in existential aspects of psychotherapy, somewhat neglected since the work of Viktor Frankl (1959) and Irvin Yalom (1980), has regained prominence. Noting the salience of existential themes in cognitive therapy, John Mack (1994) claims that being "creator of one's life . . . is essential to the sense of self" (178). Similarly, Chris Brewin and Mick Power (1999) assert, "There is little question that issues of meaning form the heart of most forms of psychopathology" (143). They also observe, however, that the mentally ill do not suffer from meaninglessness per se, but rather from a plethora of pernicious meanings such as self-hatred and radical mistrust of others. What psychotherapy calls for, perhaps even more than the interpretation of hidden realities, is the imagination of alternative possibilities.

The advocacy of psychotherapy has links to the resistance against what are widely perceived as hegemonic tendencies within medical psychiatry that result in the "loss of the personal" (Wiggins and Schwartz 1999): concentration on efficiency and cost, increasingly standardized clinical understanding, and a related preoccupation with pharmacology. Managed care and evidence-based medicine run the risk of distorting basic values of human self-understanding. In her apologia for psychoanalysis, Elisabeth Roudinesco (1999) argues that the claims of the critics of psychotherapy rest on questionable assumptions about human nature, such as the desirability of smoothing over conflict and difference. Meanwhile, mindless cost control measures produce a vision of human beings as generic and interchangeable, which A. Donald (2001) has termed "the Wal-Marting of American psychiatry."

The ascendancy of psychopharmacology within psychiatry has generated the most unease. Cultural critics such as Carl Elliott (2000) and James Edwards (2000) maintain that medication is too readily prescribed for patients experiencing what are really spiritual crises about how to live. A recent report by the President's Council on Bioethics (2003) strongly cautions against possible misuses of so-called "mood brightening" medications. These critiques implicate not only psychiatrists but also patients, many of whom are lured by culturally ambient promises of painless fixes for human problems.

The gist of these accounts is that the value of psychotherapy cannot be captured economically, by simpleminded standards of cost, efficiency, and generic symptomatology. Like literature, the endeavor often leads to clearly positive outcomes, but even when it does not, it may produce subtle changes in development and outlook, progressions in self-examination and agency, that have a spiritual aspect. Obviously, psychotherapy is no panacea, just as literature is not. But two individuals who have reached the same quantitative improvement on a depression-rating scale, one with Prozac and the other with psychotherapy, are not indistinguishable: only one has had an experience as well as a result.

This broad existential and spiritual view—a minority one in psychiatry today—contrasts with mainstream efforts to preserve psychotherapy. For instance, the American Council on Graduate Medical Education has mandated that psychiatry residents exhibit competence in five forms of psychotherapy (Yager, Kay, and Mellman 2003). While such efforts are certainly not without merit, their dependence on objectively verifiable skills and techniques learned from manuals follow from the reductive view of human functioning that has resulted from managed care and a pharmacological mindset. As I have argued previously (2004), conceptions of psychotherapy that rely primarily on the criteria used to judge biological interventions—observable brain changes, statistically measured trends in standardized rating scales—risk losing the spirit of the enterprise: the exploration of human experience and possibility. Psychotherapy should be more than that, of course, and true clinical improvement and therapist accountability are crucial, but the process remains a *human* encounter—with its inescapable idiosyncrasy and unpredictability—at the very least.

VALUES COMMON TO READING AND PSYCHOTHERAPY

Of course, literature and psychotherapy are not interchangeable endeavors, and there are many human problems for which neither is necessary or even helpful. However, the arguments reviewed above suggest that they share a quartet of essential values, which I would identify as *autonomy, complexity, curiosity,* and, for lack of a better term, *patience*. Such qualities are perpetually endangered, it seems to me, in both medical and psychiatric training and practice.

Many readers would argue that literature nourishes the *autonomous* self, promoting self-understanding and awakening one to new possibilities. Most importantly, great literature is endlessly eye-opening, resisting encapsulation by wider systems of explanation. For the postmodernist Jean-François Lyotard (1979), it is revolutionary and liberating inasmuch as it challenges totalizing social influences. From an entirely different perspective, yet analogously, Harold Bloom (2000) decries the "multicultural" trend in literary studies, which seeks to democratize the literary canon, precisely because he feels it stunts the possibilities of reading.

Psychotherapy at its best is likewise fundamentally empowering. Certainly, biological treatment may also remove impediments to human freedom, just as psychotherapy that is rigid or inept may do the opposite. However, psychotherapy not only overcomes internal barriers; it also sets in motion an exploration and challenge to the ideals of sameness and productivity that are latent but widespread in both contemporary psychiatry and Western culture. (In alternative cultures or subcultures, psychotherapy may dispute quite different values.) Like the best literature, the best psychotherapy takes nothing for granted; it fundamentally unsettles.

Books and therapists also share the presumption of human depth and *complexity*, the notion that experience is not reducible to a finite number of meanings. Both resist the idea that understanding is a matter of "sound bites" or that mental life can be entirely captured by diagnoses. Both acknowledge a deep ambiguity that makes people uncomfortable and is in principle impervious to elimination by scientific advances. To appreciate the complexity of human well-being is to recognize that there is no adequate way to quantify it, by rating scales or otherwise; depth and nuance are inevitably lost in the process. An essential aspect of such complexity—captured much more fully in the unfolding of stories or psychotherapeutic relationships than in the relatively static worlds of medication and objective understanding—is the necessarily developmental nature of human knowledge and experience.

Complementary to complexity is *curiosity*, the basic human impulse to understand and experience the foreign, the other. The curious mind seeks out literature because time and space crucially limit how much can reasonably be experienced firsthand in a lifetime. Literature not only depicts aspects of reality one might never otherwise come into contact with but can also, by means of imagination, propose alternatives to the currently real. Some types of literature may satisfy a hunger for sheer data, whether historical, cultural, or psychological, but even more germane to this discussion is the desire for experience, the inexhaustible debate over how one should live. Similarly, psychotherapy, while aiming for changes in behavior or relief of distress, would not provide a compelling alternative to medication if it did not entail an exploration of those aspects of the self that can be viewed as other. Like the philosopher, the psychotherapist must believe that the unexamined life is not worth living.

Finally, I use *patience* to express the notion, increasingly foreign in a frenetic culture, that it takes *time* to engage with issues of autonomy and complexity. In medicine as in society in general, it grows difficult to question the demands of efficiency and productivity. Reading and psychotherapy both undermine the seductive distinction between ends and means by proposing that to *be* is as important as to *do*. Immersed in a maelstrom, both medical students and patients are likely to struggle when asked to slow down, to take time to attend to subtle details within and around them. Indeed, this is *difficult*. It is often easier (at least superficially) for people to stop at simpleminded labels, to reduce the world to tidy bits of information, and to engage in hectic but unthinking activity. Both literature and psychotherapy draw attention to unpleasant, even horrible aspects of experience in the hope that suffering, when properly contained and considered, may widen one's vision.

Critics of these views might argue that we have plenty of autonomy, complexity, and patience as it is, and that these ideals too easily mutate into rootless individualism, gratuitous complication, and idle self-absorption. To be sure, both reading and psychotherapy can be perverted into sterile theory, emotional escapism, and avoidance of actual problems. And naturally, both literature and psychotherapy have other, less ambitious functions at times, such as entertainment and support, respectively. These are not necessarily trivial functions, but I would suggest that the unique significance of the two practices, the reason why they rouse such strong feelings pro and con, is the distinctive vision of human possibility they share. As Helen Vendler (2004) has written of those who study the arts, "Critics and scholars are evangelists, plucking the public by the sleeve, saying, 'Look at this,' or 'Listen to this,' or 'See how this works'" (28). Indeed, those of us dedicated to literature or to psychotherapy have a spiritual conviction that whole realities of meaning and of experience exist but are invisible to those too careless or too hurried to attend to them.

Admittedly, I have not addressed practical issues. Psychotherapy should not, after all, be a way of life; therapists, as opposed to writers, should have the goal of rendering themselves unnecessary. And for those of us lacking independent means, there is the question of how much the government or third-party payers ought to subsidize the autonomy, complexity, and patience cultivated by psychotherapy. The matter goes well beyond this discussion, but it is worth pointing out that there is an approximate parallel in the persistent debate over the relative importance of the humanities and the sciences in education. My argument is that tax dollars are supporting similar values whether applied to a high school English class or to a Medicare patient's psychotherapy. Just as the former does more than train the future work force, the latter aims at more than symptom relief.

LITERATURE FOR PSYCHOTHERAPISTS?

Life is like a story, but of course it is infinitely more than that to the one living it. So therapy may be viewed as a kind of existentially charged narrative experience. Commentators such as Robert Coles (1989) and Samuel Shem (1991) have sought a tie between psychotherapy and literature by alluding to patients who shared their literary passion. But this is a rare happenstance, as the great majority of patients, like most people in general, have no active interest in serious literature. If bibliotherapy were enough, then professional therapy would not be in such perennial demand, and there is much more to therapeutic technique than narrative competence. Furthermore, great literature is obviously not ipso facto redemptive. Ernest Hemingway and Sylvia Plath, among others, authored enduring works yet ultimately succumbed to despair.

Lest there be concern that a paradigm of narrative significance leads to detachment from the "story" of the patient, I would argue that the relation of the therapist to the therapy is preeminently an ethical and not an aesthetic one. Rather, it is the patient who bears an aesthetic relation to the therapy, who seeks a transformation of the life story. After all, it is the patient and not the therapist who is free, within reason, to drift in and out of therapy much as one might browse in a treasured book over time.

Certainly one *can* use literature to teach psychiatry residents and medical students some of the cognitive nuts and bolts of psychotherapy, such as interpretation of meaning and motivation. That is, authors and fictional characters can be made into clinical subjects of a kind. But I want those I teach not merely to gain a clinical "pearl" or two, but rather to come to *care* about literature and the values it embodies, and to see that these values also underlie the mixed status of psychiatry as both liberal art and science. In other words, I think that literature does more to strengthen the spirit of the endeavor than to convey specific techniques. Just as literature can be a safe and convenient way vicariously to "try out" various forms of life, it can also put us into the right frame of mind for exploring the possibilities of persons.

Although it is unlikely that reading *Pride and Prejudice* will provide specific ideas for clinical interventions, I suggest that literature can animate, enliven, and restore psychiatrists in a supremely subtle manner. Indeed, I would consider a wide-ranging engagement with literature to perform a function analogous to that of ongoing supervision: both defend against fatigue and narrowmindedness. In his essay "The Noble Rider and the Sound of Words" (1941), Wallace Stevens wrote that the imagination "seems, in the last analysis, to have something to do with our self-preservation; that, no doubt, is why the expression of it, the sound of its words, helps us to live our lives" (36). I would argue that such imagination makes better psychotherapists as well.

The parallel debates over narrative medicine and psychotherapy are therefore not primarily—and certainly not merely—empirical in nature. The colloquial notion of "culture war," if rather too belligerent in this context, nonetheless conveys the often irreconcilable differences between those who see and those who fail to see the worth of serious reading and listening. Particularly at the level of medical school or residency, the values that drive the two practices cannot be imposed, but only insinuated or intimated. Similarly, we obviously cannot compel patients to engage in psychotherapy. Those who care about such things should continue to carry on, unencumbered by the fantasy that there is some ultimate justification, as yet undiscovered, that will magically open the eyes of the indifferent.

NOTE

1. A representative sampling would include Charles Radey's (1992) linking of literature and practical wisdom (*phronesis*), Rita Charon's (2000) review of the narrative epistemology shared by literature and medicine, and Anne Hudson Jones's (1997) account of a uniquely narrative ethics.

REFERENCES

Baxter, Lewis, et al. 1992. Caudate glucose metabolic rate changes with both drug and behavior therapy for obsessive-compulsive disorder. *Archives of General Psychiatry* 49:681–89.

Beveridge, Allan. 2003. Should psychiatrists read fiction? *British Journal of Psychiatry* 182:385–87.

Birkerts, Sven. 1999. *Readings*. St. Paul: Greywolf Press.

Bloom, Harold. 2000. *How to read and why*. New York: Scribner.

Brewin, Chris, and Mick Power. 1999. Integrating psychological therapies: Processes of meaning transformation. *British Journal of Medical Psychology* 72:143–57.

Charon, Rita. 2000. Literature and medicine: Origins and destinies. *Academic Medicine* 75:23–27.

Coles, Robert. 1989. *The call of stories: Teaching and the moral imagination*. Boston: Houghton Mifflin.

Danto, Arthur. 1986. *The philosophical disenfranchisement of art*. New York: Columbia University Press.

Dewey, John. 1934. *Art as experience*. New York: Minton, Balch, and Co.

Donald, A. 2001. The Wal-Marting of American psychiatry: An ethnography of psychiatric practice in the late 20th century. *Culture, Medicine, and Psychiatry* 25:427–39.

Edwards, James. 2000. Passion, activity, and the "care of the self." *Hastings Center Report* 30, no. 2:31–34.

Elliott, Carl. 2000. Pursued by happiness and beaten senseless: Prozac and the American dream. *Hastings Center Report* 30, no. 2:7–12.

Fish, Stanley. 1998. Truth and toilets: Pragmatism and the practices of life. In *The revival of pragmatism: New essays on social thought, law, and culture*, ed. Morris Dickstein, 418–33. Durham: Duke University Press.

Frankl, Victor. 1959. *Man's search for meaning: An introduction to logotherapy*. Washington, DC: Washington Square Press.

Gabbard, Glen, and Jerrold Kay. 2001. The fate of integrated treatment: Whatever happened to the biopsychosocial psychiatrist? *American Journal of Psychiatry* 158:1956–63.

Gabbard, Glen, John Gunderson, and Peter Fonagy. 2002. The place of psychoanalytic treatments within psychiatry. *Archives of General Psychiatry* 59:505–10.

Geertz, Clifford. 1997. Art as a cultural system. In *Aesthetics*, ed. Susan L. Feagin and Patrick Maynard, 109–18. Oxford: Oxford University Press.

Heidegger, Martin. 1950. The origin of the work of art. Trans. Albert Hofstadter. In *Philosophies of art and beauty: Selected readings in aesthetics from Plato to Heidegger*, ed. Albert Hofstadter and Richard Kuhns, 650–700. Chicago: University of Chicago Press, 1964.

Holmes, Jeremy. 1996. Values in psychotherapy. *American Journal of Psychotherapy* 50:259–73.

Johnson, Eric, and Steven Sandage. 1999. A postmodern reconstruction of psychotherapy: Orienteering, religion, and the healing of the soul. *Psychotherapy* 36:1–15.

Jones, Anne Hudson. 1997. Literature and medicine: Narrative ethics. *Lancet* 349:1243–46.

Llosa, Mario Vargas. 2002. Why literature? In *The Best American Essays 2002*, ed. Stephen Jay Gould, 295–308. Boston: Houghton Mifflin.

Lyotard, Jean-François. 1979. *The postmodern condition.* Trans. Geoff Bennington and Brian Massumi. Minneapolis: University of Minnesota Press, 1985.

Mack, John. 1994. Power, powerlessness, and empowerment in psychotherapy. *Psychiatry* 57:178–98.

Manguel, Albert. 1996. *A history of reading.* New York: Viking.

Nussbaum, Martha. 1990. *Love's knowledge: Essays on philosophy and literature.* Oxford: Oxford University Press.

President's Council on Bioethics. 2003. *Beyond therapy: Biotechnology and the pursuit of happiness.* Washington, DC: President's Council on Bioethics.

Radey, Charles. 1992. Imagining ethics: Literature and the practice of ethics. *Journal of Clinical Ethics* 3:38–45.

Rorty, Richard. 1989. *Contingency, irony, and solidarity.* Cambridge: Cambridge University Press.

Roudinesco, Elisabeth. 1999. *Why psychoanalysis?* Trans. Rachel Bowlby. New York: Columbia University Press, 2001.

Santayana, George. 1955. *The sense of beauty: Being an outline of an aesthetic theory.* New York: Dover.

Sartre, Jean-Paul. 1948. *What is literature and other essays.* Trans. Bernard Frechtman. Cambridge: Harvard University Press, 1988.

Scheurich, Neil. 2004. Psychotherapy and somatic treatment: What's the difference? *Psychiatric Times* 21, no. 3:39–40.

Shem, Samuel. 1991. Psychiatry and literature: A relational perspective. *Literature and Medicine* 10:42–65.

Smith, Barbara Herrnstein. 1991. *Contingencies of value: Alternative perspectives for critical theory.* Cambridge: Harvard University Press.

Sontag, Susan. 1964. Against interpretation. In *Against Interpretation and Other Essays*, 3–14. New York: Farrar, Straus and Giroux, 1966.

Stevens, Wallace. 1941. The noble rider and the sound of words. In *The necessary angel: Essays on reality and the imagination*, 1–36. New York: Vintage Books: 1951.

Vendler, Helen. 2004. The ocean, the bird, and the scholar: How the arts help us to live. *The New Republic*, July 19, 27–32.

Wiggins, Osborne, and Michael Schwartz. 1999. The crisis of present-day psychiatry: The loss of the personal. *Psychiatric Times* 16, no. 8:8.

Yager, Joel, Jerald Kay, and Lisa Mellman. 2003. Assessing psychotherapy competence: A beginning. *Academic Psychiatry* 27:125–27.

Yalom, Irvin. 1980. *Existential psychotherapy*. New York: Basic Books.

FIFTEEN

Uncertain Truths

Resistance and Defiance in Narrative

SCHUYLER W. HENDERSON

ONE

WHAT DO WE LEARN from a narrative that does not just deny illness and pathology, but is written or spoken against the illness—where the "patient" is not simply saying, "I don't have this particular illness," but, "I don't see this as an illness at all"? This attitude is not unusual in medicine and is particularly contentious in the field of mental health. Opposition to standard medical illness narratives has produced some forceful counternarratives to the prevailing hegemonies and, when harnessed to a movement such as Mad Pride (*Adbusters* 2002), can have potent political and clinical clout.

To some extent, counternarratives can be incorporated into the psychoanalytic domain as "resistant" texts. For example, the authors of these narratives are said to be in denial about their illness; they are projecting their anger, anxiety, and internalized moral disapprobation about the illness onto the physician; they are displacing a sense of illness onto others. In other words, they allegedly make use of defense mechanisms, enact the phenotype of fractured selves or otherwise engage in distorting reality to protect themselves from the disturbing knowledge of their illness. Indeed, by speaking out against their "illness," they are unintentionally opening up the narratives to interpretation: the very act of rebellion, their outrage, their resounding "no" can be placed on the couch where they refuse to lie.

On the other hand, counterhegemonic authors might argue that resistance, rather than being a function of defenses, is better understood as an act of defiance, first against the pat interpretations and reductive insights provided by health care providers, and second against the power vested in the physician as an arbiter of sickness and health. Thus, defiance erupts from the concern that life experiences, with all their multifactorial volatility, will be reduced to textbook interpretations, and from the not unfounded fear that those who do not acquiesce in the treatment prescribed may even be forced to do so.

The presumed "we" in my opening question is constituted by those within the fields of narrative medicine and the medical humanities who wish to engage with counternarratives seriously and attentively. The issue then becomes how they can be read within the overarching metanarrative of medical interaction without appropriating or diluting the defiance but while maintaining a critical ear to the nuances of resistance. The psychoanalytic perspective will be particularly important here, not in order to conquer any text with foreordained readings but as a means of grappling with the uncertainty inherent in narrative. One of the most powerful challenges facing both psychoanalysis and narrative medicine is how to comprehend uncertainty. Both fields seek answers in listening, so they must at some point choose an interpretive path through the thickets of the unknown. To do so requires that the listener commit to hearing some things and not others, thus provisionally giving credence to a particular perspective by making an interpretation or a diagnosis. Despite this impetus to recover a measure of certainty, both psychoanalysis and narrative medicine are more accommodating of uncertainty than are most other approaches to the medical encounter, in part because they focus on the actual process of interaction between patient and physician.[1]

TWO

Glen Gabbard (2000) defines resistance as the "wish to preserve the status quo, to oppose the treater's efforts to produce insight and change" (14). Resistance is central to the therapeutic process because if insight and change were not difficult to attain, there would be little need for therapy in the first place. Although the patient is presumably motivated to seek treatment because of the suffering or conflicts in his or her life, the status quo is more familiar and, intrinsically, more defended than the unknown parts of the self. Gabbard goes on to say that all resistance "has in common an attempt to avoid unpleasant feelings, whether anger, guilt, hate, love (if directed against a forbidden object such as the therapist), envy, shame, grief, anxiety or some combination of these" (15). If we can agree that these "unpleasant feelings" may be contributing to whatever is disrupting the patient's equilibrium, then we can see why Freud (1916–1917) argued that "the overcoming of resistances is the essential function of analysis and is the only part of our work which gives us an assurance that we have achieved something with the patient" (291).

Viewed positively, however, resistance is also an essential function of identity. It is resistance that maintains integrity and constancy to the self in the face of the demands imposed by an always-shifting world. From this standpoint, resistance is natural and often beneficial. Indeed, a lack of resistance marks its own pathology, the *as if* personality.

Nevertheless, the concept of resistance tends to provoke antipathy in counternarratives. The very characterization of a patient's behavior or words as "resistance" implies a phenomenon open to interpretation by the analyst, but mystifying to the patient. When what is at stake is nothing less than the self, it is particularly alarming to put the power of knowledge in the hands of another (McHugh and Slavney 1998). For something to be classified as resistance, moreover, it must warrant skepticism on the part of the interpreter. A patient's tardiness may be related to an uncomfortable insight that was emerging in the previous session, but it can also be attributed to what Freud calls "chance events" (1916–1917, 291)—a broken alarm clock, a stalled train, an urgent deadline at work. But what the patient may deem to be a sufficient explanation, the psychoanalyst considers circumstantial. Such hermeneutic disagreements can be frustrating not simply for therapists but also for those whom they label as resistant.

One of the earliest accounts of resistance in psychoanalysis occurs in Freud's (1905) case history of Dora:

> My expectations were by no means disappointed when this explanation of mine was met by Dora with a most emphatic negative. The "No" uttered by a patient after a repressed thought has been presented to his conscious perception for the first time does no more than register the existence of a repression and its severity; it acts, as it were, as a gauge of the repression's strength. (58)

There are, in this passage, echoes of Gertrude's comment, "The lady doth protest too much, methinks" (*Hamlet*, 3.2.230). Like Gertrude, Freud suggests that the louder the patient says "no," the more the analyst should suspect she really means "yes." Infuriatingly, resistance can thus appear to be a Catch-22, placing the patient in a double bind, in which the very doubt she expresses about its existence becomes further evidence of its existence.

In *The Eden Express* (1975), an autobiographical account of his experience with mental illness, Mark Vonnegut writes: "If you fail to benefit from psychotherapy, you stand a better than even chance of being accused of 'resisting therapy.' As if things weren't bad enough already, you are now accused of subconsciously or even consciously wanting them that way" (209). Mark Vonnegut shares with his novelist father a precision in tone and syntax, and wields with surprising gentleness the sharp blade of his wit. Given the author's anti-authoritarian stance, however, *The Eden Express* is surprisingly sympathetic toward mental health services, and Mark Vonnegut himself subsequently went to medical school. And yet, in both the quoted sentences Vonnegut uses the word *accused*. One is *accused* of resistance as though it were a crime. Although this is not the analyst's conscious intention, the patient may feel as though he is being arraigned. What is worse, this arraignment is occurring at a time when he is already feeling vulnerable and facing the potentially catastrophic consequences of mental illness.

Vonnegut's statement is a measure of the antipathy found in counter-narratives toward the concept of resistance. So let us assume that despite its voracious appetite, resistance is not all-consuming, and that sometimes "no" *does* mean no. Let us assume further that those chance events Freud dismisses did make the patient late. From another perspective, let us also stipulate that there is more to the tension between therapist and patient than the patient's own psychology. Then we have defiance. Defiance is an ideological position. At its most supple, it respects psychology and the complexities of psychodynamics, but it will also draw upon anthropology and sociology, politics and culture—and, therefore, on an analysis of power relations. Above all, it will focus on the power relation between doctor and patient, or between the teller and the interpreter of the story; and it will contest the notion that this inter-subjective struggle over the meaning of an illness narrative can be subsumed into the patient's own pathology.

THREE

One need look no further than the accolades he has received, the debate his work has inspired, and the lawsuit against him for defaming Islam to see that the French novelist and literary *enfant terrible* Michel Houellebecq has polarized the reading public. Having previously won the Grand Prix National des Lettres, Houellebecq gained further success and notoriety with his two recent novels *Atomized* (1999a) and *Platform* (1999b): the former garnered the Prix Novembre, while the latter was the basis for the failed lawsuit.[2]

Atomized chronicles the lives of two half-brothers: Michel, a reclusive molecular biologist, and Bruno, who seems to live in a shadowland of frustrated desire. The novel traverses the end of the twentieth century, an epoch described as the "suicide of the West" (284). This process is marked by the understanding "that humanity must disappear, that humanity would give way to a new species which was asexual and immortal, a species which had outgrown individuality, individuation and progress" (371). *Atomized* is replete with dreary details and lacks any rush of excitement or ecstasy, least of all in the descriptions of physical climax. Although the novel is often sadistic without any compensatory frisson, its very dullness has much to offer the discerning reader, particularly one with a psychological bent.

Houellebecq's narrator explicitly derides psychiatry and psychoanalysis. He divulges his contempt in numerous passing comments, as when he likens talking to someone who is not listening to "talking to a wall, or a psychiatrist" (199). The narrator parallels psychotherapy with New Age spiritualism, describing both as refuges where the wounded and pathetic can seek artificial solace and superficial escape. Psychoanalytic conventions are seen as contrivances that draw on nebulous abstractions to try to pin down the human experience with meaning. Although the narrator mocks New Age platitudes and eccentricities, their proponents at least possess actual bodies. Houellebecq's psychiatrists are devoid of physicality, as bland as a blank wall, a true *tabula rasa*. What is more, "Mantras and tarots may be stupid, but they're a lot cheaper than therapy" (175).

To rebut these condemnations, one might return to Freud, who, in listing the external events that can be deployed by the patient in the service of resistance, includes "every comment by a person of authority in [the patient's] environment who is hostile to analysis" (1916–1917, 291). Houellebecq, however, being well aware of Freud (or at least popular Freudianism), appears to relish baiting readers with juicy morsels demanding an analytic interpretation, only to disappoint them. Throughout the novel, the narrator describes dreams that are excruciatingly boring, as if daring us to dismiss them. In an unusually explicit confrontation with the psychoanalytic perspective, Bruno tells his psychiatrist about the summer he turned eighteen:

> Sometimes Bruno altered or refined the details, but this is his standard version: . . . "I went into her room. They were still asleep. I hesitated for a moment or two and then pulled the sheet off them. My mother moved and for a minute I thought she was going to open her eyes; her thighs parted slightly. I knelt down in front of her vagina. I brought my hand up close— a couple of inches away—but I didn't dare touch her. Then I went outside and jerked off. There'd always been cats around the house, mostly strays. A black cat lay sunning itself on a rock. The land around the house was stony, white and forbidding. The cat looked over at me from time to time while I was wanking, but closed its eyes before I came." (1999a, 81–82)

He then picked up a rock, and the "cat's skull shattered and some of its brains spurted out" (82).

We never hear the psychiatrist's response. That there should be a "standard version" to such an outrageous story reveals that it has been told before, to other therapists, who have provided neither insight nor a sense of closure. If Freudians cannot work with this overtly oedipal material, what can they do? The passage ironically attacks the perceived ubiquity of the Oedipus complex, as if this grotesque, violent scene were, in psychoanalytic discourse, "standard." At the end of the passage, Houellebecq forestalls any foray into the psychology of the forbidden: "Bruno jumped, afraid that his mother had been awake that morning as he was staring at her vagina. In fact his mother's remark was banal: the incest taboo is well documented in the animal kingdom, especially among mandrills and grey geese. The car sped towards Saint-Maxine" (83). This appeal to birds, which are rarely considered to have complex psychologies, is amusingly bathetic. If human experience can be compared to that of geese, it hardly warrants soul-searching or the convoluted dynamics of therapy.

Throughout the novel, aspects of the characters' development that could be understood in psychological terms are portrayed solely as biological processes. For example, when Bruno loses his grandfather, Houellebecq writes: "His grandfather died in 1967. In temperate climates, the body of a bird or mammal first attracts species of flies (*Musca*, *Curtoneura*), but once decomposition has begun to set in, these are joined by others, particularly *Calliphora* and *Lucilia*" (42). As in the passage on incest, the narrator conflates animals and birds, and individual experience is subsumed to a natural cycle of decay. This reduction extends to sexual arousal, "The shaft of the clitoris and the glans of the penis are covered in Krause's corpuscles, rich in nerve endings. When touched, they cause a powerful flow of endorphins in the brain" (168), as well as to death and indeed a whole host of topics.

But the narrator is not simply arguing that humans are animals and offering biology as the sole alternative to psychology. He also contends that what makes humans different from animals is better explained by sociology and physics than it is by psychology: "Many years later Michel proposed a theory of human freedom using the flow of superfluid helium as an analogy" (108). Just as Houellebecq devotes long passages to dissecting biological events where one might have expected an affective explanation, so too he recontextualizes other experiences, such as romantic love, in social and historical terms:

> His only goal in life had been sexual, and he realized that it was too late to change that now. In that, Bruno was characteristic of his generation. While he was a teenager, the fierce economic pressures which France had suffered for two hundred years had abated. The prevailing opinion was that economic conditions tended towards a certain equality. (73–74)

In chapter 12, following on the description of the summer when Bruno turned eighteen, we read a devastating parody of the psychiatric interview:

> The psychiatrist was less interested in the part of the story that followed, but Bruno thought it was important and had no intention of passing it over. After all, he was paying the bastard to listen to him, wasn't he? . . . When he had finished his story, Bruno paused for a moment. The psychiatrist cleared his throat and said, about nothing in particular, "Good." Depending on how much of the hour had elapsed, he would prompt Bruno again, or would simply say, "We'll leave it there for today?" rising a little to make it a question. As he said this, his smile was polished and effortless. (85–87)

Therapy is a rote experience and a commercial transaction, a fifty-minute farce with only a clock for a prop. The finely observed mannerisms of the psychiatrist make this scene a far more caustic critique of his profession than the casual slanders elsewhere in the novel.

The blankness and lack of physicality of the therapist, especially by contrast with the New Age mystics, mock the notions of transference and countertransference, which depend on nonverbal as well as verbal communication. The same chapter begins with an epigraph:

> In revolutionary times, those who accord themselves, with an extraordinary arrogance, the facile credit for having enflamed anarchy in their contemporaries fail to recognize that what appears to be a sad triumph is in fact due to a spontaneous disposition, determined by the social situation as a whole. (Auguste Comte— Philosophie Positive, Leçon 48) (79)

In light of what follows, this may be aimed at Freud and his centrality to psychoanalysis, or indeed at the hero-worshiping tendencies of psychoanalysts in general. Such critiques are consistent with the novel's thrust that not the individual but the grinding evolution of society as a whole brings about change if not progress. Psychology, like New Age mysticism, is a fairy tale, veiling the brute biological and physical reality. And both psychoanalysis and New Age cults manifest their greatest insipidity in their celebration of founding gurus.

It is not just the content but the style of *Atomized* that strong-arms any would-be psychological tacklers. In what may be an ironically self-referential commentary on Houellebecq's part, Bruno says to Michel:

> "His writing is pretentious and clumsy, his characters bland ciphers, but he had one vital premonition—he understood that evolution of human society had for centuries been linked to scientific progress and would continue to be. He may have lacked style or finesse or psychological insight, but that's insignificant compared to the brilliance of the original concept." (188)

Bruno is talking about Aldous Huxley. Houellebecq's next novel, *Platform* (1999b), was severely criticized—and indeed sued—for the boorish way in which he used his characters (including a nameless "dark-skinned" Egyptian) as ciphers for lambasting Islam. He gets some practice for his political incorrectness in *Atomized*, where the female character, Christiane, attacks feminists: "Stupid bitches always going on about the washing up" (1999a, 173).

There are, to be sure, pleasures to be had in Houellebecq's style; amid the gravel, one finds gems: "He does not know it yet, but the infinity of childhood is a brief one" (34). Elsewhere, comic bathos is used amusingly to bring the high low. For the most part, however, he limits the range of affect with an austerity that refuses to yield any emotional crescendos: "The canary [Michel's pet] was dead, its cold white body lying on the gravel. He ate a Monoprix ready-meal— monkfish in parsley sauce, from their Gourmet range—washed down with a mediocre Valdepeñas" (14). One might say that there is a schizoid quality to the narrative that defies empathy. Most superficially but most sensationally, Houellebecq provokes his readers with an impolite cruelty. By muting our emotional reverberations, the novel reduces psychology to baroque decoration, as incongruous as a gargoyle adorning the façade of a skyscraper.

In Houellebecq's counternarrative, with its dismissal of psychic agency, people move as a herd. Those who object are not portrayed as self-actualized individuals, but merely as atomized fragments. Where does this resistance to and defiance of the values of psychoanalysis lead us? The privileging of the individual, along with his or her experience and narrative, is understood to be historically derived and socially sanctioned through therapy and cults, as well as by the advent of confessional writing, which here becomes a parody of self-disclosure. Houellebecq's narrators' lurid racism and sexism may likewise partake of the impulse of people to congregate into groups that imagine themselves to be somehow superior to the mass of outsiders.

What is perhaps most surprising is that with the novel's dismissal of the psychological comes the abolition of moral judgment. There is no superego, benign or punitive, in *Atomized*. Michel imagines an implacable determinism where "no one is to blame" (104). Many of the characters have anxiety or guilt ascribed to them, but only in abstract terms. One could call this an isolation of affect, were it not that the whole novel engages in such a defense. Object relations are hollow, capable of arousing no sense of abuse, and there is thus nothing to judge or condemn. One of the therapist's traditional roles is to be a non-judgmental figure, yet the novel suggests that the exercise of judgment inheres in psychological understanding. Houellebecq thus exploits the discrepancy between the psychologically minded, who pride themselves on being nonjudgmental, and the counternarrativists, who protest that they are being judged.

In *Atomized*, the language and affect of psychology cannot be dissected without confronting the fallacy of individualism and the terror of expulsion from the herd. What the narrator terms "confused and arbitrary" concepts are the ideals of "personal freedom," "human dignity," and "progress" that also happen to be the central tenets of a psychological perspective. Rather than being celebrated, however, they are invoked to "explain why human history from the fifteenth to the twentieth centuries was characterized by decline and destruction" (371). Thus, psychology and therapy, rather than offering a solution, are themselves seen as part of the problem. Sexual transgressions that are forbidden by society may actually be reified when therapy amounts to no more than a particularly fruitless form of role playing.

A final surprising twist awaits us in the epilogue, which reframes the novel as a dystopian "fiction" (369) written long after Michel's death by the cloned progeny of his scientific theories who have overcome "the monstrous egotism, cruelty and anger" (378–79) of humanity. The alternative perspective opened up by this revelation provides Houellebecq with the loophole that the entire novel is supposed to be *wrong*. Read as an inverted science fiction—where the present has become the past described from the standpoint of a scientifically advanced future—the novel's bizarre quality becomes roguishly ironic at the sincere reader's expense, much as the prophecies of our time found in the science fiction of the nineteenth or twentieth centuries now seem comically quaint and inaccurate. Houellebecq exploits the conventional norms of the genre to show how a future free from the psychological values of our time might imagine this age. The novel as a whole may be a mournful testimony to where we are headed.

Houellebecq, whose opening to *Platform* rewrites that of *The Stranger*, is the bastard offspring of Camus's existentialism. Although he disowns Freud as a sire, he may yet be a tragic Cassandra, speaking a truth that remains inaudible in these times. Despite being an exemplary counternarrative, resisting and defying analytic interpretation at every turn, *Atomized* nonetheless invites an antithetical reading. Even when it is polemical, art refuses to stoop to propaganda where brute force overpowers the subtleties and contradictions of lived experience.

FOUR

John Kennedy Toole's Pulitzer Prize–winning novel *A Confederacy of Dunces* (1980) has an unusual and tragic provenance. Brought to the attention of Walker Percy by Toole's mother after her son's suicide, it was published posthumously to critical acclaim. As Percy aptly puts it in his introduction, "The tragedy of the book is the tragedy of the author—his suicide in 1969 at the age of thirty-two. Another tragedy is the body of work we have been denied" (Toole 1980, 9).

If this book set in New Orleans is a sepulcher at once to its author and to a city that has now been washed away, it embalms a character type that once found a home in The Big Easy. Ignatius Reilly, with his outlandish clothing and bizarre mannerisms, his obstinate perseveration on Boethius and on his own "valve," smacks of Axis II, and perhaps even Axis I, psychopathology. But though Reilly can be tagged with a host of labels—schizoid, schizotypal, narcissistic, body dysmorphic, and somatizing, among others—he remains one of the towering figures in twentieth-century literature.

Undeniably, those around Reilly are quick to ascribe mental illness to him. In Toole's syrupy New Orleans dialect, George calls him a "nut" (173), while Darlene identifies him as "that big crazyman" (360). His mother's friend, Santa, tells her:

> "If you had any sense, you woulda had that boy locked away at Charity Hospital a long time ago. They'd turn a hose on him. They'd stick a letrit socket in that boy. They'd show that boy. They'd make him behave. . . . They'd make him listen. They'd beat him in the head, they'd lock him up in a straitjacket, they'd pump some water on him." (276–77)

Despite these threats, Reilly emerges from the novel as a hero with his strangeness intact. He rides off into the sunset with Myrna, his partner-in-pathology. Reilly is victorious on his own terms. He doesn't gain any insight—his delusions remain unchanged—or undergo moral improvement. As is clear from the comments by George, Darlene, and Santa, Toole furnishes the material for a psychiatric analysis both of the text and of Ignatius Reilly, but this possibility is simply rejected. Toole's posture is one of defiance, and he does not seek to explain Reilly's idiosyncracy with either grand theories (such as those favored by Houellebecq) or facile romanticization.

Whereas resistance locates the source of conflict internally, in the individual's personal history, defiance is directed toward the external world, with its collective pressures. A historical figure who may be counted as one of Reilly's ancestors, James Tilly Matthews, was a Welsh pauper held for much of his life as a lunatic in Bedlam following a public outburst. According to Michael Jay's *The Air Loom Gang* (2003), as Lord Liverpool spoke in the House of Commons, on December 30, 1796, Matthews stood up in the galleries and shouted "Treason!" (18). Jay, who ironically subtitles his biography *The Strange and True Story of James Tilly Matthews and his Visionary Madness*, relates Matthews's story less as a pathography of lunacy than as an ambiguous synthesis of psychosis with personal and public history. Matthews, it emerges, played an active role in political intrigue and espionage in the years leading up to the French Revolution, suggesting a possible basis in reality for his charge against Lord Liverpool. What is more, his bizarre behavior dovetailed with the scientific upheavals of the epoch including Mesmerism, Priestley's discovery of oxygen ("dephlogisticated air"), and the emergence of psychiatry, or "mad-doctoring," in the confines of Bedlam. Matthews's florid delusions and the treatment he received at the hands of Bedlam's resident apothecary, John Haslam, add up to an early tale of resistance and defiance. Attempting to disentangle the strands, Jay speculates on the etiology of Matthews's behavior and his psychological motivation; but, like Toole, he refuses to allow this normative discourse to reinstitutionalize his subject.

What we see in *A Confederacy of Dunces* and *The Air Loom Gang* alike is a critique of how psychiatry is recruited into the service of social control. Both Jay and Toole first dissect this process; they then, generously and quietly, release their "patients" from the grasp of institutions. Whereas resistance serves to maintain the status quo, Jay and Toole show that the function of defiance is to recognize how much is at stake in the psychiatric encounter, that the nexus of therapist and patient is not formed solely by personal transferences and countertransferences, but is charged with social and political consequences. Even while celebrating the paradigm of defiance in *Confederacy*, however, one cannot disregard Toole's suicide. Whether Toole might have been saved by psychiatric intervention can never be known, just as one can only speculate whether he might have then written an encore to his comic masterpiece. Yet honesty compels us to temper any rush to the barricades with somber reflection on the twin tragedies identified by Walker Percy.

FIVE

How do the resistance and defiance in counternarratives contribute to our understanding and practice of medicine? For one thing, they refuse to diminish the anger and despondency that cannot be expressed in words such as "anhedonia," "gout," or "rheumatoid arthritis." At the same time, they celebrate mold-breakers such as Ignatius Reilly and James Tilly Matthews without forcing them to submit to authority. A common thread running through narrative medicine and psychoanalysis is the need for just such a deepened understanding of illness, but the resistant/defiant text highlights the importance of confronting the experience of the ill person on his or her own terms.

By extension, counternarratives introduce a schism between the physician's perception of himself or herself as caring and nonjudgmental and the distrustful patient's perception of the physician as self-absorbed and punitive. Dialectically, they shed light on the resistance and defiance of health care providers themselves. Robert Whitaker's *Mad in America* (2002), for instance, provocatively asks why people with schizophrenia not only do not do better in the United States than they do in other countries, but are currently worse off here than they were thirty years ago.

These claims may be shocking to readers of medical journals and standard texts, which often include optimistic retrospectives and prognostications such as the one provided by Daniel E. Casey, MD, in his introduction (2003) to a volume of CNS *Spectrums: The International Journal of Neuropsychiatric Medicine* (funded by an "unrestricted educational grant" from Pfizer):

> The introduction of clozapine in 1989 and additional antipsychotics during the past decade has ushered in a new era of optimism for physicians who treat patients with schizophrenia. Unlike older agents, the atypical antipsychotics effectively treat a broad spectrum of symptoms with a reduced liability for extrapyramidal side effects. (4)

Mad in America, however, has a different story to tell:

> One of the enduring staples in mad medicine has been the rise and fall of cures. Rarely has psychiatry been totally without a remedy advertised as effective. Whether it be whipping the mentally ill, bleeding them, making them vomit, feeding them sheep thyroids, putting them in continuous baths, stunning them with shock therapies, or severing their frontal lobes—all such therapies "worked" at one time, and then, when a new therapy came along, they were suddenly seen in a new light, and their

shortcomings revealed. In the 1990s, this repeating theme in mad medicine
occurred once again. New "atypical" drugs for schizophrenia were brought
to market amid much fanfare, hailed as "breakthrough" treatments, while
old standard neuroleptics were suddenly seen as flawed drugs, indeed.
(Whitaker 2002, 253–54)

Whitaker goes on to describe the development and marketing of atypicals in
a more critical historical perspective than the one commonly provided in the
medical literature.

It should be noted that both the efficacy of atypical antipsychotics and
the damaging side effects of these same medications have been chronicled in
the clinic, both anecdotally and in scientifically controlled studies. But one
has to confront Whitaker's crucial question: Why are people with schizophrenia doing so poorly if psychiatry has such good pharmaceuticals? As
Jeremy Laurance (2003) notes, "[W]e are more tolerant of some kinds of dangerous behavior—driving fast, drunkenness—than of the irrationality associated with mental illness" (43), and this may be why "we will still tolerate provision in mental health that we would not tolerate in other branches of
medicine" (16). Like Houellebecq's *Atomized*, *Mad in America* casts doubt on
the very notion of progress that is integral to many medical narratives.

Homelessness, the incarceration of drug users, mental illness in prison
populations, maternal infanticide, the disenfranchisement of people with
mental illness, and some thirty thousand suicides annually in the United
States: these are public health problems—even public health disasters—that
face mental health practitioners and health care providers. Psychiatry and
psychoanalysis cannot resolve these problems alone, even with the best
intentions. The extent to which psychiatry, psychoanalysis, and public health
interventions fail—and, more bitingly, the extent to which they may actually
contribute to these problems—is chronicled not in peer-reviewed journals and
textbooks but in resistant and defiant narratives. Rejection of these narratives could be interpreted as showing the resistance of physicians themselves
in action.

Resistance and defiance manifest themselves in other fields of medicine
besides psychiatry. The "noncompliant" patient has been the bane of many
treating physicians. Instead of voicing the dispirited refrain, "Why is that
patient so *noncompliant?*" as though it were merely a rhetorical question, it
might be more useful for physicians to take the time to try to sort out the elements of resistance and defiance in their patients' behavior. Such a perspective would lead to a search for the reasons for the difficulty in the patient-
physician relationship, and serve as a cautionary reminder that the
breakdown is something for which both parties are likely to be responsible.

There is reason to hope that a better understanding of modes of protest
will shed light on the racial and cultural disparities in the provision of

health care. The feminist counternarrative to the medicalization of menopause, for example, has been vindicated by several reputable studies published in medical journals, leading Katha Pollitt (2004) to include in her catalogue of recent feminist victories, "Hormone replacement therapy was further debunked." On the other hand, "alternative" medicine frequently presents itself as a benign contrast to "Western medicine" (a term often used pejoratively and that excludes the contributions of "non-Western" scientists and doctors). But what if the counternarrative of the proponents of alternative medicine were actually motivated by a powerful *resistance* to allowing their own products and practices to be tested by double-blind, placebo-controlled experiments? At least in part, might not this self-righteous posture of "defiance" be an attempt to protect their own multimillion-dollar sector of the health care industry?

SIX

Counternarratives are problematic above all because we are unsure what to do with them: where do they fit, given that they insist upon not fitting? How does one view them when they dispute the legitimacy of the viewer's perspective? There are points of irrevocable impasse. For example, many of the claims made by the Church of Scientology about mental health and the history of psychiatry (Citizens Commission on Human Rights 2004) are simply irreconcilable with any narrative that a licensed psychologist or psychiatrist would propose (Dain 1994).

Simply by virtue of entering into a dialogue, counternarratives run the risk of being appropriated. Whenever resistant texts are incorporated into the medical curriculum, this may have the effect of sanitizing them, like pathological specimens floating in amber formaldehyde, leading to their recuperation as hegemonic narratives. This happens when clinicians listen for the Axis I pathology or the history of an arrhythmia hidden in a patient's description of his or her experience with illness. The counternarrative loses its subversive power; it is tamed and reframed. What is defiance in one context can be resistance in another. Indeed, despite the topographical metaphors that seem to suggest they occupy different spaces, in reality they are two sides of the same Möbius strip.

To see how this is so, let us conclude by considering a magazine that strives to provide a counternarrative to mainstream media. *Adbusters* takes on the influence of advertising and the ideology of consumerism in the United States; its artists and activists have a masterful knack for shifting contexts. In one number, *Adbusters* (2004) reproduces the advertisements for pharmaceuticals such as Zoloft that pose a set of questions serving to diagnose panic disorder according to DSM-IV criteria. Shifted out of the clinic into the pages of the magazine, the questions about the fear of dying, shortness of breath, and sweating become lethally mundane. Does one really need medicine for *this*? Who *wouldn't* qualify for a trial of Zoloft? The reframed messages pose even more far-reaching questions: what sort of complicity is at work when an advertisement reproduces a physician's protocol? Or are the physician's questions simply parroting the advertiser's sales pitch?

Ultimately, resistance constitutes an obstacle to insight, while defiance seeks to provide an obstacle to abuse. But how can we maintain this distinction when resistance is tinctured with defiance, and defiance is a side effect of resistance? In his inexhaustible yet outrageous case history of Dora, Freud writes, "[W]e shall not be far from solving" many mysteries "when we realize that thoughts in the unconscious live very comfortably side by side, and even contraries get on together without disputes—a state of things which persists often enough even in the conscious" (1905, 62). As narrative medicine writes its own history and makes its way into the curriculum, it would do well to set an example for other branches of medicine by learning how to appreciate the defiance and analyze the resistance both in its own texts and in those that it scrutinizes.

NOTES

1. Applying the concepts of resistance and defiance to a written text is problematic. Not only is reading a book different from conducting a human relationship, literary narratives are hardly free associations, the optimal discourse from the perspective of psychoanalysis. Even a novel as attuned to the ebbs and flows of mental life as *Ulysses* was toiled over for a decade by Joyce, and cannot be analyzed naively. This question has been addressed fruitfully by others (Holland 1993); for the purposes of this chapter, however, we can seek insight into resistance and defiance wherever we may find it.

2. Although the published translation spells *Atomised* in the English manner, I have altered the "s" to a "z" in conformity with standard American usage.

REFERENCES

Adbusters. 2002. *Mad pride*. No. 41.

———. 2004. *Distorted info*. No. 51.

Casey, Daniel E. 2003. Introduction. Optimizing treatment for patients with schizophrenia: Targeting positive outcomes. *CNS Spectrums* 8, no. 11:4.

Citizens Commision on Human Rights. 2004. Psychiatry—A global failure. Available at: http://www.cchr.org/failure/eng.

Dain, Norman. 1994. Reflections on antipsychiatry and stigma in the history of American psychiatry. *Hospital and Community Psychiatry* 45:1010–14.

Freud, Sigmund. 1905. *Fragment of an analysis of a case of hysteria*. In *Standard edition of the complete psychological works* (hereafter S.E.), ed. and trans. James Strachey et al., 7:3–122. London: Hogarth Press, 1953–1974.

————. 1916–1917. *Introductory lectures on psychoanalysis*. S.E., vols. 15 and 16.

Gabbard, Glen O. 2000. *Psychodynamic psychiatry in clinical practice*. Third ed. Washington, DC: American Psychiatric Association Press.

Holland, Norman. 1993. Psychoanalysis and literature—Past and present. *Contemporary Psychoanalysis* 29:5–21.

Houellebecq, Michel. 1999a. *Atomized*. Trans. Frank Wynne. London: Vintage, 2001.

————. 1999b. *Platform*. Trans. Frank Wynne. London: Heinemann, 2002.

Jay, Michael. 2003. *The air loom gang: The strange and true story of James Tilly Matthews and his visionary madness*. London: Bantam.

Laurance, Jeremy. 2003. *Pure madness: How fear drives the mental health system*. London: Routledge.

McHugh, Paul R., and Phillip R. Slavney. 1998. *The perspectives of psychiatry*. Second ed. Baltimore: The Johns Hopkins University Press.

National Alliance for the Mentally Ill. 2004. Available at http://www.nami.org.

Pollitt, Katha. 2004. Good news for women. *The Nation*. January 12. Available at http://www.thenation.com/doc.mhtml?i=20040112&s=pollitt.

Toole, John Kennedy. 1980. *A confederacy of dunces*. New York: Grove Weidenfeld.

Vonnegut, Mark. 1975. *The Eden express*. New York: Praeger.

Whitaker, Robert. 2002. *Mad in America: Bad science, bad medicine, and the enduring mistreatment of the mentally ill*. Cambridge, MA: Perseus.

SIXTEEN

Narrative and Beyond

GEOFFREY HARTMAN

WHAT CHARM, in the strong sense of that word, which intimates a quasi-magical or medicinal effect, does storytelling have? In general, narrative forms of representation, in fiction or nonfiction, are a steady source of comfort for both author and reader (presenter and listener), though "comfort" may not be an adequate descriptive term. Homer and Virgil are not afraid to have their warriors shed tears when hearing of past adventures and tribulations, tears that satisfy deeply.

Stories about illness and loss, however, should they portray persons reduced to suffering in a passive way, at most furnish moral examples of endurance. Or, as in Richard Selzer's (1982) eloquent vignettes of painful and diseased bodies, they show how ugliness can become, through the doctor's eye and the writer's touch, a strange source of beauty.

Yet it almost needs a conversion experience to value a redeeming change of this kind. It is hard to believe that such consoling depictions are not a mirage. Especially since the sufferer's pain is often heightened by a specific mental anguish, a conception of fault or trespass, as in the Prometheus legend, or Dante's Inferno, or the testing of Job.

Today, for the most part, we no longer assume that mortal ills reveal the (hidden) fault of individuals, or of the human as such. We also shy away from accepting Cicero's definition of the philosopher as one who studies death (not unlike the medical doctor in this), or whose entire life, like that of Socrates, is but a preparation for how to make a good end.

Heroism, nevertheless, is not always absent from scenes of an extreme suffering, though except for faction or fiction we try to confine such scenes to hospice and hospital. An implicit dramatic conflict between acceptance and defiance is often sensed, not only in the suffering person but also in the vulnerable observer.

I do not say this in order to invest suffering with an illegitimate interest. It is not the novelistic or TV potential that prompts a reflection of this sort but the practical task of care giving: what is psychically necessary in order to face this ultimate labor.

Passion narratives, of course, which depict a suffering humanity, have a long religious as well as literary tradition. Prometheus, Dionysus, and Christ are gods. At present, narratives about death, illness, madness, persecution, and calamity serve as demotic and increasingly popular versions of the genre. In proliferating TV biopics, for example, they have become formulaic parts of a celebrity's journey from (often) humble beginnings to a breakthrough to fame, then via crisis and suffering to recovery, maturity, and even greater fame.

Selzer's doctor stories are more complex. Their linkage of passion and pathology creates, as I have mentioned, a transfigurative realism, one that overrides aesthetic scruples previously limiting the serious portrayal in art of bodily deformity and its accompanying anguish. In his fictive Grand Rounds, moreover, Selzer does not present his all-too-human types as victims: in their very agony or debility, and their relations with the surgeon, they are larger than life, and even the impact of their death can have a haunting poignancy.

An early perspective on the specific affect of narratives that involve suffering, both physical and mental, is found in Aristotle's *Poetics*. Despite the sacred origins of Greek drama, his analysis remains entirely secular. Pity and fear, according to him, are purged or purified by the art of tragedy. His theory of catharsis continues to perplex because it posits a powerful emotional, but also satisfying, response to the representation of a painful subject matter. The formal care, therefore, with which the tragic story is told, and which Aristotle analyzes authoritatively, must have some bearing on that emotional uplift. Even when there is no possibility of a cure, or of a reversal of fortune, we would like to believe that art's cathartic effect (intense in the genre of tragedy but not restricted to it) lifts the spirits of those depressed by ills that flesh is heir to.

Empirically, though, it remains to be shown that stories, like music, can succeed, as Milton says in *Comus*, in "smoothing the raven down / Of darkness" (Hughes 1957, 96). So far we have no poetics of narrative medicine. The claims made for this interesting new discipline are eminently practical and humane rather than overreaching. Narrative medicine is still very much a work in progress, and its having carved out a space in medical school for teaching and reflection is already an achievement.

⁂

What is it we have learned, up to this point, about the relevance of studying literature in medical school? The following is a disorderly anatomy of the subject by an outsider, fragments or *membra disjecta* of what could go into an overview. It will be obvious that such remarks are based on my own limited roles of teacher, reader, and occasional interviewer of Holocaust witnesses.

1. As Rita Charon (Charon and Montello 2002) has emphasized, listening is not only indispensable (everybody agrees with that) but it can be, must be, developed. Influenced, like Charon, by literary studies, I have a prejudice that close reading and close listening are related. This is certainly one direction to be explored in training a medical staff.

Close reading, moreover, goes with close writing: with thinking about style (Selzer admits he does this obsessively). We are talking here about self-presentation, certainly; yet no less about presentation of the other. A morally sensitive problem makes itself felt: How can I create a new kind of holistic chart for the patient (during the illness, or as a sustained reflection on it afterward), and not be distracted by the confessional egotisms necessary for an honest account of my experience as it becomes an I/Thou encounter?

2. There is an instinctive aspect to listening. This watchfulness of the ear may come from the link between apprehending and being apprehensive. But as a creative flair it contributes to that "delight in imitation" deemed to be universal by Aristotle. A thoughtful replay of one's own or another's experience, however difficult the experience may have been, gives pleasure to both presenter and listener because the mimetic talent has found an aim, becoming mimicry in the service of mastery—yet also something more significant.

Indeed, I would like to emphasize that which cannot be subsumed under the notion of mastery. There is, on the one hand, the doctor's perspective, and, on the other, the patient's. Their typical narratives differ. It is important, as Arthur Frank makes clear in his remarkable *The Wounded Storyteller* (1995), that we recognize the variety of illness narratives that exist. But also that the claim of a "sovereign consciousness" may have to be given up. Frank quotes Jean Améry, who writes (brought to that realization by Nazi torturers), "there are situations in life where our body is our entire self and our fate" (ix).[1] Today, however, the main tendency is for cultural and commercial influences to favor what Frank calls "restitution narratives" whose storyline reinforces "the expectation that for every suffering there is a remedy" (25).

3. The sense that storyline and lifeline are connected is more than literary palmistry. Sheherazade kept an Emperor awake; her 1,001 suspenseful tales suspend a death that had been decreed. We, as patients, have to keep the doctors awake. Not a lesser task, given present health care conditions . . .

A hospital is full of stories, then; but they remain, most of them, doctor stories adjusted for the good of future patients and caregivers. Stories from the other side, by powerless observers, may seem useless. The vocabulary of agency predominates in our professional discourses. It is hard to draw sustenance or communicable lessons from situations such as the deathbed watch depicted in Ingmar Bergman's *Cries and Whispers*, a morbid film that only just avoids the *non plus ultra* of passive despair, and so a flight (not always restrained in other Bergman films) into spiritualistic fantasy.

More bearable, somehow, is a further extreme situation (also not absent from films): when friends keep a comatose patient alive. Hope in a "resurrection" then becomes tangible through talking and touching and nonabandonment—through projecting a watchful, caring presence. The lifeline here takes the form of stories read to a seemingly unconscious person, or a refusal to let the latter's immobility and silence abort the stream of talk. Some mourners carry on that conversation even after a loved one's death.

4. Narrative medicine encourages eliciting a history from every patient, however word-shy or afflicted by elective mutism. This potential dialogue needs time to develop, and the modern hospital or consulting room has little time. So that the often inarticulate story inside the patient gets to be abbreviated rather than fully told. Still, the physician-listener must assume that something of the (call it) gestalt of the person treated can be glimpsed in the brief time allotted. This requires not only the doctor's interpretive patience, strengthened by what Charon calls "narrative competence," but also an avoidance of acting out. (Such acting out is described by Selzer, who admits to quirky lapses under the pressure of a surgeon's "mad" vocation.) The aim should be a sympathetic absorption of each person's words and demeanor, so that no one is too quickly classified, shunted into a diagnostic type, frozen into a symptomatic category.

The physician, then, despite the constraint of time, cultivates an empathy that, ideally, seeks to bring forth the patient's own understanding, even self-discovery. Healing, or minimally the will to be healed, begins with the hope of reaching, by means of words, what Paul Celan (1958) has called the shoreline of a heart.

Thus, what seems of paramount importance is the element of trust. The patient should feel able to rely for support on the hospital staff's "affective community." In that sense all medicine is family medicine.

5. The physician too needs a measure of reciprocal satisfaction. This cannot often come from the person being treated, who is still in pain, and necessarily self-absorbed. It has to come from a quality of self-awareness in the doctor, a learning curve that is more than quantitative: as in teaching, where one draws on classroom encounters previously thought about, and which now help the teacher to proceed in ways that lessen the sheer opacity or resistance of the human text.

6. *The human text.* Is that an unfeeling metaphor for the living or dying human being? Not if we—teachers, doctors, observers—are part of the text, if we have to read also in ourselves. That figure of speech is not meant to promote a one-way, distancing objectification, a professional deformation satirized by John Donne's "Hymne to God my God, in my Sicknesse":

Whilst my Physitians by their lore are growne
   Cosmographers, and I their Mapp, who lie
Flat on this bed, that by them may be showne
   That this is my South-west discoverie
Per fretum febris, by these streights to die . . .
(Grierson 1968, 1:368)

Donne's bravado in sickness is extraordinary. In *Devotions upon Emergent Occasions* (1624), his meditations (a habitual, formal exercise, practiced by him in sickness or in health) on a medical crisis and the recovery from it are the kind of narrative that rivals exemplary modern instances in its self-conscious imaginative reach. The author "reads" the behavior of the physicians and the course of the disease, and ranges, by means of hyperbolic analogies, from the little world of man, and the close prison of the sickroom, to macrocosmic regions beyond the sun and just shy of God.

7. Two difficult issues, finally, must be broached. One is: How can empathy be taught? Culture as "kulcha" is a fallible instrument of humanization. The lover of music or literature can use that cultured sensibility to become blind to the suffering of others and even, in the very name of culture, to murder. We have experienced this massively in our time.

As we come to know more about brain physiology, we also learn what biochemicals are involved when persons are consistently unfeeling. But this does not answer the question of how, absent a chemical intervention, people can be brought to feel for other people; or, in diagnostic terms, what causes a severe emotional deficit, a callous or "beautiful" indifference.

Is such behavior linked to panic about a potential loss of status or self-identity? To speculate further: Could that panic be triggered by boundary problems, a compulsive tendency to overidentify? Short of pharmaceutical treatment, then, can there be empathy management, as we now have pain management? And what role could the arts play, in the dubious light of our notorious ability to compartmentalize feelings?

Still, one cannot rule out the contagious effect of a sensibility such as Tolstoy's. His sympathetic yet unsentimental understanding of the characters he presents can be exemplified by "Master and Man" (1895), a story in which the distance between the educated, classy master and his peasant sled driver is gradually worn down during a catastrophic snowstorm in which, finally, both attempt to save each other by sharing their bodily warmth.

These large questions need to be broken down into manageable bits. But even one of those bits, how to increase the sensitivity of health care professionals—or to renew it, since it is always being worn away—may need the refreshing detour of literature or other types of innovative experimentation, and that has started in the emerging field of the medical humanities.

The second issue concerns human experimentation, the possibility of a scientific study of such problems. Science is not pursued in a vacuum; the scientific method has its own problematic. The Milgram (1983) experiment, which precisely is about willingness to inflict pain in the name of science, had an elegant simplicity as well as a devastating lesson to impart.[2] Since ethical questions bearing on medical decisions are now taken very seriously, and the bioethicist has become a fixture in most schools, the kind of discussion common to literary seminars should seem less extraordinary. Such a discussion has always covered silences as well as words, indirect modes of expression, the relation of all components—narrative, symbol, metaphor, point of view—to one another, as well as the emotional or ideological complexities in the characters represented. It is surely a propaedeutic boon to have the time to think freely, to explore the very process of interpretation, without having to do it in a state of emergency.

But to return to the Milgram experiment: it may harbor unexplored implications. Does it point to the well-known mechanism of identification with the aggressor?[3] Why should such an impulse, however, outweigh a possible identification with the victim or person in pain? The issue, therefore, of how to cultivate empathy and judgment together, and whether professional literary study could help this endeavor, remains to be explored.

ﻉ

Let me describe a humane experiment, an ongoing project with intriguing relevance for the medical humanities, including narrative medicine. The project, so far, has helped those who suffered a traumatic assault that violated every habitual norm, exceeded the understanding, and attempted to dismantle, in the groups targeted, their human dignity and very sense of self. I am referring to the extreme case of victims of the Holocaust.

After the war, some find a refuge in Israel. They are safe, or are they? Memories remain—traumatic memories. In Israel the unsympathetic attitude of many sabras (or aspiring sabras) was: you should have known to emigrate earlier, to leave a corrupt diaspora. Now get on with your life.

A survey in 1993, almost fifty years after liberation, found that a large number of elderly Holocaust survivors were chronic patients in mental hospitals.[4] These survivors, according to the author (see Laub 2005, 258) of a recent report,

> had not been treated as a specialized group, and at least their trauma-related psychopathology [may have been] to some degree not fully addressed in their chronic treatment since their arrival in Israel following their Holocaust experience. They [the researchers] document that in one of Israel's largest mental health centers, nearly 67% of the 74 psycho-geri-

atric patients were Holocaust survivors (strikingly, almost all of them women) with 30% having experienced chronic hospitalization since the Holocaust. In a large number of these patients, it was reported that the medical chart contained no information of the patient's persecution experience during the Holocaust.

Ten years later a group of psychiatrists finally receives permission to employ videotaped interviews in order to decide the proper care for these patients. As part of such rehabilitation, they investigate "the effects of addressing long-term post-traumatic sequelae." The survivors are encouraged to tell their story, however belatedly. The question not fully answered, but which haunts this effort, is whether survivor patients would "experience relief to some extent had they been able or enabled to more openly share their severe persecution history." The experiment, basically and belatedly, tries a story cure or, more precisely, a testimony cure. Testimony about the Holocaust, as well as the victim's subsequent life, is to create a videotaped autobiography that can be studied by others in addition to being viewed by the patients themselves.

I should add a disclaimer before continuing. That I focus on this experiment does not imply in any way that Holocaust survivors have a greater need for psychiatric care than others who have experienced extreme trauma, or that the testimony archive Yale has been building up for twenty-five years was motivated by anything except giving witnesses a chance freely to tell what they had seen and heard, and what their present reflections are. Yale's testimony archive set out to record Holocaust memories and realities by means of oral history. This effort has a value independent of any therapeutic effect, which may or may not occur. Its importance for the future will be helped by its open and unstructured character, that it did not pursue any agenda, since that might foreclose questions from succeeding generations.

The Israeli Hospital project I have described employs recognized scientific parameters; and my choosing it is a necessity, given the difficulty of finding careful humanistic experiments with implications for health care. So far the results of using a video testimonial method on patients long neglected have been encouraging, at least for the nonpsychotic survivors. The experiment justifies thinking about the method's relevance to more usual cases of post-traumatic stress. The participant doctors are led to the following optimistic remark that points clearly to the potential of narrative medicine:

> It has been suggested that the testimonial method alleviates many chronic symptoms by transforming the painful trauma story into a cathartic experience and document which could be useful to other people. In this way some of the response which the extremes of suffering would have created in the survivor could be channeled and elaborated upon in a constructive manner. The video testimonial event is framed by its purpose, the creation of an

autobiographical document that has as its centerpiece the traumatic experience. It is a collaborative venture, during which the interviewer recedes much more into the background and the patient is said to be assisted by means of the narration of personal experience into a new social context (see Strous et al. 2005, 2288).

I want to end by suggesting that more could be done in the medical humanities with different aspects of literature, not only its narrative component. I am sometimes uneasy with how narrative as a concept has taken over (in literary studies, too). While there is no need to fuss about the habit of using "narrative" and "story" as synonyms, it should be clear that "story," in this medical context, points to a mode of presentation that involves a distinctively engaged rather than detached or omniscient observer.[5] That is also why "bearing witness" and "testimony"—not carrying, necessarily, a religious overtone—enter the discussion. "Narrative" remains appropriate, however, because it is a term giving weight to both the (potential) expressiveness of the person in pain and the scientific, cognitive side of the clinician's professional work.

The problem comes from such generalizations as "No moral theory can be adequate if it does not take into account the narrative character of our experience" (Johnson 1993, 105). A striking aphorism, but on the face of it false. Yes, the narrative turn in medicine is also an ethical turn. But is experience intrinsically narrative (let alone ethical)? It may have that character retrospectively, or when planned in advance and executed according to plan. Yet experience usually involves something hidden, oblique, unresolved, something that follows a precarious and uncertain path. Hence the suspense, as well as vacillations in the reader's empathic response.

Storytelling's internal progress, from purpose to passion (in which bearings are lost) to perception, reveals other determinants: the intervention of chance, for example, and various nonteleologic elements.[6] The narrative flow halts, digresses, turns this way and that, seems to lose its way—just like the protagonist. What often affects us, especially in the "passion" or crisis phase, is a mental or bodily short-circuiting, a turbulence swirling around a fixed idea that potentially darkens Shelley's definition of love as "a going out of our own nature and an identification of ourselves with the beautiful which exists in thought, action, or person not our own" (1821, 487). Here is where symbol and other strong poetic figures come into play as forceful condensations. The literary shows its existential rather than conventional side and points to the link between symptom and symbolic action. The body tries to speak: the physiologic or psychic marker that challenges the physician should also shield the patient from being considered a passive medical object.

In sum, there is a thinking with stories as well as about stories (see Morris 2002). This has already produced a multitude of memoirs in our autobiographical culture. The point is not, of course, to have every serious illness end as a book.

That would be a sterile move. The call is for a thinking that encourages the physician to "follow the patient's narrative thread" (Charon and Montello 2002, ix), to negotiate pathways illumined by an expanded concept of narrative poetics. It is to be sensitive also to non-narrative, apparently inconsequential or lyrical moments, surprises in the narrator's mood and mode. One learns to respect fragments of speech, abrupt figurations, shifts, jump-cuts, mixed genres. It also means, while synthesizing all these features and having them accord with, or even alter, "the professional narrative voice of medicine" (Poirier 2002, 57), to respect what does not fit.[7] For there may be more than one story struggling to emerge, as in a multiple birth.

NOTES

1. On the difference between doctor and patient stories, or between those originating in very different cultures dealing with illness, death, and therapy, see also Kathryn Hunter's fine chapter on "Narrative Incommensurability" (1991, 123–47).

2. This is based on experiments carried out by Milgram at Yale from 1961 through 1962. They demonstrated how ingrained obedience/submission to authority was (in this particular case, the authority of an experimenter claiming a scientific justification for inflicting physical pain) in a large majority of people tested, consisting of New Haven volunteers.

3. Milgram disqualifies the argument from an instinct of aggression in chapter 13 of his book, but he does in effect describe obedience as motivated by identification with a social order that is viewed as a necessary source of authority.

4. My quotations from the study of Holocaust survivors are drawn from a pre-publication manuscript sent to me by Dori Laub. The corresponding passages in the published papers I have cited are worded differently.

5. Julia Connelly differentiates between the object of discourse (the story) and the discourse itself (narrative knowledge): "Narrative knowledge—comprehension of the specific, unique, detailed, and situated individual story" (2002, 139). From a Saussurian perspective, the relationship of story to narrative could be viewed in the light of the *parole/langue* distinction.

6. I am recalling categories used by Francis Fergusson in *The Idea of a Theater* (1949). Since the medical interview, or the sustained conversation to which it may lead, is a duologue, an element of the theatrical (or performative) does enter.

7. See Poirier's entire essay in *Stories Matter*. This question of the professional stylization or authoritative tone has also been raised in the field of history, when the topic is social and political suffering.

REFERENCES

Celan, Paul. 1958. Speech on the occasion of receiving the Literature Prize of the Free Hanseatic City of Bremen. In *Collected prose*, trans. Rosemarie Waldrop, 33–36. Riverdale-on-Hudson, NY: Sheep Meadow Press, 1990.

Charon, Rita, and Martha Montello, eds. 2002. *Stories matter: The role of narrative in medical ethics*. New York: Routledge.

Connelly, Julia E. 2002. In the absence of narrative. In Charon and Montello 2002, 138–46.

Donne, John. 1624. *Devotions upon emergent occasions*. Ed. Anthony Raspa. Montreal: McGill-Queen's University Press, 1975.

Fergusson, Francis. 1949. *The idea of a theater*. Princeton: Princeton University Press.

Frank, Arthur W. 1995. *The wounded storyteller: Body, illness, and ethics*. Chicago: University of Chicago Press.

Grierson, Herbert J. C., ed. 1968. *The poems of John Donne*. 2 vols. Oxford: Oxford University Press.

Hughes, Merritt Y., ed. 1957. *Complete poems and major prose of John Milton*. Indianapolis: Odyssey Press.

Hunter, Kathryn Montgomery. 1991. *Doctors' stories: The narrative structure of medical knowledge*. Princeton: Princeton University Press.

Johnson, Mark. 1993. *Moral imagination: Implication of cognitive science for ethics*. Chicago: University of Chicago Press.

Laub, Dori. 2005. From speechlessness to narrative: The cases of Holocaust historians and of psychiatrically hospitalized survivors. *Literature and Medicine*, 24:253–65.

Milgram, Stanley. 1983. *Obedience to authority: An experimental view*. New York: Harper/Collins.

Morris, David. 2002. Narrative, ethics, and pain: Thinking with stories. In Charon and Montello 2002, 196–218.

Poirier, Richard. 2002. Voice in the medical narrative. In Charon and Montello 2002, 48–58.

Selzer, Richard. 1982. *Letters to a young doctor*. New York: Harcourt Brace.

Shelley, Percy Bysshe. 1821. *A defense of poetry*. In *Shelley's Poetry and Prose. Authoritative Texts, Criticism*, ed. Donald H. Reiman and Sharon B. Powers, 478–508. New York: Norton, 1977.

Strous, Rael D., Mordechai Weiss, Boris Finkel, Moshe Kotler, and Dori Laub. 2005. Video Testimony of Long-Term Hospitalized Psychiatrically Ill Holocaust Survivors. *American Journal of Psychiatry*, 162:2287–94.

Tolstoy, Leo. 1895. Master and man. Trans. Louise and Aylmer Maude. Boulder: NetLibrary.

Material and Metaphor

Narrative Treatment for the Embodied Self

RITA CHARON

The self—should it exist—dwells within a body that catapults it into the world. Between the body and that which lies external to it obtains a commerce of perceptions, an exchange of substances, and a flow of representations. As the copulative term between self and world, the body can donate metabolism, sensation, motion, and consciousness, thereby making possible language, action, emotion, and thought. What gets called into question at the border between psychoanalysis and narrative medicine is the body's relation to meaning.

I brooded on this question in my presentation at the outset of the "Psychoanalysis and Narrative Medicine" conference. The other papers delivered there have led me to ruminate further on the nature of the contact between the selves housed in different bodies in the clinical setting, whether medical or analytic, putting into play notions of proximity and distance, similarity and strangerliness, and narrative and the ill body. The hypothesis that generated itself in the course of my writing is that disease opens the body to proximity, and that the material proximity of illness can herald intersubjective proximity. The enabling link between these two forms of proximity is found in language, in the telling and listening to stories of self, which are themselves enabled by illness. This contact, of course, differs in the cases of medicine and psychoanalysis, and to reflect on *how* they differ is likely to be instructive for both fields.

Psychoanalytic theory and practice have established, at least as convention if not empirically verified fact, that the body's storehouse of corporeal instincts and appetites is the ground for developing intimacy in human relationships and discovering meaning in personal experience. That which the body endures and enjoys is a substrate for identity, while that which the body registers in memory is constitutive of autobiography. Having been dismissed in the centuries following Descartes, the contributions of the body to *who one is* have been celebrated lately in realms as diverse as continental phenomenology, experimental neural science, and postmodern fiction.

Psychoanalytic practice erects a filter of meaning between the body and the self of the patient as well as between the patient and doctor. Physical contact, of course, is disallowed, although by no means does this prohibition preclude passion. Throughout the treatment, at least that conducted on classical Freudian lines, the analyst does not reveal much about himself or herself but rather provides a blank and generative screen on which the analysand projects wishes, fears, and reflections. The blankness of the screen is required for transference to proceed. The analyst learns to deflect curiosity and mute opinion. Where one goes in August ought not be discussed. Whether one is ill or grieving or gay or straight ought not matter, and indeed the patient's curiosity about these aspects of the analyst's person is subject to interpretation. Playing a transformative role of great power, the analyst operates on the metaphorical and not the material level. The analyst develops this power by virtue of standing for someone else.

The medical doctor, by contrast, enters the lives of patients guilelessly, open-faced, as himself or herself. Of course, there may well be an aura of importance or authority surrounding the doctor, especially in times of acute sickness or dramatic episodes of illness. One doesn't wait for the neurosurgeon to emerge from the OR bearing news of dicey surgery as if waiting for the milkman. Some patients may always be reserved in addressing or interacting with their doctors, but more often than not the doctor becomes a staple of life, an every-third-month ritual, an entity known for itself. The doctor typically displays pictures of his or her kids in the office, hangs framed diplomas from specialty boards on the walls, and talks with relish about vacations upon return. Because patients can call us at home and often get our spouses or children on the line, they know, sort of, what kinds of lives we lead and with whom we might share them. I remember, as an intern, calling an attending physician at home about an acutely ill patient of his I had just admitted to hospital. It was around two or three a.m. On the second ring, the phone was answered by a woman's crisp voice announcing, "Dr. Hamel's office." The impression I received, as I imagined the receiver being handed over from one side of the double bed to the other, of his home life, marriage, and work life was indelible.

There is nothing wrong with this. It pleases me when my patients ask after my husband or grandchildren. I recall my mother dispensing medical advice to my father's patients over the telephone at home, knowing what he would have said to do, and I appreciate it when my husband talks gently with a distraught patient looking for me at home. The relationships I develop with my patients are ordinary ones, based on routines of life—helpful, practical, vectored relationships. No doubt, patients look to their medical doctors for assurance and steadfastness and comfort. They look to us for expert knowledge and signs of hope or defeat. But unlike analytic relationships, ours are grounded in materiality; the body roots them in matter.

The matters at hand—heart failure, tuberculosis, an earache—are *material* ones and as such can be described, examined, and compared to others of the same kind. More saliently, these material things offer themselves as triangulating entities that unite the doctor and the patient in the concrete world. The doctor and the patient can gaze together at the lung cancer or the diabetes or the miscarriage, and this gazing together at something material forms the basis for their relationship. As part of the patient's body, these triangulating things are not neutral objects outside the dyadic charge between doctor and patient. It is not as if they are together gazing at a malfunctioning carburetor or an aphid-ridden fern. The bodily part in trouble is both physical object and proxy for the patient's self. Somehow, though, the body's existence as physical object braces the relationships founded on its behalf.

This is not to say that illnesses or symptoms are always only things or events. The elevated LDL, the darkening mole, the late period, the blood in the stool count as substance in space or occurrence in time while they point to other things. They have meanings in excess of their materiality. Material *and* metaphorical, these symptoms function in the lives of the patients they afflict with both concrete and symbolic import.

The essays in this volume urge us collectively to turn a corner in considering human health and illness. Vera Camden's eloquent and mournful description of the singular experiences of one woman in her care attests to the depth of this analyst's investment in her patient. Overcoming the revulsion initiated by Mrs. F's abhorrent dreams and passive-aggressive behavior, Camden persevered in the effort to piece together the meanings latent in the not merely metaphorical wastes accumulating on her couch. Staying the course demanded stores of skill and imagination, as well as a faith that, somehow, the patient had it in her to get better, and to improve by virtue of their collaborative decoding of the personal meanings inherent in these powerful images of violence and death.

John Sassall, the "fortunate physician" whose virtues are celebrated by Fred Griffin, and the internist depicted by Lisa Schnell in her poignant memoir of the life and death of her infant daughter, are doctors of a more familiar sort. They do not set out to function as transferential objects for their patients. They take aim at the congestive heart failure or the tremor. That these physical states ultimately point beyond themselves—the heart failure confronted by Sassall to his elderly patient's apology to her family, and

Schnell's tremor to her identification with her gravely ill daughter—does not negate their having originated from within. These doctors are led to uncover levels of familial and emotional meaning through an initial engagement with the patient's material body.

Having brooded on the overlaps and disidentity between narrative medicine and psychoanalysis, and now with the aid of these chapters and the thoughts that spring from them, I find myself able to see more clearly some of what clinicians in these two fields might be able to accomplish. I can also begin, by virtue of putting them side by side, to reenvision some aspects of what, in fact, we do, and then to envision a future of shared work for both groups of caregivers.

My practice in internal medicine is becoming more and more interior as I get better at being an internist. Recently in the office, I realized that a forty-two-year-old man who came in for a checkup had been badly abused as a child. I don't know if he knows this, and I don't know exactly *how* I know it, but I do. I referred him to a very skilled family therapist who might be able to accompany this man through what will most likely be a long ordeal of discovery. The patient agreed to see the therapist when I said that it struck me that he had a lot that needed to be told. I will continue to see him regularly for his medical care, but I think my contribution to his health is to have recognized the existence of an as yet unspoken trauma.

Several months ago, I saw a new patient with joint pain and depression who had been working in lower Manhattan in the fall of 2001. I asked him on his second visit to me if he knew anyone who had been at the World Trade Center on September 11. He was there. He then told me, in thirty minutes of uninterrupted, stuttering, stirring, tearful monologue, about being trapped in the Broad Street subway station when the first explosion occurred, being herded by the police over the Brooklyn Bridge away from Manhattan, turning to see the flaming towers fall, and then reaching home in the far Bronx after walking stunned all day to an ecstatic family who had taken him for dead. I didn't think to ask the first time I saw him, and he would not have told me without my prompting. But this is what he was there for.

I am no longer surprised to find that my work in internal medicine requires such acts of witnessing from me. I have taken to calling my specialty "interior medicine," for gradually I see how being a doctor exposes me, requisitions all of me, impresses me, sparing nothing. I cannot choose to remain out of reach and do the medicine well. It is not as if one can practice medicine with only a portion of oneself, blindfolded or with one hand tied behind one's back. Many, of course, do try—practicing with detachment, with coolness, with only ideas and so-called facts—and then their medicine fails and they know not why.

Like the analyst, the ordinary doctor is confronted by materiality saturated with metaphor and usually cannot tell—in the first few years anyway—

which is which. The obese young woman who turns up in emergency room after emergency room with chest pain, back pain, and shortness of breath and has only "negative evaluations" to show for it is *after* something. No one can yet tell what. It is my first task to reach her with the realization that she is on a search, to get beyond the draining and boring and pointless diagnostic interventions toward letting her tell me what it is she needs to tell. A woman with lupus has, during decades in my practice, let me in on many aspects of her illness and her life—her major depression (under good psychiatric care), her childhood loss of her father's presence, her unachievable professional dreams, her clinging and punitive mother, her alcoholic boyfriend, the early death of her sister of gynecological cancer, her adopting of her nieces and nephews. All these factors are not extraneous to her lupus, nor is her lupus a magical consequence of them. These physical and emotional and social dimensions of her life interinanimate one another, and none can be approached in isolation. If pelvic pain occurs on the anniversary of her sister's death, I know enough to get an ultrasound to reassure her that she will not soon die of the same tumor.

In the face of serious illness, so much needs to be said and heard, yet suffering sometimes cannot be declared openly but can only be fitfully intimated by another. This is true, of course, of internal medicine, whose diseases often do not show. Not dermatologists or orthopods are we who have to divine, imagine, follow allusions to what the matter is. I remember caring for an elderly Jewish man, now dead, who came to the office feeling unwell.

"Do you have chest pain, Mr. Rubin?"
"No-oo."
"Do you feel short of breath?"
"No-oo."
"Are you nauseated?"
"No-oo."
"Do you feel *shvach*?" [in Yiddish, translates roughly into "worn out"]
"Yes!"

It seemed to me that a discursive leap was necessary, across cultures, for contact with the body, for the intimation of practice.

Sometimes, it is as if internist and patient are alien planets, aware of one another's trajectories only by traces of stray light and strange matter. "We catch a glimpse of something, from time to time," writes poet and physician William Carlos Williams in his *Autobiography*, "which shows us that a presence has just brushed past us, some rare thing—just when the smiling little Italian woman has left us. For a moment we are dazzled. What was that?" (1951, 360). Both partners in the dyad can feel like valuable but inscrutable objects of admiration for one another, each trying to penetrate the other's secrets. With what pregnant wonder we meet, trying to divine all that is being emitted by the other, sometimes unconsciously. Does the trilobite *know* what truths are transposed on his stony ridges? Do the Pleiades realize what they transmit to earth? Does the dancer whose body is represented on the funerary vase buried with the Egyptian king understand the yield of her gestures? We sit in one another's presence, silenced by the mystery, its plenitude, its alterity, in suspense, waiting.

We stay in the presence of this freight of meaning, filled not only with gratitude that we can, now, see it, but also with satisfaction that we have helped the meaning to be apprehended. Knowing something about the body grants us the license to draw near to another. Touching the patient's body in all the ways we touch it admits us at least to the forecourt of the self of the other and, by reflection, of our own selves. We push, we palpate, we hug, we invade, we incise, we touch in the most intimate ways one can imagine. And yet, physician and patient remain alien to one another, each able only to intuit the other's moods, beliefs, desires, symptoms. When a patient describes a migraine headache, the doctor has no more than imagination on which to base an impression. There is no identity. There is no evidence. Whatever familiarity or *knowingness* we might sense is based on conjecture.

We are at the same time *alone* and *with*, strange and intimate. The presence of the other is both mysterious and known. We are simultaneously excluded by the obscurity and enveloped within the familiarity of another's being. Like planets in a solar system, we revolve around and are warmed by a common sun while hosting lives of absolute distinction. In the end, we live with one another as best we can, trying to pick up the signals our patients emit while they try to convey these all but unutterable thoughts and feelings and fears. Indeed, we are revolving bodies, held aloft by the gravity of our common humanity. In our efforts to tune our receivers, we attend to all the languages of our patients—the language of symptom, the language of pleasure, the language of loss, the language of life. We represent—for their sake and ours—what we perceive them to endure, giving expression to that which we barely know. And we affiliate into sturdy working units, whirring galaxies—with hosts of patients, with interlocking teams of health care providers, with ourselves.

If you were to extend my metaphor to the analytic setting, you might make the analysand the planet and the analyst the sun. A dynamic system without ordinary congress, it is based on gravity, utter integrity, and alien attachment. At regular intervals, each of an analyst's patients is suspended in orbit. They pass in the ether of the waiting room, nodding silently, making way. They respond to the same cosmic shifts. This cluster of planets circles around its lodestar, with seasons marked by relative warmth and coolness, as when in winter the earth's northern hemisphere slants farther away from its sun on its diagonal axis than during the summer. In both the medical and the analytic universes, heavy bodies hurtle through space, undergoing tremendous yet often imperceptible interior changes while traversing the paths that identify them, with stasis the ultimate threat.

I think what narrative medicine can learn from psychoanalysis is how to let the body be the portal that admits the doctor to the inner sanctum of the patient, to appreciate that he or she has an absolutely unique planetary *life*, and that this thing we do, our proximity to illness and health, grants us the immeasurable privilege to behold another person's atmosphere and logic and meaning. With proper training, the ordinary doctor could be equipped with the skill and motivation to solicit and honor narratives of illness that are not restricted to physical symptoms but that attend to body and life, emotion and self. Such a practice would *activate* what amounts to a primitive analytic presence in every person's experience, fostering mutual recognition of what doctor means to patient and what patient means to doctor.

Conversely, I think that the dividend of narrative medicine for psychoanalysis might be to offer our workaday consulting rooms as unpretentious models for the heightened interior transformations effected by analytic practice. The humdrum routines of medical practice and the instrumental nature of the transferences we elicit provide a natural laboratory for observing and understanding how analytic contact takes place in everyday life. This "small-scale" study has the potential to shed light on the ubiquity of the human need for therapeutic relationships and how the provision of such contacts over an extended period of time serves to promote health. There may also be a bonus for analytic thinking in amplifying a sense of the corporeal in clinical transactions, not only as unconscious fantasy but also as biological reality, both to inform treatment of analysands with physical illnesses and to take advantage of contemporary notions of the body's relation to self.

The intersection of psychoanalysis and narrative medicine promises to pay compounding dividends—for practitioners, for theorists of the self and body, and for the patients under our planetary aegis. Exponentially more persons might be said to profit from analytic intervention than are generally allowed if we were to "count" such versions of transference as occur in the medical and pediatric settings. When seen by physicians imbued with both psychoanalysis and narrative medicine, patients would be the beneficiaries not only of diagnostic accuracy and appropriate medical management but also of recognition and company on their journeys of illness. Our bodies, being human, are indeed our common lot; our proper selves, being all we *are*, can only be found through telling, and only if that telling is heard.

REFERENCE

Williams, William Carlos. 1951. *Autobiography*. New York: Random House.

Notes on Contributors

JEFFREY BERMAN is Professor of English at the University at Albany. He has written a series of books on pedagogy, *Diaries to an English Professor: Pain and Growth in the Classroom* (1994), *Surviving Literary Suicide* (1999), *Risky Writing: Self-Disclosure and Self-Transformation in the Classroom* (2001), and *Empathic Teaching* (2004), all published by the University of Massachusetts Press, as well as a tribute to his late wife, Barbara, *Dying to Teach: A Memoir of Love, Loss, and Learning*, published in 2007 by SUNY Press.

VERA J. CAMDEN is Professor of English at Kent State University and Training and Supervising Psychoanalyst at the Cleveland Psychoanalytic Center. She is the founding chair of the Committee on Research and Special Training (CORST) Essay Prize Committee of the American Psychoanalytic Association. She is coeditor of *American Imago* and past president of the John Bunyan Society. She has edited *Compromise Formations: Current Directions in Psychoanalytic Criticism* (1989), *The Narrative of the Persecutions of Agnes Beaumont* (1992), special issues of *Bunyan Studies* and *American Imago*, and *Trauma and Transformation: The Political Progress of John Bunyan*, published in 2007 by Stanford University Press.

RITA CHARON is a general internist and literary critic at Columbia University, where she directs the Program in Narrative Medicine. She was the coeditor of the journal *Literature and Medicine* from 1999 to 2007, is coeditor of *Stories Matter: The Role of Narrative in Medical Ethics* (Routledge, 2002), and author of *Narrative Medicine: Honoring the Stories of Illness*, published in 2006 by Oxford University Press.

ED COHEN teaches gender and cultural studies at Rutgers University. He is the author of *Talk on the Wilde Side: Towards a Genealogy of a Discourse on Male Sexualities* (Routledge, 1993), as well as numerous articles on the history and theory of gender and sexuality. He is currently completing a book entitled A *Body Worth Defending: "Immunity" and the Bio-politics of Modern Medicine*, which traces the transformation of immunity from a 2000-year-old legal and political concept into a biomedical framework at the end of the nineteenth century.

SANDER L. GILMAN is Distinguished Professor of the Liberal Arts and Sciences at Emory University, where he is the Director of the Program in Psychoanalysis as well as of the Health Sciences Humanities Initiative. A cultural and literary historian, he is the author or editor of more than seventy books. His Oxford lectures, *Multiculturalism and the Jews*, appeared in 2006; his most recent edited volume, *Race and Contemporary Medicine*, appeared in 2007. He is the author of the basic study of the visual stereotyping of the mentally ill, *Seeing the Insane*, published by John Wiley and Sons in 1982 (rpt. 1996), as well as of the classic *Jewish Self-Hatred*, published by The Johns Hopkins University Press in 1986. For twenty-five years he was a member of the humanities and medical faculties at Cornell University, where he held the Goldwin Smith Professorship of Humane Studies. For six years he held the Henry R. Luce Distinguished Service Professorship of the Liberal Arts in Human Biology at the University of Chicago, and then for four years he was a Distinguished Professor of the Liberal Arts and Medicine and creator of the Humanities Laboratory at the University of Illinois at Chicago. During 1990–1991, he served as the Visiting Historical Scholar at the National Library of Medicine, Bethesda, MD; 1996–1997, as a fellow of the Center for Advanced Study in the Behavioral Sciences, Stanford, CA; 2000–2001, as a Berlin prize fellow at the American Academy in Berlin; and 2004–2005, as the Weidenfeld Visiting Professor of European Comparative Literature at Oxford University. He has been a visiting professor at numerous universities in North America, South Africa, the United Kingdom, Germany, and New Zealand. He was president of the Modern Language Association in 1995. He has been awarded a Doctor of Laws (*honoris causa*) at the University of Toronto in 1997 and elected an honorary professor of the Free University in Berlin.

FRED L. GRIFFIN is Associate Professor in the Department of Psychiatry at the University of Alabama School of Medicine and a Training and Supervising Psychoanalyst at the Birmingham-New Orleans Psychoanalytic Center. His interests include the clinical practice and teaching of psychodynamic psychotherapy and psychoanalysis; the use of imaginative literature to illuminate the nature of the physician-patient relationship in general medicine, psychiatry, and psychoanalysis; and the role of writing in the life of the professional.

GEOFFREY HARTMAN is Sterling Professor Emeritus of English and Comparative Literature at Yale and the Project Director of its Fortunoff Video Archive for Holocaust Testimonies. *The Geoffrey Hartman Reader*, selected from fifty years of writing, was published by Fordham University Press in 2004 and won the Truman Capote prize for literary criticism.

SCHUYLER W. HENDERSON completed a clinical fellowship in pediatric psychiatry at Columbia University, an adult psychiatry residency at Bellevue/New York University, and an internship in pediatrics at Yale. He has published in *Literature and Medicine*, *Journal of Medical Humanities*, *JAMA*, and *Academic Medicine*, as well as coauthoring several chapters and presenting research on refugee mental health at the American Psychiatric Association and the International Society of Traumatic Stress Studies.

RICHARD LEWIS HOLT graduated from New College with a degree in English and American Literature in 1991. Afterward, he spent two years in Mali, West Africa, as a Peace Corps Volunteer and another year in Ecuador as a second grade teacher. He received his MD from the University of Florida in 2003 with highest honors, and is currently chief resident in psychiatry at the Medical University of South Carolina.

TERRENCE E. HOLT is an Assistant Professor in the Department of Social Medicine and the Division of Geriatric Medicine at UNC-Chapel Hill. He holds the MA, MFA, and PhD degrees in English from Cornell University, and the MD from the UNC School of Medicine; he received his residency training in internal medicine and subspecialty training in geriatrics at the UNC hospitals. His research interests include narrative medicine, the cultural mythology of aging, and linguistic markers of disease. He is a contributing editor to *Men's Health* and is currently completing a collection of narratives about medical training. His short fiction has appeared in *O. Henry Prize Stories*, the *Beacon Best of 2000*, and *Best of Zoetrope*.

JEAN S. MASON is Associate Professor in the Department of Professional Communication, Faculty of Communication and Design, at Ryerson University in Toronto. Her research into tuberculosis pathographies is prompted by her interest in the multifarious connections between writing, learning, creativity, and health, as well as by her experience growing up in Saranac Lake, New York, where she experienced firsthand the legacy of this therapeutic community and came to know many people and artifacts connected to the tuberculosis-curing initiative. Her current research project is funded by a three-year grant from the Social Sciences and Humanities Research Council of Canada.

KIMBERLY R. MYERS is Associate Professor in the Department of Humanities at Penn State College of Medicine. In 2002, she was one of twenty-five National Endowment for the Humanities Fellows in the Summer Institute on "Medicine, Literature, and Culture." Her essay, "Coming Out: Considering the Closet of Illness," appeared in the Fall 2004 issue of *Journal of Medical Humanities*, and her "Patient Pathography #8" was a finalist for the 2004 *Journal of General Internal Medicine* national creative writing prize. Her edited volume, *Illness in the Academy: A Collection of Pathographies by Academics*, published in 2007 by Purdue University Press, is her first book-length contribution to the field of medical humanities. Professor Myers has won numerous awards for university teaching, including the President's Award for Excellence in Teaching and Distinguished University Educator for the state of Montana, where she taught prior to joining the faculty at PSU.

PETER L. RUDNYTSKY is Professor of English at the University of Florida, an Honorary Member of the American Psychoanalytic Association, and the editor of *American Imago*. He is the author of *Freud and Oedipus* (Columbia, 1987), *The Psychoanalytic Vocation: Rank, Winnicott, and the Legacy of Freud* (Yale, 1991), *Psychoanalytic Conversations: Interviews with Clinicians, Commentators, and Critics* (Analytic, 2000), and *Reading Psychoanalysis: Freud, Rank, Ferenczi, Groddeck* (Cornell, 2002), for which he received the 2003 Gradiva Award. Among his previous edited and coedited volumes is *Psychoanalyses/Feminisms*, likewise arising from a conference he organized in Gainesville and published by SUNY Press. In 2004, he was the Fulbright/Sigmund Freud Society Scholar of Psychoanalysis in Vienna.

JANET SAYERS is Professor of Psychoanalytic Psychology at the University of Kent in Canterbury, where she also works as a psychotherapist, both privately and for the National Health Service. Her books include *Mothers of Psychoanalysis* (Norton, 1991), *Freudian Tales* (Vintage, 1997), *Divine Therapy* (Oxford, 2003) and, most recently, *Freud's Art: Psychoanalysis Retold* (Routledge, 2007).

NEIL SCHEURICH is Associate Professor of Psychiatry at the University of Kentucky College of Medicine in Lexington. His clinical interests include treatment-resistant mood disorders and electroconvulsive therapy, while his research interests center on the interfaces of ethics, literature, and spirituality with psychiatry. He has published articles in *Perspectives in Biology and Medicine*, *The American Journal of Psychotherapy*, and the *Hastings Center Report*.

LISA J. SCHNELL is Associate Professor of English at the University of Vermont. Having spent most of her scholarly career to date working on the literature of seventeenth-century England (she has published papers on various women writers of the period and a book, together with Andrew Barnaby, titled *Literate Experience: The Work of Knowing in Seventeenth-Century English Writing*), she is now at work on a manuscript that explores her personal and intellectual experience of grief surrounding the brief life of her second child, Claire. In 2000 she was the recipient of a Humanities Fellowship from the Open Society Institute's Project on Death in America. She lives with her husband Andrew Barnaby and their children Emma and Ian in Burlington, VT.

BENNETT SIMON is Training and Supervising Psychoanalyst at the Boston Society and Institute and Clinical Professor of Psychiatry, Harvard Medical School at the Cambridge Hospital. He has long been interested in issues of trauma as they arise in literature, in clinical practice, and in the arenas of war and persecution. He is the author of *Mind and Madness in Ancient Greece: The Classical Roots of Modern Psychiatry* (Cornell, 1978) and *Tragic Drama and the Family: Psychoanalytic Studies from Aeschylus to Beckett* (Yale, 1988), coeditor, with Roberta J. Apfel, of *Minefields in Their Hearts: The Mental Health of Children in War and Communal Violence* (Yale, 1996), coauthor, with Elizabeth Lunbeck, of *Family Romance, Family Secrets: Case Notes of an American Psychoanalysis, 1912* (Yale, 2003), and coauthor, with Michael Puett, Adam Seligman, and Robert Weller, of *For Ritual: An Essay on the Limits of Sincerity* (Oxford, in press).

Index

Made in the USA
Middletown, DE
23 December 2020